THE
RADIOLOGY
WORD BOOK

THE RADIOLOGY WORD BOOK

Theresa Indovina RMA, CMA

Instructor
Highline Community College
Des Moines, Washington

Wilburta Q. (Billie) Lindh CMA

Program Director, Medical Assisting Department
Highline Community College
Des Moines, Washington

F.A. Davis Company • Philadelphia

NOTE: As new scientific information becomes available through basic and clinical research, recommended treatments and drug therapies undergo changes. The author(s) and publisher have done everything possible to make this book accurate, up-to-date, and in accord with accepted standards at the time of publication. However, the reader is advised always to check product information (package inserts) for changes and new information regarding dose and contraindications before administering any drug. Caution is especially urged when using new or infrequently ordered drugs.

Library of Congress Cataloging-in-Publication Data

Indovina, Theresa.
    The radiology word book / Theresa Indovina, Wilburta Q. Lindh.
        p.   cm.
    ISBN 0-8036-4856-1
    1. Radiology, Medical—Terminology.   2. Radiography, Medical—
Terminology.   3. Medicine—Terminology.   I. Lindh, Wilburta Q.
II. Title.   III. Title: Radiology word book.
    [DNLM: 1. Radiology—terminology.   WN 15 I41r]
    RC78.A3I53 1990
    616.07′57′03—dc30
    DNLM/DLC
    for Library of Congress   89-25983

DEDICATION

Theresa Indovina

To my husband, Joseph; children, Patrick, Monica, and Michael; and our family members for the love and support I have felt.

Wilburta Q. Lindh

To my husband, DeVere, and our family for their support and encouragement.

PREFACE

The Radiology Word Book is designed to be used primarily by medical radiology transcriptionists. However, many other professionals such as radiology personnel, radiology technicians, nurses, ward clerks, medical records administrators, insurance company personnel, purchasing personnel, supply and billing personnel, educators, students and other allied health professionals will find the book an excellent reference source.

Well over 30,000 terms are incorporated within the text, to ensure that this is the most comprehensive radiology resource guide to date. Entries are cross-referenced to facilitate ease and speed in locating terminology.

Although this is an extensive list, the authors realize that new developments in the field of medical technology occur daily. Therefore, this publication must be updated on a regular basis to provide the most current terminology and techniques. The authors welcome and encourage comments, identification of overlooked terms, suggestions for inclusion of new terminology, or perhaps discrepancies found within the current printing.

HOW TO USE THIS BOOK

The format of the book is based on that of a standard dictionary. It is extensively cross-referenced for ease in locating terminology. There are several categories listed both as primary entries and as cross-referenced subentries by category. Examples of such categories are bones, catheters, contrast media, diseases, methods, and syndromes.

As a specific example, if one were to look for "Amipaque" and did not realize it was a contrast medium, it would be found in the regular alphabetical listing. However, if one already knew it to be a contrast medium, turning to the list of contrast media would reveal the correct spelling of "Amipaque" as a secondary entry under contrast media.

In the cross-referencing of entries by category, the category name is repeated only by the first letter and a period. For example:

cartilage
    septal c. *(The c. stands for cartilage.)*
    c. hair hypoplasia syndrome *(The c. stands for cartilage.)*

There are some main headings in which one will not find the category name listed before or after the entry. Such headings include: bones, contrast media, muscles, radioisotopes, radionuclides, and radiopharmaceuticals. For example:

radioisotopes		radioisotopes
gold (Au) 198	NOT	gold (Au) 198 r.

Abbreviations: Standard abbreviations for entries are included and are also listed alphabetically throughout the text. Their meanings are in parentheses. For example:

AAMT (American Association of Medical Transcription)

Also listed as:

American Association of Medical Transcription (AAMT)

A transcriptionist would not normally use abbreviations, except when specifically dictated by a physician. Medical abbreviations can have many interpretations and, therefore, should be avoided in medical records. The transcriptionist should not interpret abbreviations encountered when transcribing without verification from the dictating professional.

Hyphenation: Many words formerly hyphenated are now listed as one word. An example is gastro-intestinal which currently is written gastrointestinal. Hyphenated words are alphabetized as if the words were joined as one. For example:

Golgi apparatus
Goltz-Gorlin syndrome
Gombault's neuritis

Use a hyphen when the prefix or suffix is joined with an abbreviation or number, or when it is necessary for clarity. For example:

post-MI   post-CABG   pre-1985 admission

Use a hyphen to join compound nouns which include a number or single letter. For example:

alpha-1   T-waves   x-rays

One may see the word x-ray written as xray, X-ray, x-ray, or X ray. Roentgenogram for the noun form and x-ray for the verb form only, have been adopted by some personnel in the medical field. However, noun or verb, x-ray is currently the accepted correct forms.

Join the suffix "like" to words without the use of a hyphen unless the word is an eponym, ends in 1 or a vowel, or has three or more syllables. For example:

slitlike   barrel-like chest   McBurney-like incision

Plural and Singular: Plurals formed by the standard English language rules are not included. Plurals formed by Latin, Greek, etc. rules are noted by putting the singular form, a comma, and then a small s. for singular. The plural form is listed as a secondary entry with a pl. listed after the term denoting plural form. These entries are cross-referenced then by the plural form as a primary entry and the singular form as the secondary entry. For example:

emboli, pl.   embolus s.
   embolus, s.   emboli, pl.

Some words may be singular or plural in usage. For example:

biceps   facies   series   data

Other terms are always plural in their usage. For example:

adnexa   feces   menses   genitalia

For clarification purposes, there are a few instances which address whether a word is a noun or an adjective. There will be a "n." or "adj." following such entries. For example:

callous, adj.   callus, n.

Preferred spelling: When there are two approaches to spelling a particular term, the preferred spelling will be given first, followed by a comma and the secondary spelling. The secondary spelling will not be cross-referenced.

Eponyms: Capitalize the eponymic names of operations, procedures, instruments, anatomic features, etc. Do not capitalize the noun with which an eponym is combined. For example:

Graves' disease
ligament of Treitz
von Saal pin

Numbers: If the number comes at the end of a word, it will not be taken into account when alphabetizing, except if there is a sequence of numbers. These entries will be alphabetized numerically. For example:

Granger's
    G.'s 17 degrees position
    G.'s 23 degrees position
    G.'s 107 degrees position

Numbers, if at the beginning of a word, will be printed at the beginning of each individual alphabetical letter by numerical order. For example:

A4 pulley
H-1H (headhunter) catheter

Medical Slang: Medical slang and jargon must be avoided when transcribing medical documents. If slang terms are dictated, translate them in full in medical reports. For example:

dictated: H. flu	transcribed: H. influenzae
dictated: dex	transcribed: dexamethasone
dictated: lytes	transcribed: electrolytes
dictated: appy	transcribed: appendectomy

Transcription Reports: A variety of transcription reports are included as reference resources. The reports contain many of the terminology phrases and/or procedures listed within the pages of the book to provide an example of just how they are utilized within a report. These reports will be useful as examples to the new transcriptionist.

Physical Constants: The physical constants of the elements are provided to assist the transcriptionist.

Computer Glossary: A glossary of computer related terms is provided.

Fractures: A listing of fracture names is provided.

REFERENCES

Many, many hours have been spent researching the terminology included in *The Radiology Word Book*. University and community college libraries have provided excellent reference materials. The use of computers to search nationwide via the Interlibrary Loan Service was an invaluable resource. Personal interview sessions with medical personnel from clinics, physicians' offices, and military facilities also produced many up-to-date entries. Journals, lectures, films, and newsletters related to the subject were also important resources.

The AAMT conference in Yakima, Washington (May, 1988) and the National Convention for Medical Transcriptionists in Scottsdale, Arizona (August, 1988) provided exposure to the most current approaches to transcription, new developments in the radiology field, up-to-date terminology, and excellent networking links with transcribers nationally.

ACKNOWLEDGMENTS

We are grateful to those colleagues and medical professionals who have provided and shared reference material; evaluated and proofread the manuscript; and were, in general, the encouragement we as authors needed to "keep on keeping on".

Our special thanks go to Jean-François Vilain of the F. A. Davis Publishing Company; Glenn Stewart, M.D. of the University of Washington; Computer by the Hour, Cheron Wittman, R.T.R.; Diane S. Heath, CMT, of the Southwest Diagnostic Imaging Center of Dallas, Texas; Caryn Finch, C.N.M.T. of Madigan Army Base, Tacoma, Washington; Valley Medical Imaging Center, Renton, Washington; and transcriptionists from all over the United States.

We want to acknowledge the invaluable help of the reviewers who read the manuscript so painstakingly and made so many suggestions for improvements: Barbara Blank, CMT, Harriette L. Carlin, CMA-AC Pat Forbis, CMT, Brenda J. Hurley, CMT, Christine Jacoby, CMT, Carolynn Logan, CMT, Sarah Lu Mitchell, CMT.

TABLE OF CONTENTS

Aa

A4 pulley
AA (aortic arch)
AAA (abdominal aortic
  aneurysm)
AAMA (American Association
  of Medical Assistants)
AAMT (American Association
  for Medical Transcription)
Aarskog-Scott syndrome
Aavala lung biopsy needle
Abbokinase (urokinase)
abdomen
abdominal
  a. abscess
  a. aneurysm
  a. angiography
  a. aorta
  a. aortic aneurysm (AAA)
  a. aortogram
  a. aortography
  a. calcification
  a. canal
  a. double-bubble sign
  a. esophagus
  a. gullet
  a. kidney
  a. lymph nodes
  a. pneumoradiography
  a. region
  a. sac
  a. shield
  a. vertebra
  a. viscera
abdominoaortic
abdominopelvic
  a. cavity
abducens
abduction
  a. position

a. projection
abductor
  a. digiti minimi muscle
  a. digiti quinti muscle
  a. hallucis muscle
  a. pollicis brevis muscle
  a. pollicis longus muscle
Abernethy's fascia
aberrant
  a. goiter
  a. subclavian artery
aberration
  chromatid-type a.
  chromosome a.
  commatic a.
  dioptric a.
  spherical a.
abetalipoproteinemia
ABF (aortobifemoral) bypass
ablation
above diaphragm (AD)
above-the-knee amputation
  (AKA)
ABPA (allergic
  bronchopulmonary
  aspergillosis)
ABR (The American Board of
  Radiology)
Abramson catheter
abrasion
  a. marks
Abrodil (methiodal sodium)
abrupt sign
abscess
  a. cavity
  abdominal a.
  acute a.
  alveolar a.
  amebic a.

abscess—*Continued*
apical a.
appendiceal a.
appendicular a.
arthrifluent a.
atom-activated a.
bartholinian a.
Bezold's a.
bicameral a.
bile duct a.
biliary a.
bone a.
brain a.
broad ligament a.
Brodie's a.
canalicular a.
caseous a.
cerebral a.
cheesy a.
cholangitic a.
chronic a.
circumtonsillar a.
cold a.
collar-button a.
cortical a.
dental a.
dentoalveolar a.
diffuse a.
Douglas' a.
dry a.
Dubois' a.
epidural a.
epiploic a.
extradural a.
fecal a.
frontal a.
fungal a.
gangrenous a.
gas a.
gingival a.
gravitation a.
gravity a.
helminthic a.
hepatic a.

hot a.
hypostatic a.
iliopsoas a.
intra-abdominal a.
intracranial a.
intradural a.
intrahepatic a.
intramammary a.
intramastoid a.
intraperitoneal a.
intrarenal a.
ischiorectal a.
kidney a.
lacrimal a.
lacunar a.
lateral a.
lateral alveolar a.
liver a.
mammary a.
manubriosternoclavicular a.
mastoid a.
mesenteric a.
metastatic a.
metastatic tuberculous a.
migrating a.
miliary a.
multiloculated a.
Munro's a.
orbital a.
palatal a.
pancreatic a.
parametrial a.
parametric a.
paranephric a.
pararenal a.
parietal a.
Pautrier's a.
pelvic a.
pelvirectal a.
periapical a.
periappendiceal a.
pericholecystic a.
pericoronal a.
perigraft a.

perihepatic a.
perinephric a.
periodontal a.
peripleuritic a.
perirenal a.
perisigmoidal a.
peritoneal a.
peritonsillar a.
periureteral a.
phlegmonous a.
phoenix a.
Pott's a.
premammary a.
psoas a.
pulmonary a.
pulp a.
pulpal a.
pyemic a.
pyogenic a.
rectal a.
renal a.
residual a.
retromammary a.
retroperitoneal a.
retropharyngeal a.
retrotonsillar a.
ring a.
root a.
sacrococcygeal a.
satellite a.
septicemic a.
serous a.
shirt-stud a.
spermatic a.
splenic a.
stercoraceous a.
stercoral a.
sterile a.
stitch a.
streptococcal a.
strumous a.
subaponeurotic a.
subareolar a.
subcutaneous a.

subdiaphragmatic a.
subdural a.
subfascial a.
subgaleal a.
subhepatic a.
submammary a.
subpectoral a.
subperiosteal a.
subperitoneal a.
subphrenic a.
subscapular a.
sudoriparous a.
superficial a.
suprahepatic a.
sympathetic a.
syphilitic a.
thecal a.
thymic a.
Tornwaldt's a.
tuberculous a.
tubo-ovarian a.
tympanitic a.
tympanocervical a.
tympanomastoid a.
urethral a.
urinary a.
verminous a.
vitreous a.
von Bezold's a.
wandering a.
Welch's a.
worm a.
abscessogram
abscopal
absent ovary
absolute
  a. field
  a. unit
absorbance
absorbed
  a. dose (AD)
  a. dose rate
  a. fraction
absorbent

absorber
absorptiometer
absorptiometry
absorption
    a. bands
    a. coefficient
    a. curve
    a. density
    a. discontinuity, edge or
      limit
    a. line
    a. spectrophotometer
    a. spectrum
    a. unsharpness
    a. x-ray spectrum
    bone radiation a.
    photoelectric a.
Abt-Letterer-Siwe syndrome
abut
abutment
abutting
AC (acromioclavicular)
ac (alternating current)
    ac generator
ACA (anterior cerebral artery)
acacia
acalculous cholecystitis
acanthiomeatal
    a. line
    b. projection
acanthion
acanthioparietal
    a. projection
acanthocytosis
acanthus
ACAPI (anterior cerebral artery
   pulsatility index)
ACAT (automated
   computerized axial
   tomography)
ACBE (air contrast barium
   enema)
accelerating potential
acceleration

accelerator
    a. urinae muscle
    atomic a.
    electronic linear a.
    linear a.
accentuation
acceptor
accessorius muscle
accessory
    a. cartilage
    a. gland
    a. ligament
    a. lobe
    a. nasal sinuses
    a. palatine canal
    a. renal artery
    a. rib
    a. spleen
accommodation
accretion line
accumulated dose equivalent
accuracy of registration
ACD (acid citrate dextrose)
ACD (annihilation coincidence
   detection)
acetabula, pl.
    acetabulum, s.
acetabular
    a. angle
    a. fossa
    a. fracture
    a. notch
acetabular cup
    Aufranc-Turner a. c.
    Crawford-Adams a. c.
    McKee-Farrar a. c.
    New England Baptist a. c.
acetabulum s,
    acetabula, pl.
acetanilidoiminodiacetic acid
   (HID)
acetate film
acetic
    a. acid

a. anhydride
Acetiodone
acetrizoate sodium
acetrizoic acid
acetylated
acetylation
acetylcysteine
ACG (angiocardiography)
achalasia
acheiria
Achilles tendon
achondrodysplasia
achondrogenesis, type II
achondroplasia
    a. atypica
acid
    a. citrate dextrose (ACD)
    a.-fast bacilli (AFB)
    a. fixing bath
    a. pulmonary aspiration
Acid blue 1
Acid blue 3
acidophilic adenoma
acinar
    a. cells
    a. nodule
    a. shadow
acinar-like
acini, pl.
    acinus, s.
acinus, s.
    acini, pl.
ACJ (acromioclavicular joint)
Ackermann
    A. biopsy needle
    A. needle
aclasis
    diaphyseal a.
    tarsoephiphyseal a.
ACMI catheter
Acmistat catheter
A-comm (anterior
  communicating) artery
aconitine tincture

acorn-tip catheter
acorn-tipped catheter
acortical
acoustic
    a. enhancement
    a. impedance
    a. labyrinth
    a. meatus
    a. mismatch
    a. nerve
    a. neurofibroma
    a. neuroma
    a. ohm
    a. radiation
    a. shadow
ACPS
  (acrocephalopolysyndactyly)
acquired
    a. diverticulum
    a. immune deficiency
      syndrome (AIDS)
    a. immunodeficiency
      syndrome (AIDS)
    a. time
acquisition
ACR (American College of
  Radiology)
acrania
acro-osteolysis
acrobrachycephaly
acrocallosal syndrome
acrocephalopolysyndactyly
  (ACPS), type I, II, III, IV
acrocephalosyndactylism
acrocephalosyndactyly, type I,
  II, III, IV, V
acrocephaly
acrochondrohyperplasia
acrodysostosis
acrodysplasia
acrodystrophic neuropathy
acroedema
acrofacial dysostosis
acromegaly

acromelia
acromesomelic
   a. dysplasia
acrometagenesis
acromial
   a. angle
   a. fracture
acromioclavicular (AC)
   a. dislocation
   a. joint (ACJ)
   a. ligament
   a. separation
acromiocoracoid ligament
acromiohumeral
acromion
   a. process
acromioscapular
acromiothoracic
acromutilation
acropachia ossea
acropachy
   thyroid a.
acropachyderma
acropectorovertebral dysplasia
ACT (axial computed tomography)
ACTH (adrenocorticotropic hormone)
actinic
   a. radiation
actinium
   a. series
actinogen
actinogenesis
actinogram
actinography
actinokymogram
actinokymography
actinomycosis
actinon
actinopraxis
actinoscopy
action spectrum

activated
   a. atom
   a. water
activation
   a. analysis
   a. energy
ACTR (American Club of Therapeutic Radiologists)
acupuncture/transcutaneous nerve stimulation (ACUTENS)
Acuson computed sonography
acute
   a. abscess
   a. bacterial myocarditis
   a. disc syndrome
   a. disseminated histiocytosis X
   a. exposure
   a. flexion
   a. flexion axial projection
   a. fracture
   a. gouty arthritis
   a. interstitial pneumonia
   a. isolated myocarditis
   a. parenchymatous jaundice
   a. radiation syndrome (ARS)
ACUTENS (acupuncture/ transcutaneous nerve stimulation)
AD (above diaphragm)
AD (absorbed dose)
ADA (anterior descending artery)
ADAC computer
adactyly
Adair-Dighton syndrome
adamantine
   a. epithelioma
adamantinoblastoma
adamantinoma
Adamkiewicz' artery

Adams' position
adaptation
adapter
    Check-Flo accessory a.
    leakproof a.
    Luer-Lok a.
    multipurpose tubing a.
    rotating a.
    side-arm a.
adaptometer
ADC (analog-to-digital
  converter)
A/D converter
addendum
Addison's
    A.'s disease
    A.'s melanoderma
    A.'s plane
address
    a. wire
    a. word
adduct
adduction
    a. position
    a. projection
adductor
    a. brevis muscle
    a. canal
    a. hallucis muscle
    a. hiatus
    a. longus muscle
    a. magnus muscle
    a. obliquus hallucis muscle
    a. pollicis muscle
    a. transversus hallucis
      muscle
adenitis
adenoacanthoma
adenoameloblastoma
adenocarcinoma
adenochondroma
adenofibroma
adenohypophyseal

adenoid
    a. cystic carcinoma
adenoidal-nasopharyngeal
  ratio
adenoleiomyofibroma
adenolipoma
adenolymphoma
adenoma
    a. sebaceum
    acidophilic a.
    basophilic a.
    benign a.
    bronchial a.
    chromophobic a.
    cortical a.
    oxyphil a.
    pituitary a.
    pleomorphic a.
    thyroid a.
    villous a.
adenoma, s.
    adenomata, pl.
adenomata, pl.
    adenoma, s.
adenomatoid
adenomatosis
adenomatous
    a. goiter
    a. polyostotic
    a. tumor
adenomyofibroma
adenomyoma
adenomyomatosis
adenomyosarcoma
adenopathy
    hilar a.
    mediastinal a.
adenorhabdomyosarcoma
adenosarcoma
adenosine
    a. deaminase deficiency
    a. diphosphate
    a. triphosphate

adenosis
adenosquamous
    a. carcinoma
adenovirus
adherent
adhesion
    banjo-string a.
    filmy a.
adhesive
    a. pain
    a. pericarditis
ADI (atlanto-dens interval)
adiabatic
    a. demagnetization
    a. fast passage
      (AFP)
adipose
    a. ligament
    a. tissue
aditus
    a. ad antrum
    a. ad pelvis
    a. laryngis
    a. orbitae
    a. vaginae
adjacent
adjuvant
adnexa, pl.
    adnexum, s.
adnexum, s.
    adnexa, pl.
ADR ultrasound
adrenal
    a. angle
    a. arteriogram
    a. arteriography
    a. capsule
    a. cortex
    a. gland
    a. hyperplasia
    a. hypertension
    a. imaging
    a. scan
    a. tumor

    Marchand's a.s
adrenergic
adrenocortical
adrenocorticotropic hormone
    (ACTH)
adrenogenital
adrenogram
adrenoleukodystrophy
Adriamycin (doxorubicin HCl)
Adrian-Crooks-type cassette
Adson's
    A.'s maneuver
    A.'s syndrome
adsorption
adult
    a. hydrocephalus
    a. respiratory distress
      syndrome (ARDS)
adventitious
adynamic
    a. ileus
Aeby's plane
AEC (Atomic Energy
    Commission)
AEG (air encephalogram)
AEG (air encephalography)
aerate
aerocele
aeroesophagography
aerohematoma
aeromammography
aerophagia
aerosinusitis
aerosol
    a. inhalation studies
aerosolized pentamide
A-F (air-fluid)
AFB (acid-fast bacilli)
AFB (aortofemoral bypass)
afferent (conducting toward)
affinity
affix
AFL (air/fluid level)
AFP (adiabatic fast passage)

AFP (alpha-fetoprotein)
African
    A. anemia
    A. lymphoma
afterglow
afterloading
    a. Heyman applicator
    a. technique
Ag (silver)
AGA (appropriate for
    gestational age)
agammaglobulinemia
aganglionosis
AgBr (silver bromide)
AGE (angle of greatest
    extension)
agenesis
    a. of pulmonary artery
agenetic fracture
agent
    contrast a.
AGF (angle of greatest flexion)
agglomerate
agglutination
aggregated
    a. radioiodinated
    a. radioiodinated albumin
      (human) I-131
    a. radiopharmaceutical
aglossia-adactyly syndrome
Agnew tattooing needle
agnogenic myeloid metaplasia
agranulocytosis
AHRA (American Hospital
    Radiolgy Administrators)
AI (aortoiliac)
AICA (anterior inferior
    cerebellar artery)
Aicardi syndrome
AIDS (acquired
    immunodeficiency
    syndrome)
    A. arthritis
    A.-related complex (ARC)

ainhum
air
    a. alveologram
    a. arthrogram
    a. arthrography
    a. bronchogram
    a. bronchogram sign
    a. bronchography
    a. bubble
    a. calibration
    a. cap sign
    a. clefts
    a. computed tomography
      (CT) cisternogram
    a. contrast barium enema
      (ACBE)
    a. contrast enema
    a. contrast radiography
    a. contrast study
    a. contrast UGI series
    a. crescent sign
    a. cystogram
    "a. dome" sign
    a. dose
    a. drift
    a. embolism
    a. encephalogram (AEG)
    a. encephalography
      (AEG)
    a. fluid loops
    a. fog
    a. insufflation
    a. monitor
    a. pocket
    a. sac
    a. saccule
    a. space consolidation
    extraperitoneal a.
    extrapleural a.
    free a.
    intraperitoneal a.
    intrapleural a.
air-bells
air-bone gap

air-containing nodule
air-core transformer
air-cystography
air-fluid (A-F)
air-fluid level (AFL)
air-gap principle
air-gap technique
air-lipiodol tragacanth
air-space disease
air-wall ionization chamber
airflow obstructive disease
AIUM (American Institute of
   Ultrasound in Medicine)
airway
   a. obstruction
   patent a.
   pulmonary a.
Åkerlund's hernia, type I, II, III
akinesia algera
akinesis
akinetic
Al HVL (aluminum half value
   layer)
ala, s.
   alae, pl.
alae, pl.
   ala, s.
alar
   a. cartilage
   a. ligament
   a. scapula
ALARA (as low as reasonably
   achievable)
Albarrán's gland
Albers-Schönberg
   A.-S. method
   A.-S. position
   A.-S. view
Albert's position
Albl's ring
Albright's
   A.'s hereditary
      osteodystrophy
   A.'s osteodystrophia
   A.'s syndrome

Albright-Hadorn syndrome
Albright-McCune-Sternberg
   syndrome
albumin
   a. microsphere
   iodinated I 125 serum a.
   iodinated I 131 aggregated a.
   iodinated I 131 serum a.
   macroaggregated a. (MAA)
   radioactive a.
   serum a.
Albumotope 125I
Alcock catheter
alcoholic myocardiopathy
aldosterone
aldosteronoma
Aldrich's syndrome
aleukemic reticulosis
Alexander's
   A.'s anteroposterior
      position
   A.'s lateral position
   A.'s method
algebraic reconstruction
   technique
algorithm
   a., CT
   Cooley-Tukey a.
alias
   a.-free image
   a. frequency
aliasing artifact
aliform
align
alignment
   a. bar
alimentary
   a. canal
   a. tract
aliquot
alkaline phosphatase test
alkaptonuria
alkaptonuric ochronosis
allantoid
Allemann's syndrome

allergic
    a. bronchopulmonary
       aspergillosis (ABPA)
Allison and Johnstone anomaly
Allison's atrophy
allobar
allobarbital
allotriodontia
allowable dose
allowed beta transition
alloxan
alloy
allylamine
Aloka (manufacturer)
    A. linear scanner
    A. ultrasound diagnostic
       equipment
alopecia
alpha
    a. activity
    a. chamber
    a. decay
    a. disintegration
    a. emitter
    a. filter
    a. particle
    a. particle spectrum
    a. radiation
    a. ray
    a. rhythm
    a. threshold
    a. wave
alpha-fetoprotein (AFP)
alphanumeric data
Alphazurine 26
Alport's syndrome
ALS (amyotrophic lateral
    sclerosis)
alternating current (a.c.)
    a.c. generator
alternating field
alternation
alum "Tans"
alumina
aluminosis

aluminum
    a. filter
    a. half value layer (Al
       HVL)
    a. step wedge or ladder
Alvarez-Rodriguez catheter
alveobronchiolitis
alveolar
    a. abscess
    a. bronchiole
    a. canals
    a. cell carcinoma
    a. cyst
    a. duct
    a. emphysema
    a. gas
    a. infiltrate
    a. lymphoma
    a. microlithiasis
    a. nodule
    a. pattern
    a. portion
    a. process
    a. proteinosis
    a. ridge
    a. sac
    a. saccule
    a. ventilation
    a. yoke
alveoli, pl.
    alveolus, s.
alveolodental
    a. periodontium
alveologram
alveololabial
alveololingual
alveolonasal
alveolopalatal
alveoloplasty
alveolotomy
alveolus, s.
    alveoli, pl.
Alzheimer's
    A.'s dementia
    A.'s disease

AMA (American Medical
    Association)
ambient
ambulatory visit groups
    (AVG)
ameba or amoeba
amebiasis
amebic
    a. abscess
    a. colitis
    a. meningoencephalitis
amelia
amelification
ameloblastic
    a. fibroma
    a. sarcoma
ameloblastoma
    melanotic a.
    pituitary a.
amenorrhea
American Association for
    Medical Transcription
    (AAMT)
American Association of
    Medical Assistants
    (AAMA)
American Board of Radiology
    (ABR)
American Club of Therapeutic
    Radiologists (ACTR)
American College of Radiology
    (ACR)
American Hospital Radiology
    Administrators
    (AHRA)
American Institute of
    Ultrasound in Medicine
    (AIUM)
American Medical Association
    (AMA)
American Medical Records
    Association (AMRA)
American Radium Society
    (ARS)

American Registry of Radiology
    Technologists (ARRT)
American Rheumatism
    Association (ARA)
American Roentgen Ray
    Society (ARRS)
American Society of Radiologic
    Technologists
    (ASRT)
americium
amethocaine lozenge
amidotrizoic acid
amine precursor uptake and
    decarboxylation cell tumor
    (APUDoma)
amino acid
aminopterin
Amipaque (metrizamide)
ammeter filament
ammogram
ammonium
    a. molybdate (Mo-99)
    a. thiosulfate
amniocentesis
amniogram
amniography
amnion
amniotic
    a. fluid
    a. sac
A-mode (amplitude
    modulation)
    A display
    A scanning
    A ultrasonography
amoeba
amorphous
amperage
ampere (amp)
Ampère's rule
amphetamine sulfate
amphiarthrodial
amphiarthroses, pl.
    amphiarthrosis, s.

amphiarthrosis, s.
  amphiarthroses, pl.
amphidiarthrodial joint
amphoric
  a. murmur
  a. resonance
amphoteric dipolar ion
Amplatz
  A. catheter
  A. dilator
  A. unit
  A. wire guide
amplification
  gas a.
amplifier
  a. buffer
  a. channels
  a. gradient power
  a. image
  gradient power a.
  linear a.
  nuclear pulse a.
  playback a.
  pulse a.
  voltage a.
amplify
amplifying fluoroscope
amplitude
  a. modulation (A-mode)
  a. wave
ampoule, also ampul or ampule
ampulla
  a. of Vater
  a. phrenica
ampulla, s.
  ampullae, pl.
ampullae, pl.
  ampulla, s.
ampullary aneurysm
AMRA (American Medical
  Records Association)
Amsterdam dwarf
amu (atomic mass unit)
amygdala

amygdaloglossus muscle
amygdaloid
  a. nucleus
amyloid
  a. liver
amyloidoma
amyloidosis
  a. of the kidneys
  interstitial a.
  pulmonary amyloidosis
  tracheal a.
amyoplasia congenita
amyotrophic lateral sclerosis
  (ALS)
anabolic steroid
anal
  a. atresia
  a. canal
  a. fascia
  a. fissure
  a. verge
analog
  a. computations
  a. computer
  a. computer tomography
  a. derandomizer circuit
  a. photo
  a. rate meter
  a. signal
analog-to-digital converter
  (ADC)
analysis
  activation a.
  base volume image a.
  chemical a.
  correlation a.
  feather a.
  least-square a.
  multigated acquisition a.
    (MUGA scan)
  neutron activation a.
  radiochemical a.
  regression a.
  saturation a.

analytic
analyzer
a. window width
multichannel a.
sequential multiple a.
(SMA)
anaphase
anaphylactic
anaphylaxis
anaplastic carcinoma
anastomoses, pl.
anastomosis, s.
anastomosis
jejunocolic a.
anastomosis, s.
anastomoses, pl.
anastomotic ulcer
anatomic
a. conjugate
a. landmark
a. position
anatomical
a. neck
a. position
a. snuff-box
anatomicoradiographic
anatomy
ancillary
anconad
anconeal
anconeus muscle
Anderson's
A.'s method
A.'s procedure
Andrén's method
Andrén-von Rosen technique
androgenic tumor
android pelvis
androstenedione
androsterone
Andrus view
anechoic
anemia
erythroblastic a.

familial splenic a.
Fanconi's a.
anesthesia
anesthetic
anesthetize
aneursymal
a. rupture
a. sac
aneurysm
a. anastomotica
a. by anastomosis
a. of sinus of Valsalva
abdominal a.
abdominal aortic a. (AAA)
ampullary a.
anterior communicating a.
aortic a.
aortic sinusal a.
arteriovenous a.
arteriovenous pulmonary
a.
atherosclerotic a.
axillary a.
bacterial a.
berry a.
brain a.
cardiac a.
cerebral a.
cirsoid a.
compound a.
congenital cerebral a.
Crisp's a.
cylindroid a.
cystogenic a.
dissecting a.
ectatic a.
embolic a.
embolomycotic a.
false a.
fusiform a.
Galen's vein a.
hernial a.
infected a.
innominate a.

intracranial a.
lateral a.
miliary a.
mixed a.
mural a.
mycotic a.
orbital a.
Park's a.
pelvic a.
poststenotic a.
Pott's a.
racemose a.
Rasmussen's a.
renal a.
Richet's a.
Rodrigues' a.
saccular a.
sacculated a.
serpentine a.
Shekelton's a.
spurious a.
suprasellar a.
syphilitic a.
thoracic a.
traumatic a.
true a.
tubular a.
varicose a.
venous a.
ventricular a.
verminous a.
worm a.
aneurysmal
    a. bone cyst
    a. dilatation
    a. murmur
    a. rupture
    a. sac
aneurysmogram
aneurysmography
Anger
    A. camera
    A. instrument
angina

a. pectoris
exudative a.
Ludwig's a.
Prinzmetal's a.
angioblastic meningioma
angioblastoma
angiocardiogram (ACG)
angiocardiography (ACG)
    first-pass radionuclide a.
    intravenous a.
    radionuclide a.
    selective a.
    venous a.
angiocath
angiocatheter
    Eppendorf a.
Angio-Conray
Angio-Conray 80
angiodysplasia
angioendothelioma
angiofibroma
angiografin (diatrizoic acid)
angiogram
angiographic
    a. catheter
    a. sylvian point
    a. triad in meningitis
    a. triad in tuberculosis
angiography
    abdominal a.
    biliary a.
    cardiac a.
    carotid a.
    cerebral a.
    digital subtraction a.
    femorocerebral a.
    first-pass isotope a.
    fluorescein a.
    four-vessel a.
    hepatic a.
    interventional a.
    magnification a.
    Medrat a. injector
    multigated a.

angiography—*Continued*
   nuclear a.
   peripheral a.
   pulmonary a.
   radionuclide a.
   renal a.
   subtraction a.
   three-vessel a.
   vertebral a.
   vertebrobasilar a.
   visceral a.
angiolipoma
angiology
angiolymphangioma
angioma
   a. capillare et venosum
      calcificans
angiomatosis
   a. cerebri
   a. encephalotrigeminal
angiomyolipoma
angiomyoma
Angiopac
angioplasty
   percutaneous
      transluminal a.
angiopneumogram
angiopneumography
angiosarcoma
angioscintigram
angioscintigraphy
Angioskop-D (equipment used
   in DSA)
angiosteohypertrophic
   syndrome
angiotensin I (125I)
Angiovist (diatrizoate
   meglumine)
angle
   a. averaging
   a. board
   a. of Citelli
   a. of greatest extension
      (AGE)

a. of greatest flexion
   (AGF)
a. of His
a. of inclusion
a. of Louis
a. sign of scurvy
acetabular a.
adrenal a.
basal a.
Bauman's a.
Boehler's a. (heel)
Bohlet's a.
Boogaard's a.
branching a.
bull's a.
calcaneal fifth metatarsal
   a.
cardiophrenic a. (CPA)
carrying a.
cerebellopontine a.
   (CPA)
Citelli's a.
costophrenic a. (CPA)
costovertebral a.
   (CVA)
flip a.
hepatic a.
iliac a.
Ludwig's a.
lumbosacral a.
Mikulicz' a.
nasopineal a.
phrenicovertebral a.
Q a.
Quatrefages' a.
radiocarpal a.
re-entrance a.
scapholunate a.
sinodural a. of Citelli
solid a.
sphenoid a.
splenic a.
sternal a.
subcarinal a.

Sutton's a.
talocalcaneal a.
target a.
tip a.
Treitz' a.
tuber a.
venous a. of the brain
Virchow's a.
Wiberg's a.
wide-a. tomography
Anglemann's syndrome
Angström unit
angular
    a. acceleration
    a. frequency
    a. gyrus
    a. membrane defect
    a. momentum
    a. notch
    a. sampling
    a. velocity
angulation
    a. of anode
    caudad a.
    cephalic a.
    lumbosacral a.
    volar a.
anguli, pl.
    angulus, s.
angulus Ludovici
angulus, s.
    anguli, pl.
ani, pl.
    anus, s.
anion
    a. gap
aniridia
anisuria
ankle
    a. joint
    a. mortise
ankylodactyly
ankylosing
    a. polyarthritis

    a. spondylitis
    a. vertebral hyperostosis
ankylosis
annihilation
    a. coincidence detection
      (ACD)
    a. radiation
    a. reaction
anode
    a. cooling curve chart
    a. thermal capacity
    hooded a.
    rotating a.
    stationary a.
anomalad
    Robin's a.
anomalies
    C syndrome of multiple
      congenital a.
anomalous bronchus
anomaly
    turmschädel a.
anonychia
anophthalmia
anorchism
anorectal
    a. lymph nodes
anorexia
anosteogenesis
anoxia
ansae insulare
antalgic
    a. gait
antebrachium
antecubital
    a. fossa
    a. joint
    a. vein
anteflexion
antegrade
    a. aortography
    a. blood flow
    a. perfusion pressure
      measurement

antegrade—*Continued*
a. pyelography
a. ureteral stent
antemesenteric
antenna array
anterior
a. arch
a. cerebral artery (ACA)
a. cerebral artery pulsatility index (ACAPI)
a. cervical joint
a. circulation projection
a. clinoid process
a. communicating (A-comm)
a. communicating aneurysm
a. descending artery (ADA)
a. diaphragmatic hernia
a. horn
a. inferior cerebellar artery (AICA)
a. inferior communicating artery (AICA)
a. intraoccipital joint
a. junctional line
a. ligament
a. lordotic position
a. malleolus fracture
a. maxillary bowing sign
a. mediastinal line
a. nasal spine
a. pararenal space
a. pituitary
a. profile projection
a. projection
a. sacral foramen
a. septum
anterior-posterior (AP)
anterior-superior iliac spine (ASI)
anterofundal placenta
anterolateral
anteroposterior (AP)
a. above-diaphragm projection
a. axial projection
a. basal projection
a. below-diaphragm projection
a. external projection
a. lordotic projection
a. oblique projection
a. odontoid projection
a. projection
a. view
anteroseptal infarction
anterosuperior (AS) view
anteversion
anthracosilicosis
anthracosis
anthropoid
anthropological
a. baseline
a. plane
anthropometry
anthropomorphic baseline
antibody-bound ligand
anticholinergic
anticoincidence
a. circuit
a. current
antigenic
antimesenteric
a. border
antimetabolic
antimonium tungstate (HPA-23)
antimony
a. trisulfide
antineutrino
antiparticle
antiproton
antithyroglobulin (ATG)

antitragicus muscle
Anton's syndrome
antra, pl.
    antrum, s.
antral
    a. gastritis
    a. remnant syndrome
    a. web
antrectomy
antritis
antrum
    a. of Highmore
    a. of Willis
    cardiac a.
    ethmoid a.
    frontal a.
    gastric a.
    Highmore's a.
    mastoid a.
    maxillary a.
    pyloric a.
    tympanic a.
antrum, s.
    antra, pl.
anular
    a. calcification
    a. lesion
    a. ligament
    a. phased arrays
    a. ring
    a. sclerosis
    a. shadow
anulus
    a. fibrosus
    a. of Zinn
anuresis
anuria
anuric
anus
    a. vestibularis
    artificial a.
    imperforate a.
    preternatural a.
    vulvovaginal a.

anus, s.
    ani, pl.
Ao (aorta)
aorta (Ao)
    a. anomalies
    abdominal a.
    ascending a.
    descending a.
    dextropositioned a.
    overriding a.
    thoracic a.
aortic (Ao)
    a. aneurysm
    a. arch (AA)
    a. arch syndrome
    a. assist balloon
        introducer
    a. atresia
    a. bifurcation
    a. bifurcation syndrome
    a. catheter
    a. dissection
    a. diverticulum
    a. flush pigtail catheter
    a. flush straight catheter
    a. insufficiency
    a. knob
    a. laceration
    a. leaflet
    a. lumen
    a. lymph node
    a. murmur
    a. nipple
    a. node
    a. pulmonic lymph node
    a. regurgitation (AR)
    a. root
    a. rupture
    a. sac
    a. septal defect
    a. silhouette
    a. sinusal aneurysm
    a. stenosis (AS)
    a. triangle

aortic (Ao)—*Continued*
    a. valve
    a. valve replacement
        (AVR)
    a. window
    femoral a. flush
    thoracic a. dissection
aortic-pulmonary
    communication
aortic-pulmonic window
aorticopulmonary
    a. septal defect
    a. window
aorticorenal
aorticoventricular tunnel
aortitis
aortobifemoral (ABF) bypass
aortocaval node
aortocoronary
    a. artery bypass graft
aortoduodenal fistula
aortofemoral
    a. arterial runoff
    a. arteriography
    a. bypass (AFB)
    a. bypass graft
    a. runoff
aortogram
    abdominal a.
    flush a.
aortographic catheter
aortography
    abdominal a.
    antegrade a.
    arch a.
    catheter a.
    lumbar a.
    renal a.
    retrograde a.
    selective visceral a.
    thoracic a.
    translumbar a.
    venous a.
    visceral a.

aortoiliac (AI)
    a. graft
AP (anterior-posterior or
    anteroposterior)
AP (anteroposterior)
    position
Apert's syndrome
Apert-Crouzon disease
apertura piriformis
aperture
    a. diaphragm
    a. grid
    detector a.
    gantry a.
apex, s.
    apices or apexes, pl.
apexes or apices, pl.
    apex, s.
aphalangia
aphthous
    a. stomatitis
    a. ulcer
apical
    a. abscess
    a. bronchus
    a. canaliculus
    a. cap
    a. diastolic murmur
    a. dystrophy
    a. granuloma
    a. impulse
    a. infection
    a. lesion
    a. ligament
    a. lordotic projection
    a. lymph node
    a. murmur
    a. pleura
    a. pleural thickening
    a. pneumonia
    a. position
    a. projection
    a. scarring
    a. space

a. view
apices or apexes, pl.
   apex, s.
apicoectomy
aplasia
   a. periostealis
   pectoral a.
aplastic infantile funicular
  myelosis
apochromatic objective
aponeuroses, pl.
   aponeurosis, s.
aponeurosis
   abdominal a.
   bicipital a.
   crural a.
   epicranial a.
   external oblique a.
   falciform a.
   lingual a.
   palmar a.
   perineal a.
   pharyngeal a.
   plantar a.
   subscapular a.
   supraspinous a.
   temporal a.
   vertebral a.
aponeurosis, s.
   aponeuroses, pl.
apophyseal
   a. articulation
   a. fracture
   a. joint
apophyses, pl.
   apophysis, s.
apophysis
   basilar a.
   cerebral a.
   genial a.
   iliac crest a.
   odontoid a.
   pterygoid a.
   ring a.

apophysis, s.
   apophyses, pl.
apophysitis
apoplectiform myelopathy
apoplexy
apparatus
   Deyerle a.
   Golgi a.
appearance
   "applecore-like" a.
   "ball-in-hand" a.
   "beaded" a.
   "beaked" a.
   "beaten brass" a.
   "beaten silver" a.
   "bone-within-bone" a.
   "bubble-like" a.
   "candle dripping" a.
   "cauliflower-like" a.
   "cobblestone" a.
   "cobra head" a.
   "coiled-spring" a.
   "cotton ball" a.
   "cotton-wool" a.
   "double-bubble" a.
   "drumstick" a.
   Erlenmeyer's "flask-like"
    a.
   "fan-shaped" a.
   "frayed string" a.
   "ground-glass" a.
   "hair-standing-on-end" a.
   "hammered brass" a.
   "hot-cross-buns" a.
   "inverse comma" a.
   "jail bars" a.
   "kernel of popcorn" a.
   "lace-like" a.
   "leafless tree" a.
   "light bulb" a.
   "moth-eaten" a.
   "mulberry" a.
   neoplastic a.
   "onion-peel" a.

appearance—*Continued*
   "onion-skin" a.
   "pancake" a.
   "panda" a.
   "picket fence" a.
   "picture frame" a.
   "popcorn-like" a.
   "pruned-tree" a.
   "punched out" a.
   "purse string" a.
   "railroad track" a.
   "renal string bead" a.
   "rugger jersey" a.
   "saber shin" a.
   "snow storm" a.
   "soap bubble" a.
   "spade-like" a.
   "spiked" a.
   "stepladder" a.
   "sun-ray" a.
   "sunburst" angiographic a.
   "swiss cheese" a.
   "tree-in-water" a.
   "trefoil" a.
   "web-like" a.
   "wine glass" a.
   "wormy" a.
appendage
appendiceal
   a. abscess
appendices, pl.
   appendix, s.
appendicolith
appendicular
   a. abscess
   a. ataxia
   a. lobe
   a. lymph node
   a. muscle
   a. skeleton
appendix, s.
   appendices, pl.
applanation
applecore constricture

applecore-like
applicator
   afterloading Heyman a.
   Burnett a.
   Burnett afterloading
     vaginal a.
   conical chrome a.
   Delclos a.
   Ernst a.
   Fletcher-Suit-Delclos
     (FSD) a.
   Mick a.
   Suit-Fletcher a.
apposing
apposition
appropriate for gestational age
   (AGA)
APT (automatic peak tracking)
APUDoma (amine precursor
   uptake decarboxylation cell
   tumor)
Aquaphor (cholesterolized
   anhydrous petrolatum
   ointment base)
aqueduct
   a. of Sylvius
   a. stenosis
   cerebral a.
aqueductus vestibuli vein
AR (aortic regurgitation)
ARA (American Rheumatism
   Association)
arachnodactyly
arachnoid
   a. canal
   a. cyst
   a. meninges
   a. space
arachnoidal
   a. granulations
   a. villi
   a. villoma
Arani catheter
Arantius, duct of

araphia
arborization
arc
    a. field
ARC (AIDS-related complex)
arc-to-arc movement
arc-to-line movement
arc-welder's disease
Arcelin's
    A.'s method
    A.'s position
    A.'s view
Arcelin-Stenver view
arch
    a. aortography
    a. bar
    abdominothoracic a.
    anterior a.
    aortic a. (AA)
    brachial a.
    dental a.
    fallopian a.
    longitudinal a.
    lumbar a.
    lumbocostal a.
    mandibular a.
    maxillary a.
    orbital a.
    palatal a.
    plantar a.
    posterior a.
    pubic a.
    subpubic a.
    superciliary a.
    tarsal a.
    transverse a.
    vertebral a.
    zygomatic a.
archenteron
archinephric canal
arcing
arcuate
    a. eminence
    a. ligaments

a. suture
arcuation
arcus aortae bicurvatus
ARDS (adult respiratory
   distress syndrome)
area
    a. monitoring
    Broca's a.
areae gastricae
areola, s.
    areolae or areolas, pl.
areolae or areolas, pl.
    areola, s.
areolar
areolas or areolae, pl.
    areola, s.
argentaffin carcinoma
argentaffinoma syndrome
argon (Ar)
Argyle catheter
Arkin's disease
arm extension position
armature
Armenian disease
armored heart
Arnold, canal of
Arnold-Chiari
    A.-C. deformity
    A.-C. malformation
array processor
arrays
    anular phased a.
    linear phased a.
    linear sequenced a.
arrectores pilorum muscle
arrhythmia
    continuous a.
    juvenile a.
    nodal a.
    perpetual a.
    phasic a.
    respiratory a.
    sinus a.
    ventricular a.

arrhythmogenicity
Arrillaga-Ayerza
  syndrome
Arrow-Howes multilumen
  catheter
ARRS (American Roentgen Ray
  Society)
ARRT (American Registry of
  Radiology Technologists)
ARS (acute radiation
  syndrome)
ARS (American Radium
  Society)
arsenate (As-74)
arsenic (As)
Arteray
arteria
    a. anastomotica auricularis
      magna
    a. lusoria
arteria, s.
    arteriae, pl.
arteriae, pl.
    arteria, s.
arterial
    a. catheter
    a. embolism
    a. embolization
    a. ligament
    a. murmur
    a. occlusion
    a. occlusive disease
    a. oxygen saturation
    a. oxygen unsaturation
    a. phase
    a. puncture
    a. spasm
    a. stenosis
    a. thrombosis
    a. venous catheterization
      needle
Arteriodone
arteriogram
    "pruned-tree" a.
    retrograde a.

wedge a.
arteriography
    adrenal a.
    aortofemoral a.
    brachial a.
    brachiocephalic a.
    carotid a.
    catheter a.
    celiac a.
    cerebral a.
    coronary a.
    digital a.
    femoral a.
    hepatic a.
    magnified a.
    magnified carotid a.
    magnified vertebrobasilar
      a.
    mesenteric a.
    percutaneous carotid a.
    peripheral a.
    "pruned-tree" a.
    pulmonary a.
    renal a.
    selective a.
    splenic a.
    superior mesenteric a.
    vertebral a.
    vertebrobasilar a.
    visceral a.
    wedge a.
arteriohepatic
arteriola, s.
    arteriolae, pl.
arteriolae, pl.
    arteriola, s.
arteriole
arteriomesenteric duodenal
  compression
arteriosclerosis
    a. obliterans
    cerebral a.
    coronary a.
    hyaline a.
    hypertensive a.

nodular a.
peripheral a.
presenile a.
senile a.
arteriosclerotic
a. kidney
arteriosum, s.
arteriosa, pl.
arteriosus
patent ductus a. (PDA)
arteriovenous (AV, also A-V)
a. aneurysm
a. angioma
a. fistula (AVF)
a. malformation (AVM)
a. pulmonary aneurysm
a. shunt
arteritis
giant cell a.
granulomatous a.
pulmonary a.
Takayasu's a.
temporal a.
artery
a. of Bernasconi and
Casinary
a. of the pterygoid canal
Adamkiewicz' a.
candelabra a.
carotid a.
circumflex a.
common iliac a.
coronary a.
descending a.
Drummond's marginal a.
external carotid a.
femoral a. (FA)
great anterior medullary a.
great anterior radicular a.
hepatic a. (HA)
Heubner's a.
inferior mesenteric a.
(IMA)
innominate a.
internal carotid a. (ICA)

Kugel's a.
left femoral a. (LFA)
left pulmonary a. (LPA)
left subclavian a. (LSA)
manubrial a.
medial striate a.
mesenteric a.
middle cerebral a. (MCA)
nutrient a.
orbital a.
pericallosal a.
posterior cerebral a. (PCA
posterior descending a.
(PDA)
posterior inferior
cerebellar a. (PICA)
posterior tibial (PT) a.
prefrontal a.
profunda femoris a. (PFA)
pudendal a.
pulmonary a. (PA)
recurrent lent a.
recurrent
lenticulostriate a.
right anterior descending
(RAD)
right common carotid a.
(RCCA)
right coronary a. (RCA)
right femoral a. (RFA)
right iliac a. (RIA)
right pulmonary a. (RPA)
right renal a. (RRA)
right subclavian a. (RSCA)
rolandic a.
thymic a.
vidian a.
Zinn's a.
arthrifluent abscess
arthritic spirochetosis
arthritides, pl
arthritis, s.
arthritis
a. deformans juvenilis
a. mutilans

arthritis—*Continued*
   a. spurring
   acute gouty a.
   AIDS a.
   Bekhterev's or
     Bechterew's a.
   cricoarytenoid a.
   crystal-induced a.
   degenerative a.
   enteropathic a.
   erosive a.
   exudative a.
   gonococcal a.
   hypertrophic a.
   Jaccoud's a.
   juvenile rheumatoid a.
     (JRA)
   Lyme a.
   proliferative a.
   psoriatic a.
   pyogenic a.
   radiocarpal a.
   Reiter's a.
   rheumatoid a. (RA)
   septic a.
   sicca a.
   subtalar a.
   suppurative a.
   syphilitic a.
   tuberculous a.
   venereal a.
   vertebral a.
arthritis, s.
   arthritides, pl.
arthro-onychodysplasia
arthro-ophthalmopathy
arthrocentesis
arthroclasia
arthrodesis
   Moberg a.
   triple a.
arthrodial joint
arthrodynia
arthrodysplasia

arthroempyesis
arthroendoscopy
arthroereisis
arthrogenous
arthrogram
   double-contrast a.
   vacuum a.
arthrography
   air a.
   double-contrast a.
   opaque a.
   vacuum a.
arthrogryposis
   a. multiplex congenita
   a. syndrome in the Eskimo
arthrokatadysis
arthrokleisis
arthrolith
arthrolithiasis
arthrology
arthromeningitis
arthroncus
arthronosos
   a. deformans
arthropathia psoriatica
arthropathy
   Jaccoud's a.
   neurogenic a.
   neuropathic a.
arthrophyte
arthropneumography
arthropneumoroentgenography
arthroscintigram
arthroscintigraphy
arthrosclerosis
arthroses, pl.
   arthrosis, s.
arthrosis, s.
   arthroses, pl.
articular
   a. capsule
   a. cartilage
   a. cortex
   a. facet

a. fracture
a. notch
a. pillar
a. process
a. rete
a. surface
a. tubercle
articularis genu muscle
articulate
articulation
apophyseal a.
atlanto-occipital a.
atlantoaxial a.
atloido-occipital a.
cervicothoracic a.
costomanubrial a.
incudostapedial a.
lumbosacral a.
sternoclavicular a.
temporomandibular a.
tibiofibular a.
artifact
aliasing a.
channel errors on CT
slices a.
clip a.
cupping a.
edge gradient a.
electrical a.
environmental density a.
geometric a.
hairspray a.
linear partial volume a.
low-density a.
mascara a.
metallic a.
motion a.
nonlinear a.
nonlinear partial volume a.
out-of-field a.
overshoot a.
partial volume a.
ring a.
rings on CT slices a.

sampling a.
segmentation a.
soft tissue a.
star a.
straight-line a.
streak a.
superimposed a.
underscan a.
view-aliasing a.
view-sampling a.
view-streak a.
"volume averaging" a.
artifactual
artificial
a. anus
a. permanent magnet
a. radioactive isotope
a. radioactivity
aryepiglottic
a. cyst
a. fold
aryepiglotticus muscle
arytenoid
a. cartilage
arytenoideus muscle
AS & E CT scanner
AS (anterosuperior)
AS (aortic stenosis)
as low as reasonably
achievable (ALARA)
asbestosis
A-scan
A. echography
ascending
a. aorta
a. cholangitis
a. colon
a. Lipiodol (iodized oil)
a. myelopathy
a. pyelography
a. urography
Aschoff-Tawara node
ascites
exudative a.

ascites—*Continued*
  loculated a.
A-scope SEG
  (sonoencephalography)
ASD (atrioseptal defect)
aseptic necrosis
ash-leaf spot
Asherman's syndrome
ASIS (anterior-superior iliac
  spine)
aspera
aspergillosis
  allergic
    bronchopulmonary a.
  bronchopneumonic a.
  pulmonary a.
asphyxia
asphyxiate
asphyxiatic dystrophy of the
  newborn
asphyxiating thoracic
  dystrophy (ATD)
aspirated foreign body
aspiration
  a. biopsy
  a. pneumonia
  a. pneumonitis
  a. syndrome
  a. transducer
  CT-guided a.
  cytologic a.
  meconium a.
  mineral oil a.
  pulmonary a.
asplenia
ASRT (American Society of
  Radiologic Technologists)
assay
  erythropoietin a.
  Factor III multimer a.
  immunoradiometric a.(IRMA)
  thyroid radioisotope a.
    (TyRIA)
assimilation sacrum

Assmann's focus
astatine-210 (At 210)
aster
asterion
asternal rib
asthenic habitus
asthma
astragali or astragaluses, pl.
  astragalus, s.
astragaloid
astragaloscaphoid
astragalotibial
astragalus or talus
astragalus, s.
  astraguli or astragaluses,
    pl.
astragaluses or astragali, pl.
  astragalus, s.
astroblastoma
astrocytoma
  juvenile pilocytic a.
asymmetrical uptake
asymmetry
asymptomatic
  a. murmur
asystole
ataxia
  equilibratory a.
  Marie's a.
  telangiectatic a.
ataxic gait
ATD (asphyxiating thoracic
  dystrophy)
atelectasis
ateliosis
atelosteogenesis
ATG (antithyroglobulin)
atherogenesis
atheromatous ulcer
atherosclerosis
atherosclerotic
  a. aneurysm
athetotic gait
athletic heart

athyreosis
ATL (Advanced Technology
  Laboratory) ultrasound real-
  time
ATL-MK500 ultrasound
  machine
atlanto-occipital
  a.-o. articulation
  a.-o. joint
atlantoaxial
  a. articulation
  a. fusion
  a. joint
atlantodens interval (ADI)
atlantoepistropheal joint
atlantomastoid
atlas (vertebra)
atloaxoid
atloido-occipital
  a.-o. articulation
atom
  a. smasher
  activated a.
  excited a.
  helium a.
  hydrogen a.
  Na a.
  stripped a.
  tagged a.
atom-activated abscess
atomic
  a. accelerator
  a. energy
  a. mass
  a. mass unit (amu)
  a. neurogenic bladder
  a. nucleus
  a. number
  a. shell
  a. spectrum
  a. theory
  " a. time clock"
  a. volume
  a. weight unit

Atomic Energy Commission
  (AEC)
atony
  a. diabetic
Atraloc needle
atresia
  a. multiplex congentia
  anal a.
  aortic a.
  biliary a.
  bronchial a.
  choanal a.
  duodenal a.
  esophageal a.
  follicular a.
  glottic a.
  intestinal a.
  mitral a.
  pulmonary a.
  pyloric a.
  tricuspid a.
atretic
atria, pl.
  atrium, s.
atrial
  a. appendage
  a. arrhythmia
  a. fibrillation
  a. flutter
  a. infarction
  a. myxoma
  a. obstruction
  a. septum
  a. valve
atrialized chamber
atriodigital dysplasia
atrio-His pathway or tract
atrioseptal
  a. defect (ASD) shunt
  a. sign
atrioseptostomy
atrioventricular (AV)
  a. canal
  a. node

atrioventricular (AV)—
  Continued
    a. septum
atrioventricularis communis
atrium, s.
    atria, pl.
atrophic
    a. arthritis
    a. cardiomyopathy
    a. fracture
    a. gastritis
    a. hydrocephalus
    a. kidney
    a. ligamentous spondylitis
    a. pyelonephritis
atrophy
    mucosal a.
    pathologic a.
    Sudeck's a.
atropinization
attenuate
attenuation
    a. coefficient
    a. deficit
    a. loss
    a. value
    decreased a.
    increased a.
attenuator
attic
attolens aurem muscle
attrahens aurem muscle
atypical chondrodystrophy
Au (gold)
    195 Au (gold)
    198 Au (gold)
    199 Au (gold)
auditory
    a. canal
    a. meatus
    a. nerve
    a. ossicle
    a. radiation
    a. tube
    a. vesicle

Auer rod
Auerbach's plexus
Aufranc-Turner acetabular cup
Auger
    A. effect
    A. electron
augmentation mammoplasty
    implant
Augustine boat nail
AUR (The Association of
    Universty Radiologists)
aural
Aurcoscan 198
Aureoloid 198
Aureotope
auricle
auricula
    a. atrii
    a. cordis
    a. dextra cordis
    a. sinistra cordis
auricula, s.
    auriculae, pl.
auriculae, pl.
    auricula, s.
auricular
    a. appendage catheter
    a. flutter
    a. ligament
    a. line
    a. point
auricularis
    a. anterior muscle
    a. posterior muscle
    a. superior muscle
auriculoinfraorbital plane
Ausab
Auscell
auscultory gap
Ausria H-125
Aus-tect test system
Austin Moore
    A. M. hip prosthesis
    A. M. nail
Autima II pacemaker

autocorrelation function
autofluoroscope
    digital a.
auto-immune
AutoLogic (manufacturer)
    A. 50 gamma counting
      system
    A. 100 gamma counting
      system
autologous
automated computerized axial
  tomography (ACAT)
automatic
    a. collimator
    a. exposure
    a. injectors
    a. line voltage
      compensator
    a. mode scan
    a. peak tracking
      (APT)
    a. processing system
    a. serial changer
autonomic
autonomous nodule
autoradiogram
    contact a.
autoradiograph
    a. technique
autoradiography
    contact a.
    dip-coating a.
    film-stripping a.
    thick-layer a.
    two-emulsion a.
Autoscan scanner
autotomogram
autotomography
autotransformer
    a. formula
auxiliary ventricle
AV (arteriovenous)
AV (atrioventricular)
avalanche
    a. ionization

    Townsend's a.
avascular necrosis (AVN)
average
    a. acoustic output
    a. deviation
    a. gradient
    a. life (mean life)
    a. power
AVF (arteriovenous fistula)
AVG (ambulatory visit groups)
aviator's astragalus fracture
avidity
AVM (arteriovenous
  malformation)
AVN (avascular necrosis)
Avogadro's number
AVR (aortic valve replacement)
avulsion fracture
avulsive cortical irregularity
axes, pl.
    axis, s.
axial
    a. computed tomography
      (ACT)
    a. cuts
    a. plane
    a. plate
    a. position
    a. projection
    a. resolution
    a. section
    a. skeleton
    a. slice
    a. supine projection
    a. transcranial projection
    a. transverse tomography
axillary
    a. aneurysm
    a. folds
    a. line
    a. lymph nodes
    a. lymphadenopathy
    a. projection
    a. region
    a. space

axiolateral
    a. position
    a. projection
axiopetrosal
    a. plane
axis
    celiac a.
    longitudinal a.
    vertical a.
    X a.
    Y a.
axis, s.
    axes, pl.

Ayerza's syndrome
Ayerza-Arrillage syndrome
Azetylpromazine
azimuth resolution
azygoesophageal recess
azygogram
azygography
azygos
    a. lobe
    a. lobe fissure
    a. lymph node
    a. uvulae muscle
    a. vein

Bb

B (Bucky)
B (magnetic induction of flux density)
B ray
B septal lines
B-27 linked spondyloarthropathy
Ba (barium)
BA (bone age)
Baastrup's syndrome
Baber's syndrome
Babinski's
    B.'s reflex
    B.'s sign
Babinski-Fröhlich syndrome
bacciform
bacillary colitis
back
    b. projection
    b. scatter factor (BSF)
    b. surface resolution
back emf (back electromotive force)
backfire fracture
backflow
background (BG)
    b. activity
    b. corrected (BG-corr)
    b. count
    b. density
    b. elimination (erase)
    b. erase
    b. radiation
    b. subtraction technique
backscatter
    b. peak
bacteria

bacterial
    b. aneurysm
    b. colitis
    b. endocarditis
    b. pericarditis
bactericide
Badgley plate
Bado's fracture
BaE or BE (barium enema)
Baer's plane
bag catheter
bagassosis
Bagshaw's massives
Bailey catheter
Baker's cyst
Bakwin-Eiger syndrome
Bakwin-Krida syndrome
BAL (bronchoalveolar lavage)
bald gastric fundus
Balkan fracture frame
ball-and-socket joint
Ball-Golden method
Ball's method
ball-type valve
ball-valve
    b.-v. carcinoid tumor
    b.-v. gallstone
Balli's sphincter
Ballingall's disease
ballistic
balloon
    b. biliary catheter
    b. catheter
    b. catheterization
    b. dilation
    b. French shaft
    b. image data

b. tuboplasty
ballooning of the sella turcica
balsa wood block
Baltaxe-Mitty-Pollack coaxial
  needle
Bamatter's syndrome
"bamboo" spine
band
    fibrous b.
    Ladd's b.
bandbox resonance
bands
    b. of density
bandwidth
banjo-string adhesions
Bankart's
    B.'s fracture
    B.'s lesion
Banti's syndrome
BAP (brightness area product)
Barclay's niche
Bard (manufacturer)
    B. bioptic gun
    B. catheter
Bardam catheter
Bardex (manufacturer)
    B. bulb
    B. catheter
    B. Foley catheter
Bardic catheter
Bard-Pic syndrome
Baridol
Bariform
Bari-O-Meal
baritosis
barium (Ba)
    133Ba (barium)
    b. carbonate
    b. column
    b. double-contrast study
    b. enema (BE or BaE)
    b. fleck
    b. fluorochloride
    b. lead sulfate

b. meal
b. meal study
b. platinocyanide
b. strontium sulfate
b. sulfate (BaSO4)
  (Barotrast)
b. swallow
b. vaginography
b. wafer
hydrophilic nonflocculating b.
barium-based
barn
Barodense (colloidal
  microbarium sulfate)
Barolius, valve of
Baroloid (microbarium sulfate)
Baropaque A, B, or C
Barosperse 5:2
Barotrast (barium sulfate)
barotrauma
Barr's triad
barrel chest
barrel-shaped thorax
barreling distortion
Barrett's
    B.'s epithelium
    B.'s esophagus
    B.'s syndrome
    B.'s ulcer
bar-ridge deformity
barrier
Bársony-Polgár syndrome
Bársony-Teschendorf
  syndrome
Bart's abdominoperipheral
  angiography unit
Bartenwerfer's syndrome
Barth
    B. biliary drainage needle
    B. needle
Bartholin's
    B.'s cyst
    B.'s ducts
    B.'s gland

Bartholin-Patau syndrome
bartholinian abscess
Barton's
    B.'s disease
    B.'s fracture
Bartter's syndrome
BAS 16
bas-fond (French fundus)
basal
    b. angle
    b. cell carcinoma
    b. cell nevus syndrome
    b. cistern
    b. foramen
    b. ganglia
    b. kyphosis
    b. neck fracture
    b. segmental bronchus
    b. skull fracture
    b. vein of Rosenthal
basalis
base
    b. density
    b. fog
    b. volume image analysis
    orbital b.
baseball
    b. bat shape
    b. finger
Basedow's
    B. disease
    B. goiter
baseline
    anthropological b.
    anthropomorphic b.
    radiographic b.
    Reid's b. (RBL)
basilar
    b. apophysis
    b. implant
    b. impression
    b. investigation
    b. position
    b. projection

    b. vein
    b. vertebra
    b. view
Basile hip screw
basilic
    b. vein
basioccipital
basion
basket cells
basketball foot dislocation
Basle Nomina Anatomica (BNA)
BaSO4 (barium sulfate)
    (Barotrast)
Basolac
basophil
basophilic adenoma
basovertical projection
Bass' syndrome
Bassen-Kornzweig syndrome
bat-wing
    b.-w. formation
    b.-w. shadow
    b.-w. sign
Bateman
    B. finger prosthesis
    B. toe prosthesis
bathrocephaly
batrachian position
Batson's plexus
battered-baby syndrome
battered-child syndrome
Baudelocque's diameter
Bauhin, valve of
Bauman's angle
bauxite worker's disease
Bayes theorem
Bayford-Autenrieth dysphagia
Bayley and Pinneau, tables of
BB or BBx (breast biopsy)
BBB (blood-brain barrier)
BBB (bundle-branch block)
BBx or BB (breast biopsy)
BCD (binary-coded decimal)
BCDDP (breast cancer

detection and demonstration
project)
BD (below diaphragm)
BD (bile duct)
BDM (border detection
method)
Be (beryllium)
BE or BaE (barium enema)
bead chain cystography
beaded ureter
beading of a vessel
beak sign
beaked pelvis
beaking
Beall prosthesis
beam
  b. barrier
  b. CT scanner
  b. edge
  b. hardening
  b. hardening correction
  b. length
  b. monitor
  b. restrictor
  b. shaping filter
  b. therapy
  b. width
  central b.
  electron b.
  useful b.
  x-ray b.
beam-bending magnet
beam-flattening filter
beam-limiting
beam-restricting
beam-splitting
beamsplitter
Beckwith's syndrome
Beckwith-Wiedemann
  syndrome
Béclère's
  B.'s method
  B.'s position
becquerel (Bq)

Becton-Dickinson
  (manufacturer)
    B-D thin-wall needle
Bedfordil
Bednar-Parrot disease
bedside radiography
beer heart
Beer-Low projection
Behnken's unit
BEI (butanol-extractable
  iodine)
Bekhterev's or Bechterew's
    B.'s arthritis
    B.'s disease
Bekhterev-Strümpell-Marie
  disease
Belevac
bell
    b. hernia
    b. shape
Bell's brachydactyly, type A, B,
  C, D, E
Bell-Dally dislocation
bell-metal resonance
Bell-Thompson rule
belladonna tincture
Bellini, ducts of
below diaphragm (BD)
below-the-knee amputation
  (BKA)
Belsey esophagram
Benadryl (diphenhydramine
  hydrochloride)
Benassi's
    B.'s method
    B.'s position
bending-forward position
bending fracture
bengal dye
benign
    b. adenoma
    b. chondroblastoma
    b. lesion
    b. paroxysmal peritonitis

benign—*Continued*
    b. tumor
Bennett
    B. fracture
    B. reverse fracture
Benoist penetrometer
bent
    b. blade plate
    b. bronchus sign
    b. fracture
Bentson
    B. cerebral curved safe-T-J guide wire
    B. cerebral straight guide wire
    B. guide
    B. introducer
Bentson-Hanafee-Wilson catheter
benzidine
benzoate
benzoic acid
Berardinelli's lipodystrophy syndrome
Bergman's sign
Bergonié-Tribondeau law
Bergstrand's disease
beriberi heart disease
berkelium
berkelium-247 (Bk 247)
Bernasconi and Casinary, artery of
Bernheim's syndrome
Bernstein-Ballantine counter
berry aneurysm
Berry clamp
Berry's syndrome
Bertel's
    B.'s method
    B.'s position
    B.'s projection
    B.'s view
Bertin's
    B.'s column
    B.'s ligament

berylliosis
beryllium (Be)
    b. granulomatosis
    b. window
Besey esophagram
Besnier-Boeck-Schaumann syndrome
Besnier-Tennesson syndrome
beta
    b. decay
    b. detection
    b. disintegration
    b. emission
    b. emitter
    b. particle
    b. radiation
    b. scan
    b. transition
    b. wave
beta-oxybutyric acids (BOBA)
beta-ray spectrometer
betatron
    b. therapy
Beuren's syndrome
BEV (billion electron volts)
bevatron
bezoar
Bezold-Jarisch reflex
Bezold's
    B.'s abscess
    B.'s syndrome
B/F (bound-to-free) ratio
bfs (blood flow study)
BG (background)
BG (bismuth germinate)
BG-corr (background corrected)
biarticular
biaxial joint
bibasilar
bicameral abscess
bicaudate catheter
biceps
    b. brachii muscle

b. femoris muscle
Bichat's canal
bicipital
  b. aponeurosis
  b. groove
  b. rib
biconcave
bicondylar
  b. joint
biconvex
bicornuate
  b. uterus
bicoudé catheter
bicuspid valve
BIDA (parabutyl IDA)
Bidirus, valve of
Biemond's syndrome
bifid
  b. patella
  b. rib
  b. thumb
bifida
  b. occulta
bifurcation
big rib sign
Bigelow screw
Bigelow's ligament
bilateral
  b. changes
  b. dysfunction
  b. function
  b. hilar adenopathy
  b. polycystic ovarian
    syndrome
bilaterality
Bilbao-Dotter
  B.-D. catheter
  B.-D. tube
bile
  b. duct (BD)
  b. duct abscess
  b. duct carcinoma
  b. leakage
  b. reflux
  b. salt breath test

Bilevac
bilharziasis or bilharziosis
biliary
  b. abscess
  b. angiography
  b. atresia
  b. calculus
  b. canal
  b. canaliculi
  b. catheter
  b. cirrhosis
  b. cirrhotic liver
  b. decompression
  b. duct
  b. obstruction
  b. rim sign
  b. stenosis
  b. stent
  b. system
  b. tract
  b. tree
biliary-enteric fistula
Biligrafin
  B. forte
Biligram
Biliodyl
bilious
Biliselektan
Bilitrast
Bilivistan
billion electron volts
  (BEV)
Billroth's operation
bilocular
  b. heart
  b. joint
biloma
Bilombrine
Bilopaque (tyropanoate
  sodium)
Biloptin
Bilospext
bimalleolar fracture
bimastoid
bimolecular

binary
    b.-coded decimal (BCD)
    b. scaler
binding energy
    b. e. alpha particle
    b. e. electron
    b. e. neutron
    b. e. nuclear
    b. e. proton
    b. e. total electron
binocular stereoscope
bioassay
    erythropoietin b.
biologic half-life
biomedical radiography
biomolecular reaction
biophysical profile
biophysics
biopsy (Bx)
    aspiration b.
    bronchial brush b.
    CT-directed b.
    CT-guided b.
    cytologic b.
    endoscopic duodenal b.
    large-bore b.
    percutaneous liver b.
Biorck-Thorson syndrome
biosynthesis
biparietal
    b. diameter (BPD)
    b. suture
bipartite diameter (BPD)
bipedal
biphasic
biplane
    b. film changer
    b. filming
    b. projection
    b. screening
    b. sector probe
    b. table
    b. view

bipolar catheter
bird's eye needle
bird-breeder's lung
bird-fancier's lung syndrome
bird-headed dwarfism
bisacodyl tannex
bishop's cap
bismuth
    b. bands
    b. carbonate
    b. germinate (BG)
    b. line
bit CT
bite-wing
bituberous diameter
biventer cervicis muscle
biventricular
    b. dilatation
    b. enlargement
Björk-Shiley prosthesis
black
    b. cardiac
    b. liver-jaundice syndrome
    b. lung
    b. pleura
black-level
Blackett-Healy
    B.-H. method
    B.-H. position
    B.-H. prone position
    B.-H. supine position
bladder
    atonic neurogenic b.
    b. calculi
    b. catheter
    b. diverticulum
    b. ears
    b. sphincter dyssynergy
    double b.
    neurogenic b.
    prolapsed b.
blade plate
blade/plate device
Blakemore needle

Blalock-Hanlen operation
Blalock-Taussig
    B.-T. operation
    B.-T. shunt
bland fluid
Bland-White-Garland
  syndrome
blast injury
Blasucci catheter
bleb
    emphysematous b.
bleeders' joint
Blegvad-Haxthausen syndrome
blepharophimosis
blind
    b. intestine
    b. loop syndrome
    b. pouch
    b. ureter
Blineau's projection
blink
    b. mode
blip
blister
    b. of bone
    b. sign
Blitt catheter
Bloch's equation
block
    alveolar-capillary b.
    b. vertebra
    balsa wood b.
    cerrobend b.
    customized b.
blockage
blood
    b. disease therapy
    b. flow measurement
    b. patch
    b. pigments
    b. pool imaging
    b. pool scan
    b. studies
    b. volume (BV)

    b. volume measurements
blood-brain barrier (BBB)
blood flow study (bfs)
    cerebral bfs
    pulmonary bfs
Bloom-German syndrome
Bloom's syndrome
blooming focal spot
Blount-Barber syndrome
Blount plate
Blount's
    B.'s osteochondrosis
    B.'s syndrome
blow-in fracture
blow-out
    b.-o. fracture
    b.-o. fracture of the orbit
    b.-o. view
blue dye
blue sclera syndrome
Blumenbach's plane
Blumensaat's line
blunting
blur
blurring motion
BMD (bone mineral density)
BMHP (bromomercurihydroxi
  propane)
B-mode (brightness
  modulation)
    B.-m. display
    B.-m. scan
    B.-m. ultrasound
BNA (Basle Nomina
  Anatomica)
BNL (breast needle
  localization)
Bo (magnetic induction field)
board
    b. angle
boat-shaped head
BOBA (beta-oxybutyric acids)
Bochdalek-Morgagni (UGI)
  syndrome

Bochdalek
  foramen of B.
Bochdalek's
  B.'s gap
  B.'s hernia
  B.'s valve
body
  b. cast syndrome
  b. composition
  b. habitus
  b. rotation method
  b. section radiography
  b. surface area (BSA)
  b. tonicity disturbance
  carotid b.
  ciliary b.
  pineal b.
  vitreous b.
  x-ray b.
body-section radiogram
body-section radiography
Boeck's
  B.'s sarcoid
  B.'s sarcoidosis
Boehler's
  B.'s angle (heel)
Boerhaave's syndrome
Bogros space
Böhler fracture frame
Bohlet angle
Bohlman pin
Bohr
  B. equation
  B. magnetron
  B. radius
  B. theory
Bolton-nasion plane
Boltzmann's
  B.'s distribution factor
  B.'s factor
bolus
  b. injection
    nephrotomography
bombardment

neutron b.
photon b.
bond
  chemical b.
  covalent b.
  valence b.
bone
  b. abscess
  b. absorption
  b. age (BA)
  b. age radiograph
  b. age radiography
  b. age—Greulich and Pyle
  b. chip
  b. density
  b. destruction
  b. dosage
  b. erosion
  b. formation
  b. fossa
  b. infarction
  b. marrow
  b. marrow scanning
  b. marrow suppression
  b. mineral analysis
  b. mineral density (BMD)
  b. of Vesalius
  b. radiation absorption
  b. scan
  b. seeker
  b. window technique
  "b.-within-bone" appearance
  cancelled b.
  cancellous b.
  compact b.
  inferior point of the pubic
    b. (IPP)
  innominate b.
  marble bs.
  os trigonum b.
  "penciling" b.
  phantom bs.
  Pirie's b.
  rider's b.

styloid b.
"sucked-candy" b.
bone-negative image
bones
    ankles (talus or
      astragalus)
        astragaloid
        astragaloscaphoid
        calcaneus (heel or os
          calcis)
        cuboid
        cuneiform,
          intermediate
        cuneiform, lateral
        cuneiform, medial
        navicular
        scaphoid
        tarsus (talus,
          calcaneus,
          navicular, cuboid,
          cuneiform)
    arms and shoulders
        clavicle (collar bone)
        humerus (upper arm
          bone)
        radius
        scapula (shoulder
          bone)
        ulna
    auditory ossicles
        incus
        malleus
        stapes
    chest
        costa, s. (costae, pl.)
        false rib
        floating rib
        manubrium
        sternum
        true rib
        xiphoid process
    cranial
        ethmoid
        frontal

        occipital
        parietal
        pterygoid
        sphenoid
        temporal
        wormian
    facial
        lacrimal
        mandible (jaw)
        maxilla
        nasal
        palatine
        turbinate (concha, s.;
          conchae, pl.)
        vomer
        zygoma (jugal, malar,
          or cheek)
    feet
        metatarsal
        phalanx, s.
          (phalanges, pl.)
        tarsal
    hands
        carpal
        metacarpal
        phalanx, s.
          (phalanges, pl.)
        tarsal
    hips (innominate)
        acetabulum
        ilium
        ischium
        pubic
    legs
        femur
        fibula
        patella (knee cap)
        tibia (shin)
    neck
        hyoid
    vertebrae
        atlanto-axial (C1-2)
        atlas
        cervical

bones—*Continued*
    cervical axis
    coccyx (4 bones fused
       into 1)
    dorsal (D1-12) same
       as thoracic
    lumbar (L1-5)
    sacrum (S1-5)
    thoracic (T1-12) same
       as dorsal
  wrists
    capitate
    carpal
    hamate
    lunate
    navicular or scaphoid
    pisiform
    trapezium
    trapezoid
    triquetrum
Bonfils' disease
Bonnano catheter
Bonner's position
bony
  b. architecture
  b. bridging
  b. deformity
  b. island
  b. labyrinth
  b. prominence
  b. ridge
  b. skeleton
  b. thorax
  b. union
Boogaard's angle
booster circuit
boot-top fracture
border
  b. detection method (BDM)
  b. sign
boron counter
Borries syndrome
Borsony-Polgar syndrome
boss

bosselated
bosselation
Bossing occipital view
Bosworth
  B. acromioclavicular screw
  B. coracoclavicular screw
  B. fracture
  B. intramedullary splint
  B. osteotomy splint
  B. procedure
  B. screw
  B. splint
Botallo
  chorda of B.
  duct of B.
  foramen of B.
  ligament of B.
botryoid
Bouchard's node
bougie
bound
  b. electron
  b. ligand
bound-to-free ratio (B/F ratio)
Bourneville-Brissaud
  syndrome
Bourneville's syndrome
boutonnière deformity
bowed tendon
bowel
  b. gas pattern
  b. impaction
  b. obstruction
  b. pattern
  b. preparation
  b. transit time
Bowman's
  B.'s capsule
  B.'s space
boxer's fracture
bow-tie filter
boxy
Boyce and Vest fistula
Boyce's position

Boyd's
    B.'s classification
    B.'s fracture
Boyden
    B. meal
    B. nomenclature
Boyd-Stearns syndrome
Bozeman
    B. catheter
Bozeman's
    B.'s position
Bozeman-Fritsch catheter
BPD (biparietal diameter)
BPD (bronchopulmonary
   dysplasia)
Bq (becquerel)
Braasch catheter
brachial
    b. arch
    b. arteriography
    b. arteritis
    b. lymph nodes
    b. plexus
brachialis muscle
brachiocephalic
    b. arteriogram
    b. arteriography
brachiocephaly
brachiocubital
brachioradialis muscle
Brachmann-de Lange
   syndrome
brachycephalic
    b. skull
brachydactyly
    Bell's b.
    Christian's b. syndrome
    Mohr-Wriedt b.
brachyesophagus
brachymelia
brachymesophalangism
brachymetacarpalia
    cryptodontic b.
brachymorphic

brachymorphism and ectopia
   lentis
brachytherapy
    stereotaxic b.
Bradford fracture frame
bradykinin
Bragg
    B. curve
    B. equation
    B. peak
    B. spectrometer
Brailsford-Morquio syndrome
Brailsford's
    B.'s line
    B.'s osteonecrosis
    B.'s peripheral dysostosis
brain
    b. abscess
    b. aneurysm
    b. scan
    b. stain sign
    b. studies
    b. trapped-air sign
brainstem glioma
branch
branched calculus
branchial
    b. arch syndrome
    b. cleft
    b. cleft cyst
branching
    b. angle
    b. decay
    b. fraction
    b. ratio
branchiogenic
    b. cyst
Brauer's syndrome
Braun's anastomosis
Brazilian type of
   achondrogenesis
breadth
breast
    b. biopsy (BB or BBx)

breast—*Continued*
    b. cancer detection and
        demonstration project
        (BCDDP)
    b. needle localization
        (BNL)
    b. self-examination (BSE)
    b. shadow
breech presentation
breeder reactor
bregma (skull)
bregmatic space
bregmatomastoid
    b. suture
brem's radiation
bremsstrahlung
    b. process
    b. radiation
Breschet's
    B.'s canals
    B.'s plexus
    B.'s sinus
    B.'s veins
Bret's syndrome
Breuerton's view
brevicollis
BRH (Bureau of Radiological
  Health)
Brickner's position
Bridges and Good syndrome
Bridgman projection
Bright's disease
brightness
    b. area product (BAP)
    b. modulation (B-mode)
brilliant blue (dye)
Brill-Symmers giant follicular
  lymphadenopathy
brim sign
brimstone liver
Brinton's disease
brisk erythema
Bristow's procedure
British thermal unit (BTU)

broad
    b. ligament abscess
    b. thumb-hallux syndrome
broad-based
broad-beam scattering
Broadbent–Bolton plane
Broca's
    B.'s area
    B.'s gyrus
    B.'s plane
Broca, retrofacial cells of
Brock's
    B.'s classification
    B.'s syndrome
Brockenbrough catheter
Broden's
    B.'s method
    B.'s position
Broder's grade
Broderick spinal strut
Brodie's
    B.'s abscess
    B.'s joint
    B.'s ligament
Brodney clamp
bromide
bromine
brominized oil
bromomercurihydroxi propane
  (BMHP)
Bromsulphalein (BSP)
  (sulfobromophthalein
  sodium)
bronchi, pl.
    bronchus, s.
bronchia, pl.
    bronchium, s.
bronchial
    b. adenoma
    b. atresia
    b. brush biopsy
    b. catheter
    b. markings
    b. meniscus sign

b. obstruction
b. pneumonia
b. rupture
b. sharp cutoff
b. tree
b. washings
bronchiectasis
    cylindrical b.
    saccular b.
bronchiectatic collapse
bronchiole
    alveolar b.
    terminal b.
bronchiolectasis
bronchioli, pl.
    bronchiolus, s.
bronchiolitis
    b. obliterans
bronchiolus, s.
    bronchioli, pl.
bronchitis
bronchium, s.
    bronchia, pl.
bronchoalveolar lavage
  (BAL)
bronchogenic
    b. carcinoma
    b. cyst
    b. diverticulum
bronchogram
    air b.
    tantalum b.
bronchography
    Cope-method b.
    inhalation b.
    percutaneous
      transtracheal b.
broncholith
broncholithiasis
bronchomalacia
bronchopleural fistula
bronchopneumonia
bronchopneumonic
  aspergillosis

bronchopulmonary
    b. dysplasia (BPD)
    b. lymph node
bronchoradiogram
bronchoradiography
bronchoscopy
    fiberoptic b.
    nonfiberoptic b.
bronchospasm
bronchospirometric catheter
bronchotomogram
bronchovesicular markings
  (BVM)
bronchus
    anomalous b.
    apical b.
    basal segmental b.
    cardiac b.
    eparterial b.
    hyparterial b.
    lobar b.
    lower lobe b.
    main stem b.
    middle lobe b.
    patent b.
    segmental b.
    subsegmental b.
    upper lobe b.
bronchus, s.
    bronchi, pl.
bronze liver
bronzed disease
Brophy plate
Broviac catheter
brow-down position
brow-up position
Brown corrugated fastener
Brown-Roberts-Wells (BRW)
    CT stereotaxic guide
brown-spot syndrome
Browning's vein
Brucella
bruit
Brunauer's syndrome

Brunner's gland
brush-like renal pyramids
BRW (Brown-Roberts-Wells)
   CT stereotaxic guide
Bryant's traction
BSA (body surface area)
B-scan
   B-s. echography
B-scope SEG
   (sonoencephalography)
BSE (breast self-examination)
BSF (back scatter factor)
B-shaped stomach
BSP (Bromsulphalein)
   (sulfobromophthalein
   sodium)
Btu (British thermal unit)
bubble
   b. ventriculography
bubble-like
"bubbly lung" syndrome
bucca
buccal
   b. cavity
   b. lymph node
   b. mucosa
   b. surface
buccinator
   b. lymph node
   b. muscle
Buck's
   B.'s fascia
   B.'s traction
bucket-handle fracture
buckle fracture
buckling
   b. of the aorta
Buckner button
buckshot
Bucky (B)
   B. diaphragm
   B. film
   B. grid
   B. ray

   B. split
   B. table
   B. tray
   B. view
   B. wallstand
   oscillating B.
Bucky-Potter diaphragm
Budd-Chiari syndrome
buddy splint
Budin joint
Budin-Chandler method
Büdinger-Ludloff-Läwen
   syndrome
BUDR (clinical radiosensitizer)
Buerger's disease
Buerhenne catheter
buffer amplifier
buffy coat
Buie's position
bulb
   b. catheter
   b. of aorta
   b. palsy
   b. ureteral catheter
   duodenal b.
bulbar
   b. fascia
   b. tract
bulbocavernosus muscle
bulbocavernous gland
bulbomedullary junction
bulbospinal tract
bulbourethral
   b. gland
bulbous
bulboventricular fold
bulging
bulk film loading
bull's
   b.'s angle
   b.'s eye lesion
   b.'s eye plot
   b.'s eye program
   b.'s eye sign

bulla
  b. mastoidea
  b. ossea
  emphysematous b.
  ethmoid b.
bulla, s.
  bullae, pl.
bullae, pl.
  bulla, s.
bulldog scalp
Bullit's method
bullous emphysema
bumper fracture
bunamidol
bunamiodyl
bundle
  b. branch block (BBB)
  b. of His
  Kent b.
bunion
bunkbed fracture
Bunt catheter
buoyancy
bur hole
Bureau of Radiological Health
  (BRH)
Burhenne tip control catheter
Burke's syndrome
Burkhart's deformity
Burkitt's
  B.'s lymphoma
  B.'s tumor
Burn's osteonecrosis
Burnett
  B. afterloading vaginal
    applicator
  B. applicator
bursa
  ischial b.
  omental b.

  subacromial-subdeltoid b.
  suprapatellar b.
  trochanteric b.
bursa, s.
  bursas or bursae, pl.
bursae or bursas, pl.
  bursa, s.
bursitis
  iliopsoas b.
  trochanteric b.
bursting fracture
Busi's sphincter
busulfan lung syndrome
butanol-extractable iodine
  (BEI)
butterfly
  b. distribution
  b. fracture
  b. lesion
  b. needle
  b. position
  b. shadow
  b. tumor
  "b." vertebra
buttock
button
  b. sequestrum
  b. sign
  Kistner's tracheal "b."
buttonhole fracture
buttress plate
buttressing callus
BV (blood volume)
BVM (bronchovascular
  markings)
Bx (biopsy)
bypass
  cardiac b.
  jejunoileal b.
byssinosis

Cc

C syndrome of multiple
  congenital anomalies
C. (coulomb)
Ca 45 (calcium chloride)
Ca fluoroscopy
CABG (pronounced "cabbage")
  (coronary artery bypass
  graft) procedure
cachexia
CAD (coronary artery disease)
Cadman's triangle
cadmium (Cd)
    c. chloride (Cd109)
    c. zinc sulfide
café au lait spots
Caffey
    tables of C.
Caffey-Kempe syndrome
Caffey's
    C.'s disease
    C.'s elongation of the
      metaphysis and the
      diaphysis
    C.'s osteonecrosis I, II
    C.'s pseudo-Hurler's
      syndrome
    C.'s syndrome
Caffey-Silverman syndrome
Caffey-Smyth disease
cage
    Faraday's c.
Cahoon's
    C.'s method
    C.'s position
    C.'s view
Cairns' syndrome
Caisson's disease
cake kidney
calcanea, pl.

    calcaneum, s.
calcaneal
    c. fracture
    c. line
    c. spur
    c. sulcus
    c. tendon
calcaneal-fifth metatarsal angle
calcanei, pl.
    calcaneus, s.
calcaneoapophysitis
calcaneoastragaloid
calcaneocavus
calcaneocuboid joint
calcaneofibular ligament
calcaneonavicular ligament
calcaneoplantar
calcaneoscaphoid
calcaneotibial
calcaneovalgocavus
calcaneum, s.
    calcanea, pl.
calcaneus (heel or os calcis)
calcaneus, s.
    calcanei, pl.
calcar
    c. femoris
    c. pedis
calcarea
calcareous
calcarine
    c. fissure
    c. sulcus
calcemia
calcific
    c. aortic stenosis
    c. carotid stenosis
    c. density
    c. shadow

calcific—*Continued*
  c. tendinitis
calcification
  abdominal c.
  anular c.
  conglomerate c.
  costochondral c.
  ectopic c.
  "eggshell" c.
  heterotopic c.
  interstitial c.
  intracranial c.
  joint c.
  "mulberry-type" c.
  non-neoplastic c.
  pancreatic c.
  "parentheses-like" c.
  pericardial c.
  "popcorn" c.
  prostatic c.
  punctate c.
  stippled c.
  thoracic c.
  thrombus c.
  valvular c.
  vascular c.
calcified
  c. granuloma
  c. lymph node
  c. pericardium
  c. renal cyst
  c. shadow
  c. thrombus
  c. uterine fibroid
calcifying
  c. cholecystitis
  c. giant cell tumor
calcimine
calcinosis
  c. universalis
calcitonin
calcium (Ca)
  c. (with scandium 47)
  c. channel blocker
  c. chloride (Ca-45)

  c. chloride (Ca-47)
  c. deposit
  c. endocrine regulation
  c. gluconate
  c. ioglycamate
  c. phosphate
  c. pyrophosphate
    dihydrate (CPPD)
  c. tungstate
  ipodate c.
  milk-of-c.
  Oragrafin c. (ipodate
    calcium)
calculated image
calculi
  staghorn c.
calculi, pl.
  calculus, s.
calculogram
calculography
calculus
  biliary c.
  branched c.
  renal c.
  staghorn c.
  ureteral c.
calculus, s.
  calculi, pl.
Caldwell's
  C.'s position
  C.'s projection
  C.'s view
Caldwell-Moloy
  C.-M. classification
  C.-M. method
calibrate
calibration
  E-dial c.
calibrator
  digital isotope c.
  radioisotope c.
calices or calyces, pl.
  calix or calyx, s.
calicified
  c. density

caliectasis or calyectasis
californium (Cf)
caliper
    direct-reading c.
    radioisotope c.
calix or calyx, s.
    calices or calyces, pl.
callodial chromic phosphate (P32)
callosal
    c. gyrus
    c. sulcus
callosomarginal
    c. gyrus
callous (adj.)
    c. formation
callum
    c. dentis
    c. femoris
callus (noun)
    buttressing c.
    exuberant c.
calvarial
    c. "doughnut" lesion
    c. osteomyelitis
    c. teratoma
calvarium
Calvé's
    C. spondylitis
    C. vertebra planum
Calvé-Perthes-Legg syndrome
calyceal
    c. crescent sign
    c. dilatation
    c. diverticulum
    c. stump
    c. system
calyces or calices, pl.
    calyx, s.
camera
    Anger c.
    c. tube
    cine c.
    Circon video c.
    data c.
    format c.

    gamma c.
    gamma scintillation c.
    Isocon c.
    laser c.
    LEM scintillation c.
    Medx c.
    multicrystal c.
    multiformat c.
    Newvicon c.
    Odelca c. unit
    Orbitome tomographic s.
    Orthicon television c.
    PHO/Gamma LEM low
        energy mobile
        scintillation c.
    PHO/Gamma V
        scintillation c.
    pinhole c.
    positron scintillation c.
    radioisotope c.
    Saticon c.
    scintillation c.
    Spectroscaler 4R
        scintillation c.
    video display c.
    Vidicon c.
    x-ray pinhole c.
Cameron
    C. fracture appliance
    Norland-C. photon
        densitometry
Cameron's
    C.'s method
Camp-Coventry
    C.-C. method
    C.-C. position
Camp-Gianturco method
Campbell catheter
Camper line
Campiodol
Camp grid cassette
camptobrachydactyly
camptodactyly
camptomelic
    c. dwarfism

camptomelic—*Continued*
  c. dysplasia
  c. hypoplasia
camptomicromelic
  c. dwarfism
Campylobacter
  C. jejuni
  C. pyloris
Camurati-Englemann
  syndrome
Canadian Association of
  Radiologists (CAR)
canal
  abdominal c.
  accessory palatine c.s
  adductor c.
  alimentary c.
  alveolar c.s
  anal c.
  arachnoid c.
  archinephric c.
  artery of pterygoid c.
  atrioventricular c.
  auditory c.
  Bichat's c.
  biliary c.
  c. of Arnold
  carotid c.
  carpal c.
  cerebrospinal c.
  cervical c.
  Cloquet's c.
  cochlear c.
  condylar c.
  craniopharyngeal c.
  crural c.
  Dorello's c.
  endocervical c.
  entodermal c.
  ethmoid c.
  eustachian c.
  external auditory c.
  femoral c.
  Guidi's c.

  Guyon's c.
  haversian c.
  Hering's c.
  Hunter's c.
  hyaloid c.
  hypoglossal c.
  infraorbital c.
  inguinal c.
  lacrimal c.
  mandibular c.
  medullary c.
  nasolacrimal c.
  nasopalatine c.
  neural c.
  Nuck's c.
  optic c.
  petromastoid c.
  portal c.
  pterygopalatine c.
  pudendal c.
  pyloric c.
  sacral c.
  Schlemm's c.
  semicircular c.
  Sondermann's c.
  sphenopalatine c.
  sphenopharyngeal c.
  spinal c.
  spiral c.
  Sucquet-Hoyer c.
  supraciliary c.
  supraoptic c.
  Theile's c.
  tubal c.
  umbilical c.
  urogenital c.
  uterine c.
  uterocervical c.
  van Hoorne's c.
  ventricular c.
  vidian c.
  Volkmann's c.
  vomerobasilar c.
  vomerovaginal c.

vulvar c.
vulvouterine c.
zygomaticotemporal c.
canalicular
    c. abscess
canaliculi, pl.
    canaliculus, s.
canaliculus
    apical c.
    c. innominatus
    mastoid c.
    tympanic c.
canaliculus, s.
    canaliculi, pl.
canalization
cancellated bone
cancelli, pl.
    cancellus, s.
cancellous
    c. bone
    c. exostoses
cancellus, s.
    cancelli, pl.
cancer therapy
cancericidal level
candela
candelabra artery
Candida osteomyelitis
candle
    "c. dripping" appearance
    c. power
    c. vaginal (radium insertion)
    foot-c.
cane, sign of
canine
caninus muscle
Cannon-Bohm sphincter
Cannon's
    C.'s level
    C.'s point
    C.'s ring
cannula
cannulate
cannulated nail

cannulating
cannulization
canthi, pl.
    canthus, s.
canthomeatal line
canthus, s.
    canthi, pl.
Cantor's tube
cap
    apical c.
    phrygian c.
capacitance
capacitive reactance
capacitor
    c. discharge system
    electrical c.
capillary
    c. blocked perfusion scan
    c. blood gas (CBG)
    c. blush
    c. fracture
    c. wedge pressure
capital
    c. epiphysis
capitate
    c. notch
capitate-hamate fusion
capitate-trapezoid fusion
capitellum
capitopedal
capitula, pl.
    capitulum, s.
capitular
    c. joint
    c. process
capitulum
    c. costae
    c. fibulae
    c. humeri
    c. mallei
    c. mandibulae
    c. ossis metacarpalis
    c. radii
    c. stapedis

capitulum—*Continued*
    c. ulnae
capitulum, s.
    capitula, pl.
Caplan-Colinet syndrome
Caplan's syndrome
capsular
    c. fibrositis
    c. ligament
    c. space
capsule
    adrenal c.
    articular c.
Bowman's c.
Crosby-Kugler c.
    external c.
    Gerota's c.
    Glisson's c.
    Heyman's c.
    internal c.
    joint c.
    prostate c.
    renal c.
    synovial c.
    Tenon's c.
    tonsillar c.
capsulotomy
captive
    c. bolus
capture
    cross-section c.
    electron c.
    gamma-ray c.
    radiative c.
    resonance c.
caput
    c. medusae
    c. succedaneum
carbon (C)
    c. 14
    c. dioxide
    c. fiber
CAR (Canadian Association of Radiologists)

carcinoembryonic antigen test (CEA)
carcinogen
carcinogenic
carcinoid
    c. syndrome
    c. tumor
carcinoidosis
carcinoma
    adenoid cystic c.
    adenosquamous c.
    alveolar cell c.
    anaplastic c.
    argentaffin c.
    basal cell c.
    bile duct c.
    bronchogenic c.
    cavitary c.
    cervical c.
    embryonal cell c.
    endometrial c.
    esophageal c.
    gastric c.
    hepatocellular c.
    islet cell c.
    jejunal c.
    laryngeal c.
    linitis plastica c.
    medullary c.
    metastatic c.
    mucinous c.
    mucoepidermoid c.
    nevoid basal cell c.
    oat cell c.
    obstructive c.
    pancreatic c.
    polypoid c.
    renal cell c.
    "spindle cell" c.
    squamous cell c.
    subglottic c.
    subungual epidermoid c.
    supraglottic c.

thyroid c.
transglottic c.
transitional cell c.
   stage A, stage B1, stage
   B2, stage C, stage D1,
   stage D2
uterine c.
vaginal c.
verrucous c.
carcinoma, s.
   carcinomata, pl.
carcinomata, pl.
   carcinoma, s.
carcinomatosis
carcinomatous
   c. pericarditis
   c. tumor
cardboard (cb)
cardiac
   c. aneurysm
   c. angiography
   c. antrum
   "c. asthma"
   c. blood pool imaging
   c. bronchus
   c. bypass
   c. catheterization
     (cc)
   c. chamber
   c. cycle
   c. decompensation
   c. effusion
   c. end of stomach
   c. failure
   c. gating
   c. herniation
   c. incisura
   c. index (CI)
   c. mensuration
   c. murmur
   c. notch
   c. orifice
   c. output
   c. shadow

c. shunt
c. silhouette
c. tamponade
c. ventricle
c. ventriculography
Cardio-Conray
Cardio-Green (dye) (sterile
   indocyanine green)
cardioangiogram
cardioangiography
   retrograde c.
cardioaortic
cardiocele
cardiochalasia
cardiocirrhosis
cardiocutaneous syndrome
cardiodiaphragmatic
cardioesophageal
   c. sphincter
cardiogenic shock
Cardiografin (meglumine
   diatrizoate)
cardiohepatic
cardiohepatomegaly
cardiokymography
cardiology
   nuclear c.
   quantitative c.
cardiomalacia
cardiomediastinal silhouette
   (CMS)
cardiomegalia
   c. glycogenica
     circumscripta
   c. glycogenica diffusa
cardiomegaly
cardiomelic syndrome
cardiomyopathy
   atrophic c.
   congestive c.
   hypertrophic c.
   obstructive c.
   restrictive c.
cardionecrosis

cardionephric
cardioneural
cardiopathia nigra
cardiopericarditis
cardiophrenic angle
    (CPA)
cardiopulmonary
cardiopyloric
cardiorenal
cardioscan
cardiospasm
cardiosplenomegaly
cardiothoracic (CT)
cardiothoracic ratio (CTR)
cardiotomy syndrome
cardiotoxicity
Cardiotrast
cardiovascular (CV)
    c. computed tomography
        (CVCT) scanner
    c. nuclear medicine
    c. ultrasonography
    c. ultrasound
cardiovasorenal syndrome
Carey-Coons stent
caries
carina, s.
    carinae or carinas, pl.
carinae or carinas, pl.
    carina, s.
carinal nodes
carinas or carinae, pl.
    carina, s.
Carlens catheter
Carman-Kirklin meniscus sign
Carman's meniscus sign
C-arm fluoroscopy unit
Carnoy's solution
Caroli's
    C.'s choledochus, type I,
        type II
    C.'s disease
    C.'s syndrome

carotid
    c. angiogram
    c. angiography
    c. arteriogram
    c. arteriography
    c. artery
    c. body
    c. bruit
    c. canal
    c. endarterectomy artery
        (CEA)
    c. gland
    c. sinus massage (CSM)
    c. siphon
    c. stenosis
carotid-cavernous fistula
carpal
    c. age
    c. angle
    c. bones
    c. bridge
    c. canal
    c. collapse
    c. dislocation
    c. fracture
    c. fusion
    c. joint
    c. ligament
    c. necrosis
    c. ossification
    c. scaphoid lag screw
    c. subluxation
    c. synostosis
    c. tunnel syndrome
    c. width
Carpenter's syndrome
carpi, pl.
    carpus, s.
carpocarpal
carpometacarpal
    c. dislocation
    c. fracture
    c. joint (CMJ)

c. ligament
carpopedal
carpophalangeal
carpoptosis
carpotarsal
carpus, s.
    carpi, pl.
Carr-Purcell-Meiboom-Gill
  sequence
Carr-Purcell sequence
carrier-free radioisotope
carrying angle
Carson catheter
cartilage
    accessory c.
    alar c.
    articular c.
    arytenoid c.
    c. inhibitor
    conchal c.
    corniculate c.
    costal c.
    cricoid c.
    cuneiform c.
    diarthrodial c.
    hyaline c.
    innominate c.
    interosseous c.
    intervertebral c.
    laryngeal c.
    semilunar c.
    septal c.
    thyroid c.
    triangular c.
    vomeronasal c.
    xiphoid c.
cartilage-hair hypoplasia
  syndrome
cartilaginous
    c. anulus fibrosis
    c. exostosis
    c. joint
    c. labrum

c. ossification
cartwheel pattern
caruncle
cascade
    c. deformity of the
      stomach
    c. stomach
Case's pad sign
caseating granuloma
caseation (n.)
caseous (adj.)
    c. abscess
    c. lymphadenitis
Caspar's ring opacity
Casselberry's position
cassette
    Adrian-Crooks c.
    Adrian-Crooks-type c.
    c. changer
    c. grid
    c. tunnel
    c. unloader
    Camp grid c.
    grid c.
    multisection c.
    Wisconsin kVp c.
cast
    "c." syndrome
    "egg" c.
    ellipsoidal c.
    fiberglass c.
    plaster c.
    plaster-of-Paris c.
    spheroidal c.
Castaneda internal-external
  drain
Castine-Kinney method
castings
    Cerrobend c.
Castleman's disease
castor oil
CAT (chlormerodrin
  accumulation test)

CAT (computer assisted tomography)
CAT (computerized axial tomography) scan
catabolism
catalyst
cataphoresis
catarrhal
    c. cystitis
    c. gastritis
    c. mastoiditis
catenary
    c. syndrome
    c. system
cathartic
    c. colitis
    c. colon
catheter
    Abramson c.
    ACMI c.
    Acmistat c.
    acorn-tip c.
    acorn-tipped c.
    Alcock c.
    Alvarez-Rodriguez c.
    Amplatz c.
    angiocatheter
    angiographic c.
    aortic c.
    aortic flush pigtail c.
    Arani c.
    Argyle c.
    Arrow-Howes multilumen c.
    arterial c.
    auricular appendage c.
    bag c.
    Bailey c.
    balloon biliary c.
    balloon c.
    Bard c.
    Bardam c.
    Bardex c.

    Bardex Foley c.
    Bardic c.
    Bentson-Hanafee-Wilson c.
    bicoudate c.
    bicoudé c.
    Bilbao-Dotter c.
    biliary c.
    bipolar c.
    bladder c.
    Blasucci c.
    Blitt c.
    bonnano c.
    Bozeman c.
    Bozeman-Fritsch c.
    Braasch bulb c.
    Brockenbrough c.
    bronchial c.
    bronchospirometric c.
    Broviac c.
    Buerhenne c.
    Buerhenne tip control c.
    bulb c.
    bulb ureteral c.
    Bunt c.
    c. à demeure
    c. aortography
    c. arteriography
    c. coudé
    c. drainage
    c. en chemise
    c. exchange curved safe-T-J guide wire
    c. exchange straight guide wire
    c.-induced thrombus
    c. needle
    c. plug
    c. tip
    c. trocar
    Campbell c.
    cardiac c.
    Carlen c.

Carson c.
Cathlon IV c.
caval c.
cecostomy c.
central venous c.
central venous pressure c.
cerebral c.
Chaffin c.
Chemo-Port c.
cholangiography c.
Chuang c.
Cobra c.
conical c.
conical tip c.
Constantine c.
Cook enforcer c.
Cook-Cope c.
Cook-Cope-type loop
  biliary drainage c.
Cook-Cope-type loop
  nephrostomy c.
Cope c.
Cope loop c.
Cordis-Ducor c.
coudé c.
coudé-tip c.
Councill c.
Cournand c.
Coxeter c.
Critikon balloon c.
Cummings c.
Cummings-Pezzer c.
CurlCath
curved c.
cut-down c.
Davis c.
Davol c.
DeLee c.
de Pezzer c.
Deseret c.
Desilet c.
Devonshire c.
disposable c.

Dormia stone-basket c.
Dotter balloon
  transluminal angioplasty
  c.
Dotter c.
double-current c.
double-J c.
double-J stent c.
double-lumen c.
drainage c.
Drew-Smythe c.
Easy c.
Edwards c.
elbowed c.
embolectomy c.
entry c.
Ependorf angioc.
Eppendorf c.
Erythroflex c.
esophagoscopic c.
eustachian c.
Evermed c.
fallopian c.
faucial c.
faucial eustachian c.
female c.
femoral aortic flush c.
femoral visceral renal
  curve c.
fenestrated c.
filiform c.
filiform-tipped c.
flexible c.
flexible metal c.
floating c.
flow-directed c.
Fogarty artery
  embolectomy c.
Fogarty balloon biliary c.
Fogarty c.
Foley c.
Foley-Alcock c.
Foltz c.

catheter—*Continued*
    four-wing Malecot retention c.
    French c.
    French Foley c.
    French polyethylene c.
    French Robinson c.
    Friend c.
    Fritsch c.
    Furniss c.
    Gambro c.
    Garceau c.
    gastroenterostomy c.
    Gensini arterial
      percutaneous c.
    Gesco c.
    Gilbert c.
    Goodale-Lubin c.
    Gouley c.
    Goutz c.
    Groll c.
    Grollman pigtail c.
    Grollman pulmonary
      pigtail c.
    Groshong c.
    Gruentzig or Grüntzig
      balloon-tip c.
    Gruentzig or Grüntzig c.
    H-1-Hc (headhunter) c.
    Hagner c.
    Hakion c.
    Hanafee c.
    Hartmann c.
    Harwood-Nash c.
    Hatch c.
    Hawkins c.
    headhunter c.
    Hemaquet c.
    Hemed c.
    hemostatic c.
    Hepacon c.
    Hickman c.
    Higgins c.
    Hilal aortogram c.

    Hilal c.
    Hilal modified headhunter
      cerebral c.
    Hinck headhunter c.
    Hinck headhunter cerebral
      c.
    Hook visceral c.
    Hryntschak c.
    ICP c.
    indwelling c.
    infant c.
    infant female c.
    infant male c.
    Ingram trocar c.
    intercostal c.
    intracardiac c.
    Intracath c.
    intraluminal c.
    intraperiosteal c.
    intraperitoneal c.
    intrauterine c.
    intravenous (IV) c.
    irrigating c.
    Itard c.
    Jackson-Pratt c.
    Jaeger-Whiteley c.
    Javid c.
    JB1 c.
    JB3 c.
    Jelco c.
    Jelm c.
    Judkins left coronary c.
    Judkins right coronary c.
    jugular venous c.
    Kaye c.
    Kerber c.
    Kerber cerebral c.
    Kerlan-Ring c.
    Kimball c.
    KISS c.
    Lane c.
    Lapides c.
    latex c.

Le Fort c.
Lehman c.
Levin c.
Levin visceral c.
Lifecath c.
Lloyd c.
lobster-tail c.
Longdwel c.
LoProfile-II balloon c.
lymphangiography (LAG)
c.
Malecot c.
Maloney c.
Manashil c.
Manashil sialography c.
Mani c.
Manhurkar c.
Mani (French) c.
Mani cerebral c.
Manu c.
mastoid c.
McCaskey c.
McGoon perfusion c.
McIntosh double-lumen c.
McIver c.
Med-Tech c.
Medina ileostomy c.
Mercier c.
metal c.
Metras c.
Mikaelsson visceral c.
mini cerebral c.
Mixtner c.
Morris c.
Mueller biliary drainage c.
Mueller c.
multi-med c.
multi-med triple-lumen
infusion c.
mushroom c.
Myler c.
nasal c.
nasogastric c.

nasotracheal c.
Neal c.
Nélaton c.
nephrostomy c.
Newton cerebral c.
NIH c.
Nutricath c.
Odman-Ledin c.
olive-tip c.
Omega C balloon
transluminal angioplasty
c.
Omega C c.
Omega NV balloon
transluminal angioplasty
c.
Omega NV c.
oval pigtail c.
Owens c.
pacemaker c.
Paceport c.
pacing c.
Paparella c.
Park Blade septostomy c.
PE Plus-II c.
pediatric Harwood-Nash
cerebral c.
pediatric Hinck
headhunter cerebral c.
pediatric pigtail c.
pediatric straight c.
penile c.
percutaneous c.
Pezzer c.
Pharmaseal c.
Phillips c.
pig-tailed c.
pigtail c.
Pilcher c.
Pilotip c.
plastic c.
plastic-sheathed needle c.
polyethylene c.

catheter—*Continued*
    polystan c.
    polystan venous return c.
    Profile Plus c.
    prostatic c.
    pulmonary artery c.
    Quinton c.
    Quinton-Mahurkar dual-
        lumen c.
    RaafCath c.
    Rabinov c.
    Rabinov sialography c.
    radiopaque c.
    railway c.
    Raimondi c.
    Raimondi ventricular c.
    Rashkind c.
    rectal c.
    red Robinson c.
    red rubber c.
    reinforced balloon dilation c.
    renal double curve
        visceral c.
    retention c.
    retrograde c.
    return flow hemostatic c.
    ring c.
    Ring-McLean c.
    Robinson c.
    Rodriguez-Alvarez c.
    Ross c.
    Ross transseptal c.
    round tip c.
    Royal Flush II high-flow
        thinwall c.
    rubber c.
    Rusch c.
    Rusch-Foley c.
    Ruschelit c.
    Salmon c.
    Schoomaker c.
    Schrötter c.
    Schwarz c.
    Seldinger c.

selective and
    superselective visceral
    c.
Seletz c.
self-retaining c.
Shaver c.
Shepherd hook visceral c.
short-arm Grollman c.
sidewinder c.
Silastic c.
Silitek c.
Simmons 1, 2, or 3 c.
Simmons cerebral c.
Simmons Newton Torcon
    c.
Simpson Artherocath c.
Skene c.
soft c.
solid-tip c.
Sones c.
Sones coronary c.
SOS c.
SOS dilation c.
spiral-tip c.
split sheath c.
Squire c.
Stitt c.
stonebasket c.
straight c.
styletted c.
suction c.
Sugg c.
suprapubic c.
Surgitek c.
Swan-Ganz c.
Tauber c.
Teflon c.
Tenckhoff c.
Texas c.
Thompson c.
Thoraflex c.
three-way c.
Tiemann c.
Tiemann-coudé c.

tip-deflecting c.
Tomac c.
toposcopic c.
Torcon balloon
  embolization c.
tracheal c.
transseptal c.
transthoracic c.
transvenous pacemaker c.
Trattner c.
triple lumen c.
trocar c.
Tuohy c.
twist drill c.
two-way c.
umbilical artery c. (UAC)
umbilical c.
umbilical venous c.
  (UVC)
ureteral c.
ureterographic c.
urethral c.
urinary c.
urologic c.
vabra c.
Vacurette c.
van Andel c.
van Andel dilatation c.
van Tessel c.
VasCath c.
Venocath c.
venous c.
vertebrated c.
vinyl c.
Virden c.
vanSonnenberg c.
Walther c.
Weber c.
whalebone filiform c.
whistle-tip c.
White c.
Wholey c.
Winer c.
winged c.

Wishard c.
Witzel c.
Witzel enterostomy c.
Wolf c.
Woodruff c.
woven silk c.
Wurd c.
Yankauer c.
Yune-Klatte c.
Yune-Klatte sialography c.
Zavod c.
catheterization
  balloon c.
  c. of bladder
  c. of duct
  c. of eustachian tube
  c. of heart
  cardiac c. (cc)
  hepatic vein c.
  Seldinger c.
catheterize
Cathlon IV catheter
cathodal dark space
cathode
  c. cable
  c. ray
  c. ray oscilloscope
  c. ray tube (CRT)
  hot c.
cation
cauda
  c. cerebelli
  c. epididymidis
  c. equina
  c. equina syndrome
  c. helicis
  c. nuclei caudati
  c. pancreatis
cauda equina, s.
    caudae equinae, pl.
cauda, s.
    caudae, pl.
caudad, (adj.)
    c. angulation

caudae equinae, pl.
  cauda equina, s.
caudae, pl.
  cauda, s.
caudal
  c. ligament
  c. projection
caudate
  c. lobe
  c. nucleus
caudocranial
Causton's
  C.'s method
  C.'s position
cava
  c. vergae
cava, pl.
  cavum, s.
caval
  c. catheter
  c. lymph node
cavernitis fibrosa
cavernolith
cavernous
  c. sinus
cavitary
  c. lesion
cavitary carcinoma
cavitation
cavity
  abdominopelvic c.
  buccal c.
  dorsal c.
  glenoid c.
  Meckel's c.
  medullary c.
  orbital c.
  pelvic c.
  pericardial c.
  peritoneal c.
  pleural c.
  tympanic c.
  ventral c.
cavogram

cavography
cavovalgus
cavum
  c. septi pellucidi
  c. septum pellucidum
    (CSP)
  c. veli interpositi
  c. vergae
cavum, s.
  cava, pl.
cb (cardboard)
CBD (common bile duct)
CBDE (common bile duct
  exploration)
CBF (cerebral blood flow)
CBG (capillary blood gas)
CBG (corticosteroid-binding
  globulin)
CC (cardiac catheterization)
CCA (common carotid artery)
CCG (cholecystogram)
CCHD (cyanotic congenital
  heart disease)
CCI (Conqvist cranial index)
CCK (cholecystokinin)
CCT (combined cortical
  thickness)
CCT (cranial computed
  tomography)
CD (common duct)
CD (computed dynamic)
CDC (chenodeoxycholic
  acid)
CDE (common duct
  exploration)
CDH (congenital dislocation of
  hip)
Ce (cerium)
CEA (carcinoembryonic
  antigen test)
CEA (carotid endarterectomy)
cecocolon
cecostomy catheter
cecum

celiac or coeliac
    c. access
    c. arteriogram
    c. arteriography
    c. axis
    c. disease
    c. lymph node
celiectomy
celiocentesis
cell
    ethmoidal air c.
    Kupffer's c.
    oat c.
    osteoprogenitor c.
    polygonal c.
    reticuloendothelial c.
    sickle c.
    spindle c.
cellule
celomic cyst
Celsius
cementifying fibroma
cementoblastoma
cementoma
cementum fracture
center
    Kerckring's c.
centigrade
centigray (cGy)
centimeter (cm)
    c. pattern of bronchial
        branching
centimeter-gram-second (cgs
    or CGS)
centimeters cubed (cm³)
central
    c. beam
    c. fracture
    c. hypoplasia
    c. line
    c. lobe
    c. lymph node
    c. ray
    c. sulcus

c. tendon
c. venous catheter
c. venous pressure
    catheter
centrencephalic
centric position
centrifugal force
centrilobular
    c. emphysema
centriole
centripetal force
centronuclear myopathy
centrosome
centrum
    c. semiovale
cephalad
    c. angled projection
cephalhematoma
cephalic
    c. angulation
    c. index
    c. projection
    c. vein
cephalocaudad
    c. instability
cephalocaudal
cephalohematoma
cephalometry
    fetal c.
    ultrasonic c.
cephalopelvic
    c. disproportion
cephalopelvimetry
cephalopharyngeus muscle
cephalopolydactyly
    Greig's c.
cephalopolysyndactyly
cerebella or cerebellums, pl.
    cerebellum, s.
cerebellar
    c. gait
    c. hemorrhage
    c. notch
    c. olive

cerebellar—*Continued*
    c. tract
    c. vermis
cerebellomedullary
    c. cistern
cerebellopontine
    c. angle (CPA)
cerebellorubrospinal
    c. tract
cerebellospinal tract
cerebellotegmental
    c. tract
cerebellothalamic
    c. tract
cerebellum, s.
    cerebellums or cerebella, pl.
cerebellums or cerebella, pl.
    cerebellum, s.
cerebra or cerebrums, pl.
    cerebrum, s.
cerebral
    c. abscess
    c. aneurysm
    c. angiogram
    c. angiography
    c. apophysis
    c. aqueduct
    c. arteriogram
    c. arteriography
    c. arteriosclerosis
    c. blood flow (CBF) study
    c. blood flow convexities
    c. catheter
    c. cortex
    c. fossa
    c. gigantism
    c. gyri
    c. hematoma
    c. hemisphere
    c. infarct
    c. metabolic rate for glucose (CMRglu)
    c. metabolic rate for oxygen (CMRO2)

c. pneumoencephalogram (PEG)
c. pneumoencephalography (PEG)
c. pneumogram
c. pneumography
c. radionuclide angiography
c. sinogram
c. sinography
c. sphingolipidosis
c. sulci
c. thrombosis
c. ventricle
c. ventriculogram
c. ventriculography
cerebrohepatorenal syndrome (CHRS)
cerebrometacarpometatarsal dystrophy
cerebroretinal arteriovenous aneurysm
cerebroside lipidosis
cerebrospinal
    c. canal
    c. fluid (CSF)
    c. tract
cerebrovascular accident (CVA)
cerebrum, s.
    cerebra or cerebrums, pl.
Cerenkov
    C. counter
    C. radiation
ceric nitrate (Ce 141)
cerium (Ce)
Cerium-141
ceroband blocks
cerrobend
    c. block
    c. castings
ceruloplasmin
cervical
    c. axis

c. canal
c. carcinoma
c. curve
c. deep fascia
c. disc, disk
c. hydrocele
c. lymph node
c. myelogram
c. myelography
c. os
c. pleura
c. prevertebral stripe, sign of
c. rib
c. rib syndrome
c. spine (CS)
c. superficial fascia
c. tunnel
c. vertebra
c. vesicle
cervicalis ascendens muscle
cervico-obturator line
cervico-occipital junction
cervico-oculo-acusticus syndrome
cervicodorsal
cervicothoracic
c. articulation
c. projection (Fletcher)
c. sign
cesarean
cesium (Cs)
c. iodide screen
c.-137 (Cs 137)
cessation
Cf (californium)
CFA (common femoral artery)
CGD (chronic granulomatous disease)
CGS or cgs (centimeter-gram-second)
cGy (centigray)
Chaffin catheter

Chagas' disease
chagasic myocardiopathy
chain
c. cystourethrogram
c. reaction
chalasia
chalky
c. bone
c. gout
chamber
air-wall ionization c.
alpha c.
atrialized c.
cardiac c.
cloud c.
extrapolation ionization c.
"free-air" c.
"free-air" ionization c.
integrating ionization c.
ionization c.
multiwire proportional c.
pocket c.
pocket ionization c.
spark c.
standard free-air ionization c.
"thimble" c.
ventricular c.
Wilson c.
Wilson cloud c.
Chamberlain's
C.'s line
C.'s method
C.'s view
Chamberlain-Towne position
champagne glass type of stomach
Chance's fracture
Chandler's disease
changeover switch
changer
Puck cutfilm c.
channel
c. blocker

channel—*Continued*
    c. errors on CT slices artifact
    c. of Lambert
    c. ulcer
channels of Lambert
Chaoul tube
Chapple's sign
Chaput, tubercle of
characteristic
    c. curve
    c. peak
    c. radiation
    c. spectrum
Charcot-Marie-Tooth disease
Charcot's
    C.'s disease
    C.'s gait
    C.'s joint
    C.'s spine
charger
    Sanchez-Perez cassette c.
Charnley hip replacement
Charnley-Mueller hip
  prosthesis
Chassard-Lapiné
    C.-L. maneuver
    C.-L. method
    C.-L. position
    C.-L. projection
Chauffard-Ramon syndrome
Chauffard-Still syndrome
Chauffeur's fracture
Chaussé's
    C.'s III method
    C.'s method
    C.'s view
    C.'s projection
CHD (common hepatic duct)
Check-Flo
    C.-F. accessory adapter
    C.-F. introducer
check ligament
Chédiak-Higashi syndrome
cheesy abscess

cheirolumbar dysostosis
cheiromegaly
cheirospasm
chelate (MPI DTPA kit)
chelated yttrium
chemical
    c. analysis
    c. bond
    c. dose
    c. dosimeter
    c. electrostatic
    c. element
    c. energy
    c. fog
    c. shift
chemodectoma
chemoembolization
Chemo-Port catheter
chemotherapeutic
chemotherapy
chenodeoxycholic acid (CDC)
cherubism
chest-abdomen sign
chest
    c. congestion
    c. position
    c. x-ray (CXR)
    flail c.
CHF (congestive heart failure)
Chiari's malformation
chiasma
    optic c.
chiasmatic
    c. cistern
chiasmatis
    c. cisterna
Chiba
    C. needle
    C. transhepatic
        cholangiography needle
Chilaiditi's
    C.'s sign
    C.'s syndrome
chip fracture

chisel fracture
chloral hydrate
chlorambucil
chloresium (chlorophyll)
chlorine
chlorine-36
chloriodized oil
chlormerodrin
    c. accumulation test (CAT)
    c. Hg 197
    c. Hg 203
    c. scan
    c.-cysteine
chloromycetin
chlorpromazine
choana, s.
    choanae, pl.
choanae, pl.
    choana, s.
choanal atresia
choke
    c. coil
choked disk, disc
cholangiocarcinoma
cholangiogram
    endoscopic retrograde c.
    intraoperative c. (IOC)
    intravenous c. (IVC)
    operative c. (OCG)
    percutaneous
      hepatobiliary c.
    percutaneous transhepatic
      c. (PTC)
    retrograde c.
    transhepatic c.
    T-tube c.
cholangiography
    c. catheter
    delayed operative c.
    direct percutaneous
      transhepatic c.
    endoscopic retrograde c.
    intraoperative c. (IOC)
    intravenous c. (IVC)

    operative c. (OCG)
    oral c.
    percutaneous
      hepatobiliary c.
    percutaneous transhepatic
      c. (PTC)
    postoperative c.
    retrograde c.
    transabdominal c.
    transhepatic c.
    T-tube c.
cholangiopancreatogram
    endoscopic retrograde c.
    (ERCP)
cholangiopancreatography
    endoscopic retrograde c.
    (ERCP)
cholangiotomogram
cholangiotomography
cholangitic abscess
cholangitis
    c. lenta
    sclerosing c.
Cholebrine (iocetamic acid)
cholecalciferol
cholecyst
cholecystangiography
cholecystectomy
cholecystic
cholecystitis
    acalculous c.
    emphysematous c.
cholecystocholangiogram
cholecystocholangiography
cholecystocolic fistula
cholecystoenteric
    c. fistula
cholecystogogue
cholecystogram (CCG)
    intravenous c. (IVC)
    oral c. (OCG)
cholecystography
    intravenous c. (IVC)
    oral c. (OCG)

cholecystokinin (CCK)
cholecystolithiasis
cholecystopaque
cholecystosonography
choledochal
   c. cyst
choledochiarctia
choledochoduodenostomy
choledochogram
choledochography
choledochojejunostomy
choledocholithiasis
choledochus
cholegram
cholegraphy
cholelith
cholelithiasis
cholepathia
Cholepulvis
Choleradiognost
cholescintigram
   radionuclide c.
cholescintigraphy
   radionuclide c.
cholestatic jaundice
cholesteatoma
   c. verum tympani
cholesterol
   c. stone
cholesterolized anhydrous
   petrolatum ointment
   (Aquaphor)
cholesterolosis
Cholestim
Cholevic
Cholevue
Cholex
Cholografin
  meglumine
  (iodipamide
  methylglucamine)
choloresis
Cholotrast
chondral
   c. fracture

chondro-osseous
chondro-osteodystrophy
chondroangiopathia calcificans
congenita
chondroblastoma
chondrocalcinosis
  (pseudogout)
chondrocostal joint
chondrodysplasia
   c. punctata
   Conradi-Hünermann c.
    punctata
   Grebe's c.
   metaphyseal c.
chondrodystrophia
   c. calcificans congenita
   c. fetalis
chondrodystrophy
chondroectodermal dysplasia
chondroepiphysitis
chondroma
   juxtacortical c.
   periosteal c.
chondroma-enchondroma
chondromalacia patellae
  (CMP)
chondromatosis
   synovial c.
chondromatous
   c. hamartoma
chondrometaplasia
chondromyoma
chondromyxoid
   c. fibroma
chondromyxosarcoma
chondroplasia
   metaphyseal c.
chondrosarcoma
chondrosternal
Chopart's
   C.'s fracture
   C.'s joint
chordo of Botallo
chordoma
choreic gait

choriocarcinoma
chorio-epithelioma
chorionic sac
choristoma
chormerodrin
    c. Hg 197
    c. Hg 203
choroid
    c. plexus
    c. plexus papilloma
choroideus muscle
Christian's brachydactyly
  syndrome
chromaffin
    c. bodies
chromaffinomatosis
Chromalbin (chromium Cr 51
  and human albumin)
chromate (Cr 51)
chromatic spectrum
chromatid-type aberration
chromatoelectrophoretic
chromatogram
chromatographic-fluorometric
  technique
chromatography
chromic
    c. chloride (Cr 51)
    c. phosphate (P 32)
Chromitope
    C. chloride
    C. sodium
      (chromate Cr
      51, sodium)
chromium (Cr)
    c. 51 labeled serum
      albumin
    c. 51 tagged red cells
    c. red cell mass
chromopertubation
chromophobe
chromophobic adenoma
chromosome
    c. aberration
    c.-type aberration

chronic
    c. abscess
    c. adhesive otitis media
    c. granulomatous disease
      (CGD)
    c. myocarditis
    c. obstructive lung disease
      (COLD)
    c. obstructive pulmonary
      disease (COPD)
chronotropic reflex
CHRS (cerebro-hepato-renal
  syndrome)
CHT (closed head trauma)
Chuang catheter
chylopericarditis
chyloperitoneum
chylopneumothorax
chylothorax
chylous
chyluria
chylus
chymopapain injection
CI (cardiac index)
Ci or c (curie)
Cibis ski needle
cicatricial
    c. kidney
cicatrix
cicatrization
CID (cytomegalic inclusion
  disease)
CIE
  (counterimmuno-
  electrophoresis)
ciliaris muscle
ciliary body
cine
    c. camera
    c. CT scan
    c. CT scanner
    c. CT unit
    c. film
    c. fluoroscopy
    c. study

cineangiocardiogram
cineangiocardiography
cineangiogram
cineangiography
cinebronchogram
cinebronchography
cinecholedochogram
cinecholedochography
cinecystogram
cinecystography
cinedensigram
cinedensigraphy
Cinefluorex
cinefluorogram
cinefluorography
cinefluoroscopy
cinematogram
cinematography
cinematoradiogram
cinematoradiography
cinephlebogram
cinephlebography
cineradiogram
cineradiography
cineroentgenofluorogram
cineroentgenofluorography
cineroentgenogram
cineroentgenography
cingulate
    c. gyrus
    c. sulcus
circle
    c. of confusion
    c. of Willis
Circon video camera
circuit
    analog derandomizer
      c.
    anticoincidence c.
    booster c.
    c. breaker
    c. diagram, x-ray
    coincidence c.
    constant-potential c.

    electronic c.
    filament c.
    integrating c.
    magnetic c.
    parallel c.
    photoelectric c.
    phototube output c.
    primary c.
    rectifying c.
    self-rectified c.
    series c.
    short c.
    three-phase c.
circuitry
circular
    c. motion
    c. movement
    c. striation
    c. sulcus of Reil
    c. tomography
circulating Tc test set
circulation time
circulatory
circumcardiac lymph node
circumcaval ureter
circumduct
circumferential fracture
circumflex
    c. artery
    c. lesion
circumflexion
circumflexus palati muscle
circumlinear
circumscribed
    c. myxedema
circumscripta
    c. cutis
    tumoral c.
circumtonsillar abscess
circumvent
cirrhosis
    biliary c.
    Laennec's c.
    macronodular c.

muscular c.
xanthomatous biliary c.
cirrhotic gastritis
cirsoid
    c. aneurysm
cistern
    basal c.
    cerebellomedullary c.
    chiasmatic c.
    interhemispheric c.
    interpeduncular c. (IPC)
    subarachnoidal c.
    suprasellar c.
    sylvian c.
    terminal c.
cisterna
    c. ambiens
    c. cerebellomedullaris
    c. chiasmatis
    c. chyli
    c. fossae lateralis cerebri
    c. interpeduncularis
    c. magna
    c. pontis
    c. venae magnae cerebri
    perinuclear c.
cisterna, s.
    cisternae, pl.
cisternae, pl.
    cisterna, s.
cisternal
    c. initis
    c. injection
    c. puncture
cisternogram
    oxygen c.
cisternography
    radionuclide c.
    RISA (radioiodinated
        serum albumin) c.
cisternomyelogram
cisternomyelography
Cistobil
Cistopac

Citelli's angle
citrate
    c. imaging
C-jun (Rad Onc)
clam shell brace
clasmocytic lymphoma
clasmocytoma
classification
    Boyd's c.
    Brock's c.
    c. of O'Rahilly
    Caldwell-Moloy c.
    Delbet's c.
    Fielding's c.
    Frykman's c.
    Garden's c.
    Gunther's c.
    Hawkins' c.
    Japanese c.
    Keith-Wagener c.
    Kiel c.
    K-W (Keith-Wagener) c.
    Ladd-Gross c.
    Lattimer's c.
    Lauge-Hanson c.
    Mason c.
    Neil-Gilmour c.
    Pipkin c.
    Salter-Harris c.
    Semb's c.
    Shopfner c.
    Sinegas c.
    Torg's c.
    Viamonte's c.
    Weber c.
clastogenic
claudication
claustra, pl.
    claustrum, s.
claustrum, s.
    claustra, pl.
clavicle (collar bone)
clavicular
    c. fracture

clavicular—*Continued*
  c. notch
claw
  c. hand
  c. toes
claw-like finger
Clayton-Johnson view
cleansing enema
clearing time
cleavage fracture
Cleaves
  C. method
  C. position
cleft
  c. palate
  c. vertebra
  laryngotracheoesophageal c.
cleidocranial
  c. dysostosis
  c. dysplasia
Cleland's ligament
Clements-Nakayama position
Cleopatra
  C. projection
  C. view
click-murmur syndrome
clinical radiosensitizer (BUDR)
clinically relevant detail
clinodactyly
  factitious c.
  traumatic c.
clinoid
  c. plate
  c. process
clinoparietal line of Taveras-
  Poser
clip artifact
clivus
cloaca
cloaking
C-loop
Cloquet's
  C.'s canal
  C.'s fascia

C.'s node
closed
  c. fist configuration
  c. fracture
  c. head injury
  c. head trauma (CHT)
  c. manipulation
closed-core transformer
closing
  c. ring of Winkler-
    Waldeyer
  c. velocity
cloud chamber
cloverleaf
  c. deformity
  c. skull
Cloward needle
Clq assay
clubfoot (talipes equinovarus)
clubfoot deformity
clubhand (talipomanus)
clump kidney
Clutton's joint
clysis
Clysodrast (bisacodyl and
  tannic acid)
cm (centimeter)
cm^3 (centimeters cubed)
CMJ (carpometacarpal joint)
CMP (chondromalacia
  patellae)
CMRglu (cerebral metabolic
  rate for glucose)
CMRO2 (cerebral metabolic
  rate for oxygen)
CMS (cardiomediastinal
  silhouette)
Co 57 bleomycin
Co 60 Schilling test
coach's finger dislocation
coagulation
coalescence
coalition
coaptation plate

coarctation of aorta
coarsening
coaxial cable
cobalt (Co)
    c. 57 (Co 57)
    c. 58 (Co 58)
    c. 59 (Co 59)
    c. 60 (Co 60)
    c. therapy
    c. w/ vitamin B_{12}
cobaltous
    c. chloride (Co-57)
    c. chloride (Co-60)
Cobatope-57 (colbaltous chloride)
Cobb's
    C.'s measurement
    C.'s method
cobblestoning
Cobra catheter
coccydynia
coccygeal
    c. joint
    c. spine
    c. vertebra
coccygectomy
coccyges or coccyxes, pl.
    coccyx, s.
coccygeus muscle
coccyx, s.
    coccyges or coccyxes, pl.
coccyxes or coccyges, pl.
    coccyx, s.
cochlear
    c. canal
    c. implant
    c. joint
    c. otosclerosis
    c. window
Cockayne's syndrome
coded-aperture imaging
codeine
"codfish" vertebrae
Codman's triangle

coefficient
    absorption c.
    attenuation c.
    c. absorption
    Compton attenuation c.
    conversion c.
    effective mass attenuation c.
    linear absorption c.
    linear attenuation c.
    mass absorption c.
    partition c.
coelom
coeur en sabot
coffin joint
cogwheel
    c. gait
    c. rigidity
coherent scattering
cohesion
coil
    crossed c.
    Gianturco c.
    Golay c.
    Helmholtz c.
    RF (radiofrequency) c.
    shim c.
    solenoid c.
    surface c.
    transformer c.
coiled
    c. position
    "c.-spring" appearance
coin lesion
coin-like
coincidence
    c. circuit
    c. counting
    c. loss
    c. sum peak
colbaltous chloride Co-57 (Cobatope-57)
Colcher-Sussman
    C.-S. method

Colcher-Sussman—*Continued*
   C.-S. technique
colchicine
cold
   c. abscess
   c. agglutinin titer
   c. area
   c. lesion
   c. nodule
   c. spot
COLD (chronic obstructive
   lung disease)
Cole fracture frame
Cole's sign
colic
   c. flexure
   c. lymph node
   c. valve
colitis
   amebic c.
   bacterial c.
   c. cystica profunda
   c. gravis
   c. polyposa
   cathartic c.
   granulomatous c.
   infectious c.
   ischemic c.
   milk-induced c.
   mucous c.
   pseudomembranous c.
   radiation c.
   ulcerative c.
   whipworm c.
colla, pl.
   collum, s.
collagen
   c. disease
   c. vascular disease
collagenosis
collapse
   bronchiectatic c.
   compression c.

contraction c.
inspiratory c.
lobar c.
obstructive c.
pulmonary c.
vascular c.
vertebral c.
collar
   "c. button" ulcers
   "c. on the Scottie dog"
collar-button abscess
collateral
   c. air drift
   c. channel
   c. flow
   c. joint
   c. ligament
   c. sulcus
   c. ventilation
COLLEAGUE computer
collecting system
Colles
   C. fracture
   C. reversed fracture
   C. space
colliculus
collimated
   c. scintillation detector
collimation
collimator
   automatic c.
   converging c.
   detector c.
   diverging c.
   focusing c.
   high-energy c.
   high-resolution c.
   high-sensitivity c.
   multihole c.
   parallel-hole c.
   pinhole c.
   single-hole c.
   slant-hole c.

source c.
thick-septa c.
thin-septa c.
Collimex
colliquationcolpostat
collision
    c. elastic
    c. inelastic
colloid
    c. cyst
    c. goiter
    c. gold
    c. technetium isotope (Tc99)
    sulfur c.
colloidal
    c. barium sulfate
    c. gold
    c. phosphorus
collum
    c. dentis
    c. femoris
    c. valgum
    c. valgumzymogen
collum, s.
    colla, pl.
coloboma
colon
    ascending c.
    c. gas
    descending c.
    iliac c.
    "lead pipe" c.
    pelvic c.
    sigmoid c.
    transverse c.
colonic
    c. angiodysplasia
    c. distention
    c. ileus
    c. lymphangioma
    c. perforation
    c. polyp
color scan

colorectal
colorimetric
colorvascular Doppler
    ultrasound
colovesical
    c. fistula
colpocephaly
columella
column
    Bertin's c.
    ilioischial c.
    iliopubic c.
    spinal c.
    vertebral c.
columnar epithelium
combined
    c. cortical thickness (CCT)
    c. transmission-emission
        scintiphoto
comedocarcinoma
commatic aberration
comminuted fracture
commissure
    habenular c.
common
    c. bile duct (CBD)
    c. bile duct exploration
        (CBDE)
    c. carotid artery (CCA)
    c. duct (CD)
    c. duct exploration (CDE)
    c. femoral artery (CFA)
    c. hepatic duct (CHD)
    c. iliac artery
    c. tendon
communicating
    c. hydrocele
    c. hydrocephalus
commutator ring
compact bone
comparison
    c. film
    c. view

compartment
  pararenal c.
  perirenal c.
  vascular c.
compartmental analysis
compatible with (c/w)
compensated gain time
compensating filter
compensator
compensatory
  c. curve
  c. emphysema
Compere
  C. modification
  C. pin
competitive protein binding
  (CPB)
complemental space
complete fracture
complex
  c. fracture
  c. mass
  c. simple fracture
  c. structure
  chlormerodrin-cysteine
    c.
  Eisenmenger c.
  Ghon c.
  Golgi c.
  Ranke c.
complexus muscle
complicated fracture
composite
  c. dorsoplantar projection
  c. fracture
  c. joint
  c. scan
  c. video signal
composite-mask subtraction
  procedure
composition
compound
  c. aneurysm
  c. fracture

  c. joint
  c. scanning
  Hurler-Scheie c.
  unsaturated c.
compression
  c. bladder
  c. collapse
  c. cone
  c. device
  c. fracture
  c. myelopathy
  c. screw
  c. technique
  digital c.
  "pancake" c.
  ureteric c.
compressor
  c. naris muscle
  c. urethra muscle
Compton
  C. absorption
  C. attenuation coefficient
  C. edge
  C. effect
  C. electron
  C. photon
  C. recoil electron
  C. scattering photon
  C. wavelength
compuscan
computed
  c. axial tomography (CAT)
  c. dynamic CT
  c. myelogram
  c. myelography
  c. tomography (CT) disc
    or disk
computer
  c.-assisted tomography
    (CAT)
  c. examination
computer display consoles
computerized
  c. axial tomography (CAT)

c. fluoroscopy
c. radiotherapy
c. tomoangiography
 (CTA)
c. tomography (CT) study
c. transaxial tomography
 (CTAT)
concavoconcave
concavoconvex
concentric
 c. pantomogram
 c. pantomography
concept
 "ring of bone" c.
concha
 ethmoidal c.
 nasal c.
 spenoidal c.
concha, s.
 conchae, pl.
conchae, pl.
 concha, s.
conchal cartilage
concomitant
concretion
concussion myelopathy
condenser
conductance
conductivity
 thermal c.
condylar
 c. canal
 c. fracture
 c. joint
 c. plate
condylarthrosis
condyle
condyli, pl.
 condylus, s.
condyloid
 c. fossa
 c. joint
 c. process
condyloma acuminatum, s.

condylomata accuminata,
 pl.
condylomata accuminata, pl.
 condyloma accuminatum, s.
condylomatous
condylus, s.
 condyli, pl.
cone
 c. epiphysis
 medullary c.
Cone needle
cone-shaped configuration
coned-down
 c.-d. projection
 c.-d. view
configuration
 closed fist c.
 cone-shaped c.
 cylindrical c.
 donut c.
 horseshoe c.
 "iceberg" c.
 "sawtooth" c.
 sigmoid-shaped c.
 "wooden shoe" c.
confluence of sinus
confluent
confusion, circle of
congenital
 c. absence
 c. adrenal hyperplasia
 c. agyria
 c. analgia
 c. anomaly
 c. cerebral aneurysm
 c. constricting bands
 c. contractural
  arachnodactyly
 c. contracture
 c. curve
 c. defect
 c. deformity
 c. dislocation of hip (CDH)
 c. fracture

congenital—*Continued*
   c. goiter
   c. hepatic fibrosis
   c. hyperuricosuria
   c. hypoplastic anemia
   c. malformation
   c. metacarpotalar
     syndrome
   c. murmur
   c. nystagmus
   c. osteoporosis
   c. pulmonary venolobar
     syndrome
   c. renal dysplasia
   c. scoliosis
   c. torticollis
congestive
   c. cardiomyopathy
   c. heart failure (CHF)
conglomerate calcification
conical
   c. catheter
   c. chrome applicator
   c. tip catheter
conjoined tendon
conjugata
   c. anatomica
   c. diagonalis
   c. vera
   c. vera obstetrica
conjugate
   anatomic c.
   c. focus
   diagonal c.
   external c.
   obstetric c.
conjunctival
   c. sac
Conley
   C. jaw replacement
   C. mandibular plate
connective tissue
conoid
   c. ligament

   c. process
   c. tubercle
Conqvist cranial index (CCI)
Conradi-Hünermann
   chondrodysplasia punctata
Conray (iothalamate
   meglumine)
   C.-280
   C.-30
   C.-325[b]
   C.-400
   C.-420
   C.-43
   C.-480
   C.-60
conservation of mass-energy
console
   direct display c.
   operator c.
consolidation
consolidative process
constant
   c. decay
   c. potential circuit
   c. potential system
   dipolar coupling c.
   longitudinal time c.
   permeability c.
   Planck's c.
   spin-lattice c.
   spin-lattice relaxation time
     c.
   spin-spin c.
   spin-spin relaxation time
     c.
Constantine catheter
constriction
constrictor
   c. pharyngis inferior
     muscle
   c. pharyngis medius
     muscle
   c. pharyngis superior
     muscle

c. urethrae muscle
contact
    c. autoradiogram
    c. autoradiography
    c. scanning
    c. shield
    c. technique
contiguous
    c. scan
    c. sections
continuous
    c. arrhythmia
    c. spectrum
    c. wave (CW)
    c. wave Doppler (CWD)
    c. wave resonance
contour
    "cupid's bow" c.
contracted kidney
contractility
contracting skull
contraction collapse
contracture
    c. postischemia
    Dupuytren's c.
    extension c.
    flexion c.
    Volkmann's c.
contralateral
contrast
    c. agent
    c. control
    c. enhanced image
    c. enhancement
    c. injection
    c. laryngography
    c. resolution
    c. study
    c. ventriculogram
    c. ventriculography
contrast media
    Abbokinase (urokinase)
    Abrodil (methiodal
      sodium)

Acetiodone
acetrizoate
acetrizoic acid
Acid blue 1
Acid blue 3
air-lipiodol tragacanth
Alphazurine 2G
amidotrizoic acid
Amipaque (metrizamide)
Angio-Conray
Angio-Conray 80
Angiografin (diatrizoic
  acid)
Angiopac
Angiovist (diatrizoate
  meglumine)
Aquaphor (cholesterolized
  anhydrous petrolatum
  ointment base)
Arteray
Arteriodone
ascending Lipiodol
  (iodized oil)
Baridol
Bariform
Bari-O-Meal
barium sulfate
Barodense (colloidal
  microbarium sulfate)
Baroloid (microbarium
  sulfate)
Baropaque A, B or C
Barosperse 5:2
Barotrast (barium sulfate)
  ($BaSO_4$)
BAS 16
Basolac
Bedfordil
benzoic acid
Biligrafin
Biligrafin forte
Biligram
Biliodyl
Biliselektan

contrast media—*Continued*
- Bilitrast
- Bilivistan
- Bilombrine
- Bilopaque (tyropanoate sodium)
- Biloptin
- Bilospext
- bisacodyl
- bismuth
- blue dye
- Bracco
- brilliant blue (dye)
- brominized oil
- bunamiodyl
- calcium
- calcium ipodate
- Campiodol
- Cardio-Conray
- Cardio-Green (dye) (sterile indocyanine green)
- Cardiografin (meglumine diatrizoate)
- Cardiotrast
- cerium (Ce)
- chloriodized oil
- Cholebrine (iocetamic acid)
- Cholepulvis
- Choleradiagnost
- Cholestim
- Cholevic
- Cholevue
- Cholex
- Cholografin meglumine (iodipamide methylglucamine)
- Cholotrast
- Chromalbin (chromium Cr 51 and human albumin)
- Cistobil
- Cistopac
- Clysodrast (bisacodyl and tannic acid)
- colloidal barium sulfate
- Conray (iothalamate meglumine)
- Conray 325[b]
- Conray-30
- Conray-60
- Conray-280
- Conray-325
- Conray-400
- Conray-420
- Conray-480
- Contrast-U
- Conturex
- Cysto-Conray
- Cysto-Conray II
- Cystografin (meglumine diatrizoate and bound iodine)
- Cystokon
- diaginol
- Diagnorenol (methiodal sodium)
- diatrizoate
- diatrizoate meglumine
- diatrizoate sodium
- diatrizoic acid
- Dijodin
- Dikol
- Dimer X
- diodine
- diodone
- Diodrast
- Dionosil
- Diorast
- diphosphonate
- diprotrizoate
- Ditriokon
- Ditrox
- Duografin
- Duroliopaque
- dysprosium
- E-Z-CAT
- E-Z-Em disposable barium enema
- E-Z-Gas
- E-Z-H-D barium sulfate

E-Z-Paque
Endobile
Endografin
Esophotrast (barium
    sulfate)
Ethiodane
ethiodized oil
Ethiodol (ethiodized oil)
Ethyl diiodo stearate
Ethyl triiodo stearate
ethyliodophenylundecyl
Evans blue
GP prep emulsion
gadolinium
Galisol
gas (myelography)
Gastriloid
Gastro-Conray
Gastrografin (diatrizoate
    methyl-glucamine and
    sodium diatrizoate)
Gastropaque
Gastroview
GBD tablets
Gelobarin
glucagon
Hexabrix
Hippodin
Hippuran
Hydrombrine
Hypaque (diatrizoate
    meglumine and
    diatrizoate sodium)
Hypaque-Cysto
Hypaque-DIU 30%
Hypaque-meglumine 60%
Hypaque-meglumine 75%
Hypaque-meglumine 90%
Hytrast
I-X barium
Intron
Intropaque (barium
    sulfate)
iobenzamic acid
iobutoic acid

iocarmate meglumine
iocarmic acid
iocetamate
iocetamic acid
Iod-Cholegnostyl
iodamic acid
iodamide
iodatol
iodecol
Iodeikon
iodide
iodipamic acid
iodipamide
iodized oil
iodoalphionic acid
Iodochlorol
Iodognost
iodohippurate
iodomethamate
iodophen
iodophendylate
iodophor
iodophthalein
iodopyracet
Iodosol
iodoxamate
iodoxamic acid
Iodoxyl
Ioduron
ioglicate
ioglicic acid
ioglucol
ioglucomide
ioglunide
ioglycamic acid
ioglycamide
iogulamide
iohexol
iomide
iopamidol
Iopan
iopanoate
iopanoic acid
Iopax
iophendylate

contrast media—*Continued*
  iophenoxic acid
  ioprocemic acid
  iopromide
  iopronic acid
  iopydol
  iopydone
  lopyracil
  iosefamate
  iosefamic acid
  iosefamide
  ioseric acid
  iosulamic acid
  iosulamide
  iosumetic acid
  iotasul
  iotetric acid
  iothalamate
  iothalamic acid
  iotrol
  iotroxamide
  iotroxic acid
  ioxaglate
  ioxaglic acid
  ioxithalamate
  ioxithalamic acid
  iozomic acid
  ipodate calcium
  ipodate sodium
  ipodic acid
  Iso-rodeikon
  ISO/Meridrin Hg197, 203
  Isopaque (metrizoate
    sodium)
  Isopaque 280
  Isopaque 370
  Isopaque 440
  Isopaque B
  isosulfan blue
  Isovue (iopamidol with
    tromethamine and
    edetate calcium disodium)
  Isovue-M (iopamidol with
    tromethamine and
    edetate calcium

  disodium)
Jodafen
Jodairal
Jodobilan
Jodosol
Jodtetragnost
Joduron
Keraphren
Kinevac (sincalide)
large particle barium
Lipiodol
Lipiodol "F"
Lipomul (corn oil
  solution)
Liquibarine
Liquid Polibar
Liquipake (barium sulfate
  suspension)
Lumoxyd
Lymphazurin (isosulfan
  blue)
Mack-Brunswick medium
magnesium (Mg)
Mallinckrodt U.S.P. barium
manganese
Medopaque
Medopaque Hond
Medopaque U
meglumine
    m. diatrizoate
    m. iodiapamide
    m. iothalamate
Methiodal Sodium
methylglucamine
    m. iodipamide
    m. iodoxamate
    m. ioglycamide
    m. iothalamate
    m. iotroxamide
    m. metrizoate
metrizamide
metrizoate
metrizoic acid
Metufan
Micropaque

Microtrast
Miokon
Mirropaque
Mixobar
Monophen [2-(4-Hydroxy-
3,5-diiodobenzyl)-
cyclohexane carboxylic
acid]
Morujodol
Mulsopaque
Myodil (ethyl
iodophenylundecylate)
Neo-Cholex
(fat emulsion
containing pure
vegetable oil)
Neo-Hydriol fluid
(viscous)
Neo-Iodipin
Neo-Iopax
Neo-Methiodal
Neo-Skiodan
Neo-Tenebryl
neostigmine
Niopam
Nosophen
Nosydrast
Nosylan
Novopaque
Nyegaard
Omnipaque (iohexol)
Oncotrac
Opacin
Opacol
Oparenol
oprocemic acid
Orabilex
Oragrafin
O. calcium (ipodate
calcium)
O. sodium (ipodate
sodium)
Oratrast (barium sulfate)
Oravue
Osbil

Osteoscan
Panorex
Pantopaque
(iophendylate,
ethyl
iodophenylundecanoate)
pantothenic acid
papaverine hydrochloride
Patent Blue V
Per-Abrodil
Per-Radiographol
Perjodal
Perurdil
Pheniodol
phenobutiodyl
phentetiothalein
Pilopaque
Polibar
potassium bromide
Praestholm
Priodax
propyliodone
prostigmin
Pychokon-R
Pyelectan
Pyelombrine
Pyelosil
Pylumbrin
Radiographol (methiodal
sodium)
Raybar 75
Rayopak
Rayvist
Redi-Flow
Reno-M-30 (meglumine
diatrizoate)
Reno-M-60 (meglumine
diatrizoate)
Reno-M-Dip (meglumine
diatrizoate)
Renografin (meglumine
diatrizoate, sodium
diatrizoate)
Renovist (diatrizoate
methylglucamine,

contrast media—*Continued*
　　sodium diatrizoate, iodine)
　Renovist II (sodium
　　　diatrizoate, meglumine
　　　diatrizoate)
　Renovue (iodamide
　　　meglumide)
　Retro-Conray
　Rheopac
　Rugar
　Salpix
　Savac
　Seidlitz 8.l:1
　Sephadex
　Shadocol
　shadow meal
　sincalide
　Sinografin (meglumine
　　　diatrizoate and
　　　meglumine iodipamide)
　Skiabaryt
　Skiodan
　Skiodan Acacia
　sodium
　　　pertechnetate Tc 99m
　　s. bicarbonate
　　s. bromide
　　s. buniodyl
　　s. carbonate
　　s. chloride
　　s. chromate (Cr 51)
　　s. diatrizoate
　　s. diprotrizoate
　　s. hydroxide
　　s. iodide (Na I)
　　s. iodipamide
　　s. iodohippurate
　　s. iodomethamate
　　s. iothalamate
　　s. ipodate
　　s. methiodal
　　s. methyglucamine
　　　diatrizoate
　　s. metrizoate

　　s. phosphate (P 32)
　　s. radioiodide
　　s. rose bengal (I 131)
　　s. sulfite
　　s. thiosulfate
　　s. thorium tartrate
　　s. tyropanoate
　　s. warfarin
Solu-Biloptin
Solutrast
Sombracol
Sombradil
Stabarium
Steripaque-BR
Steripaque-V
Syntetragnost
tantalum (Ta)
Telebrix
Telepaque (iopanoic acid)
Teridax
tetrabromophenolphthalein
tetraiodophenolphthalein
Thixokon
thorium
　　t. dioxide
　　t. tartrate
Thorotrast
toluidine blue
TomoCat (CT barium
　　sulfate)
Triabrodil
triiodoethionic acid
Triiodyl
Triopac
Triosil (sodium
　　metrizoate)
Triurol
Trixobar
tyropanoate
tyropanoic acid
Ultrapaque B, C
Umbradil
Umbrathor
Unibaryt C

Unibaryt rectal
Uriodone
Urografin
Urografin 45
Urografin 60
Urografin 76
Urokon
Urombrine
Uromiro
Uropac
Uroselectan B
Urotex
Urotrast
Urovision
Urovist
Vascoray
Vasiodone
Vasobrix
Vasoselectan
Veri-O-Pake
Veripaque
Visciodol
X-Baryt
X-iodol
Xumbradil
contrast media, pl.
    contrast medium, s.
contrast medium, s.
    contrast media, pl.
contrast-enhanced
  visualization
Contrast-U
Control-Release needle
Conturex
contusion pneumonia
conus
    c. arteriosus
    c. medullaris
convergence
converging collimator
conversion coefficient
converter
    analog-to-digital c.
    (ADC)

digital-to-analog c.
image c.
convex
convexobasia
convexoconcave
convexoconvex
convolution back projection
convolutional pattern
convulsive fracture
Cook
    C. enforcer catheter
    C. modified percutaneous
        entry needle
    C. percutaneous entry
        teflon catheter needle
    C. winged percutaneous
        entry needle
Cook-Cope catheter
Cook-Cope-type loop biliary
    drainage catheter
Cook-Cope-type loop
    nephrostomy catheter
cool area
Cooley's erythroblastic anemia
Cooley-Tukey algorithm
Coolidge
    C. transformer
    C. tube
Coons
    C. guide
    C. interventional wire
        guide
    C. stent
Copan wire
COPD (chronic obstructive
    pulmonary disease)
Cope
    C. catheter
    C. loop
    C. loop catheter
    C. mandrel or mandril
        guide wire
    C. nephrostomy tube
    C. stents

Cope-method
    C.-m. bronchogram
    C.-m. bronchography
copper (Cu)
    c. half-value layer (Cu
      HVL)
    c. T intrauterine device
    c. wire
copper-7 intrauterine device
  (IUD)
coprecipitation
coprolith
copy film
cor
    c. adiposum
    c. biloculare
    c. bovinum
    c. dextrum
    c. pendulum
    c. pulmonale
    c. sinistrum
    c. triatriatum
    c. triloculare
    c. triloculare biatriatum
    c. triloculare uniatriatum
    c. venosum
    c. villosum
coracoacromial ligament
coracobrachialis muscle
coracoclavicular ligament
coracohumeral ligament
coracoid
    c. notch
    c. process fracture
Corbin technique
cord
    hepatic c.
    lumbosacral c.
    medullary c.
    spermatic c.
    umbilical c.
cordate
cordiform

cordis sarcoidosis
Cordis-Ducor catheter
core iron
corkscrew
    c. esophagus
    c. pattern
cornal
    c. orientation
    c. reconstruction
corniculate cartilage
cornu, s.
    cornua, pl.
cornua, pl.
    cornu, s.
cornucommissural tract
coronal
    c. plane
    c. suture
coronarography
coronary
    c. angiogram
    c. arteriogram
    c. arteriography
    c. arteriosclerosis
    c. artery bypass graft
      (CABG) (pronounced
      "cabbage")
    c. artery disease (CAD)
    c. cineangiogram
    c. cineangiography
    c. circulation
    c. occlusion
    c. spasm
    c. sulcus
    c. tendon
    c. thrombosis
coronoid
    c. fossa
    c. process
corpora, pl.
    corpus, s.
corpus
    c. callosum

c. luteum
c. striatum
c. uteri
corpus, s.
    corpora, pl.
corpuscle
corpuscular radiation
CORRELATE system
correlation analysis
correlative imaging
corresponding ray
corrosive gastritis
corrugator
    c. cutis ani muscle
    c. supercilli muscle
cortex
    adrenal c.
    homotypical c.
    piriform c.
    subchondral c.
cortex, s.
    cortices or cortexes, pl.
cortexes or cortices, pl.
    cortex, s.
cortical
    c. abscess
    c. adenoma
    c. bone loss
    c. buckle fracture
    c. hyperostosis
    c. labyrinth
    c. lucency
    c. obliteration
    c. sclerosis
    c. screw
    c. striation
cortices or cortexes, pl.
    cortex, s.
corticobulbar tract
corticocerebellar tract
corticomedullary junction
corticoperiosteal
corticopontine

corticorubral
corticospinal tract
corticosteroid-binding
    globulin (CBG)
corticothalamic tract
Cortioids test set
Cortisol (hydrocortisone)
Corvisart's disease
cosmic
    c. radiation
    c. ray
cosmotron
costa, s.
    costae, pl.
costae, pl.
    costa, s.
costal
    c. bone
    c. cartilage
    c. chondritis
    c. groove
    c. margin
    c. notch
    c. pleura
    c. pleurodiaphragm
    c. process
Costen's syndrome
costicartilage
costispinal
costochondral
    c. calcification
    c. joint
    c. junction
costochondritis
costoclavicular ligament
costocolic ligament
costocoracoid ligament
costomanubrial articulation
costophrenic
    c. angle (CPA)
    c. sinus
    c. sulcus
costopleural

costosternal
costotransverse
    c. joint
    c. ligament
costovertebral
    c. angle (CVA)
    c. joint
    c. ligament
costoxiphoid
Cotrel-Duboussett
  instrumentation
Cotrel's traction
Cotton's fracture
cotyledon
cotyloid
    c. cavity
    c. joint
cotylopubic
cotylosacral
coudé
    c. catheter
    c. tip catheter
cough
    c. fracture
    c. resonance
coulomb (C.)
Coulomb's
    C.'s force
    C.'s law
Coulter counter
Councill catheter
count
    c. (radiation
      measurements)
    c. density
    c. rate meter
counter
    boron c.
    c. electromotive force
    Cerenkov c.
    Coulter c.
    gamma well c.
    gas-flow c.

    Geiger c.
    Geiger-Mueller c.
    proportional c.
    radiation c.
    resolving time c.
    scintillation c.
    self-quenched c. tube
    whole-body c.
counterimmunoelectrophoresis
  (CIE)
counterpulsation balloon
    intra-aortic c. b. (IACB)
counting rate meter
counts per minute (cpm)
counts per second (cps)
coupling
Cournand
    C. catheter
    C. needle
courvoisier
Courvoisier's gallbladder
Coutard's method
covalent bond
Cowden's syndrome
Cowper's duct
coxa
    c. magna
    c. malum senilis
    c. plana
    c. valga deformity
    c. valgus
    c. vara
    c. vara deformity
coxa, s.
    coxae, pl.
coxae, pl.
    coxa, s.
Coxeter catheter
Coyle's trauma position
CPA (cardiophrenic angle)
CPA (costophrenic angle)
CPB (competitive protein
  binding)

cpm (counts per minute)
CPPD (calcium pyrophosphate dihydrate)
cps (counts per second)
Cr 51 (chromate)
Cr 51 (chromium)
Cr 51-RBC (chromium-51 tagged red blood cells)
cracked-pot resonance
Craig needle
craniad
cranial
    c. computed tomography (CCT)
    c. suture
    c. vertebra
craniectomy
cranioacrominal
cranioaural
craniocarpotarsal
    c. dysostosis
    c. dysplasia
craniocaudal
    c. projection
    c. view
craniocele
craniocerebral
cranioclasis
cranioclast
cranioclasty
craniodiaphyseal dysplasia
craniodidymus
cranioectodermal dysplasia
craniofacial
    c. dysostosis
    c. dysplasia
    c. fracture appliance
craniofenestria
craniognomy
craniology
craniomalacia
craniomeningocele
craniometaphyseal dysplasia

craniometer
craniometric
craniometry
craniopharyngeal
    c. canal
craniopharyngioma
craniophore
cranioplasty
craniopuncture
craniorachischisis
craniosacral
cranioscopy
craniostenosis
craniostosis
craniosynostosis
craniotabes
craniotelencephalic dysplasia
craniotelencephaly
craniotome
craniotomy
craniotrypesis
craniovertebral junction
cranium
crater
    ulcer c.
Crawford-Adams acetabular cup
crease
    inframammary c.
    simian c.
cremaster muscle
crepitation
crepitus
crescendo murmur
crescentic
crest
    c. voltmeter
    iliac c.
    intertrochanteric c.
cretinism
cri-du-chat syndrome
cribriform
    c. fascia

cribriform—*Continued*
    c. plate
cricoarytenoid
    c. arthritis
    c. joint
cricoarytenoideus
    c. lateralis muscle
    c. posterior muscle
cricoesophageal tendon
cricoid
    c. cartilage
    c. ring
cricopharyngeal ligament
cricothyroid
    c. joint
    c. ligament
cricothyroideus muscle
cricotracheal ligament
crinkle mark
Crisp's aneurysm
crisscross heart
crista
    c. falciformis
    c. galli
    c. lacrimalis
    c. transversa
critical mass
Critikon balloon catheter
CRL (crown-rump length)
Crohn's
    C.'s disease
    C.'s granulomatous enteritis
cromalbin
Cronqvist's cranial index
Crookes
    C. space
    C. tube
Crosby-Kugler capsule
cross-fire treatment
cross-scatter
cross-section capture
cross-sectional
    c.-s. echocardiogram (ECHO)
    c.-s. plane

    c.-s. transverse projection
    c.-s. view/projection
crosstable
    c. lateral position
    c. lateral view
    c. view
crossed
    c. coil
    c. ectopy
crossfill attempt
crosshair
crosshatch grid
Crouzon's
    C.'s dysostosis
crown glass
crown-rump length (CRL)
CRT (cathode ray tube)
cruces, pl.
    crux, s. (heart)
cruciate ligament
cruciform ligament
crura, pl.
    crus, s.
crural
    c. aponeurosis
    c. canal
    c. ligament
crureus muscle
crus, s.
    crura, pl.
Crutchfield's skeletal traction
Cruveilhier's joint
crux, s. (heart)
    cruces, pl.
cryogenic
cryoglobulinemia
cryomagnet
cryostable magnet
cryostat
crypt
    Morgagni's c.
cryptococcosis
cryptodontic
    brachymetacarpalia

cryptophthalmos
cryptopodia
cryptorchidism
cryptoscope
    Satvioni c.
cryptoscopy
crypts
    c. of Lieberkühn
    c. of Luschka
crystal
    c. photomultiplier tube
    c. scanner
crystal-induced
    c.-i. arthritis
    c.-i. arthropathy
crystalline phosphor
    detector
CS (cervical spine)
Cs 137 (cesium-137)
CSF (cerebrospinal fluid)
CSM (carotid sinus massage)
CSP (cavum septum
    pellucidum)
CSRT (The Canadian Society
    of Radiological
    Technicians)
CT (cardiothoracic)
CT (computed tomography)
    CT aspiration
    CT body scanner
    CT directed biopsy
    CT disc or disk
    CT gantry
    CT raw data
    CT reconstruction
    CT scanner
    CT slice
    CT slice thickness
    CT stereotaxic guide
      (BRW)
CT-guided aspiration
CT-guided biopsy
CTA (computerized tomo-
    angiography)

CTAT (computerized transaxial
    tomography)
CTE 100 neurodiagnostic
    scanner
CTR (cardiothoracic ratio)
CT/T computed tomography
    system
cubital
    c. fossa
    c. joint
    c. lymph node
    c. patella
    c. tunnel
cubitocarpal
cubitoradial
cubitus
    c. valgus
    c. varus
cuboid
cuboideonavicular
    c. joint
    c. ligament
cuff
    musculotendinous c.
    rotator c.
cuffing
Cu HVL (copper half value
    layer)
cuirass
cul-de-sac
Culiner's theory
culla
Cumming catheter
Cummings-Pezzer catheter
cumulative dose
cuneate lobe
cuneiform
    c. cartilage
    intermediate c.
    lateral c.
    medial c.
cuneocuboid joint
cuneometatarsal joint
cuneonavicular ligament

cuniculi, pl.
    cuniculus, s.
cuniculus, s.
    cuniculi, pl.
Cunningham's solution
cup-and-spill stomach
cuplike
cupola
cupping artifact
cupric acetate (Cu 64)
cupula
curiage
curie (Ci or c)
curium
CurlCath
curling
Curling's ulcer
current
    alternating c. (a. c.)
    anticoincidence c.
    c. density
    direct c. (d. c.)
    eddy c.
    effective c.
    filament c.
    ionization c.
    pulsating c.
    rectified c.
    saturation c.
    scaling c.
    single-phase c.
    three-phase c.
    tube c.
    unidirectional c.
Curry needle
curvature
curve
    Bragg c.
    c. of carus
    cervical curve
    characteristic c.
    compensatory c.
    congenital c.
    Hurter and Driffield
      photographic c.

    idiopathic c.
    isodose c.
    kyphotic c.
    lordotic c.
    neuromuscular c.
    thoracic c.
    thoracolumbar c.
    time density c.
curved catheter
curvilinear
CUSA ultrasonicator
Cushing's
    C.'s syndrome
    C.'s ulcer
customized block
cut
    thin-section c.
    tomographic c.
cut-down catheter
cut-off sign
cutaneous suture
cutdown
Cutie Pie
cutis
cutoff
cuvette
CV (cardiovascular)
CVA (cerebrovascular
    accident)
CVA (costovertebral angle)
CVCT (cardiovascular
    computed tomography
    scanner)
c/w (compatible with)
CW (continuous wave)
CWD (continuous wave
    Doppler)
CXR (chest x-ray)
cyanocobalamin Co 57, Co 58,
    Co 60
cyanocobalamin solution
cyanotic
    c. congenital heart disease
      (CCHD)
    c. kidney

c. spleen
CYBER 170/720 (Cybex
  ergometer)
Cybex
    C. ergometer (CYBER 170/
      720)
    C. test
cycle
    cardiac c.
    Krebs c.
    pentose c. (PC)
    QRS c.
cycles per second
cyclophosphamide
cyclotron radiation
cylinder
cylindrical
    c. bronchiectasis
    c. configuration
cylindroid aneurysm
cylindroma
cyst
    alveolar c.
    arachnoid c.
    aryepiglottic c.
    Baker's c.
    branchial cleft c.
    branchiogenic c.
    bronchogenic c.
    calcified renal c.
    choledochal c.
    colloid c.
    Dandy-Walker c.
    dentigerous c.
    dermoid c.
    diaphragmatic c.
    echinococcal c.
    enterogenous c.
    ependymal c.
    epidural c.
    gastrogenic c.
    hemorrhagic c.
    hydatid c.
    intracranial c.
    intramedullary c.

    intrapericardial c.
    leptomeningeal c.
    lymphangiectatic c.
    multilocular renal c.
    neurenteric c.
    pancreatic c.
    parenchymal c.
    perinephric c.
    pilonidal c.
    porencephalic c.
    primordial c.
    radicular c.
    retention c.
    sebaceous c.
    Stein-Leventhal c.
    subchondral c.
    subglottic c.
    synovial c.
    theca-lutein c.
    thyroglossal duct c.
    unifocal c.
    urachal c.
    vitelline c.
cystadenocarcinoma
cystadenoma
cysteine
cystic
    c. angiomatosis
    c. bronchiectasis
    c. differentiated
      nephroblastoma
    c. duct
    c. duct obstruction
    c. fibrosis
    c. gastritis
    c. kidney
    c. lymphangioma
    c. pattern
    c. structure
    c. tumor
cysticercosis
cystinosis
cystitis
    c. cystica
    c. emphysematosa

cystitis—*Continued*
   c. follicularis
   c. glandularis
   c. papillomatosa
   catarrhal c.
cysto (cystogram)
Cysto-Conray
Cysto-Conray II
cystocele
cystogenic aneurysm
Cystografin (meglumine
  diatrizoate, bound iodine)
cystogram (cysto)
   postvoiding c.
   triple-voiding c. (TVC)
cystography
   bead chain c.
   radionuclide c.
   retrograde c. (RC)
   triple-voiding c. (TVC)
Cystokon
cystometrogram
cystoperitoneal
   c. shunt
cystosarcoma phylloides
cystoscope
cystoscopy

cystostatic
cystoureterogram
cystoureterography
cystourethrogram
   chain c.
   expression c.
   isotope voiding c.
    (IVCU)
   micturition c.
   radionuclide c.
   retrograde c.
   voiding c.
cystourethrography
   "chain" c.
   expression c.
   iosotope voiding c.
   micturition c.
   radionuclide voiding c.
   retrograde c.
   voiding c. (VCUG)
cytologic
   c. aspiration
   c. biopsy
cytomegalic inclusion disease
  (CID)
cytoplasm
cytostatic

Dd

DAC (digital-to-analog
    converter)
dacryocystogram
dacryocystography
dacryosialocheilopathia
dactyledema
dactylitis
    tuberculous d.
dactylium
dactylolysis spontanea
"dagger" sign
Dalkon shield intrauterine
    device
Dameshek's syndrome
Dandy's vein
Dandy-Walker
    D. cyst
    D. malformation
    D. syndrome
Danielius-Miller
    D. modification of Lorenz
        method
    D. position
Danlos syndrome
dark-field examination
DAS (data acquisition system)
dashboard
    d. fracture
    d. injury
data
    alphanumeric d.
    d. acquisition system
        (DAS)
    d. camera
    d. reduction system
    ferrokinetic d.
    raw d.

Daubenton's plane
daughter
    d. element
    d. nucleus
    d. nuclide
David's disease
Davis catheter
Davis method
Davol catheter
daylight system
db or dB (decibel unit)
d.c. (direct current)
DC defibrillator
DCP plate
DDC (direct display console)
DE (dose equivalent)
de Bois normogram
de Broglie's
    d.'s wavelength
De Martini-Balestera
    syndrome
de Morsier syndrome
de Pezzer catheter
de Quervain's
    d. Q.'s fracture
    d. Q.'s thyroiditis
de Toni-Caffey syndrome
de-excitation
dead
    d. man switch
    d. space
    d. time
deafness-onychodystrophy-
    osteodystrophy retardation
    (DOOR) syndrome
Debré-Sémélaigne syndrome
debris

decade scaler
decay
    alpha d.
    beta d.
    branching d.
    d. constant
    d. curve
    d. mode
    d. product
    d. scheme
    d. series
    exponential d.
    free-induction decay
    isometric d.
    nuclear d.
    positron d.
    radioactive d.
deceleration
decibel unit (db or dB)
deciduous
deciliter (dl)
deck plate
decompression sickness
decon (decontamination)
decontamination (decon)
decortical position
decreased attenuation
dector collimator
decubitus
    d. position
    d. projection
    d. ulcer
    d. view
decussation
deep
    d. roentgen ray therapy
    d. sella
    d. vein thrombosis (DVT)
    d. venous
        thromboscintigram
        (DVTS)
    d. x-ray (DXR)
defecogram
defecography

defect
    atrioseptal d.
    congenital d.
    fibrous cortical d.
    filling d.
    film d.
    mass d.
    "napkin ring" d.
    osseous d.
    septum primum d.
    sinus venosus atrial septal
        d.
    ventriculoseptal d. (VSD)
defervesce
defervescence
defervescent
defibrillator paddles
deficiency
    glucose-6-phosphatase
        dehydrogenase d.
    transverse d.
deflation
deflection
deformans
deformity
    "applecore" d.
    Arnold-Chiari d.
    bar-ridge d.
    "bayonet" d.
    bony d.
    boutonnière d.
    Burkhart d.
    cascade d. of the stomach
    cloverleaf d.
    clubfoot d.
    congenital d.
    coxa valga d.
    coxa vara d.
    "egg-in-the-cup" d.
    Erlenmeyer's "flask-like" d.
    familial form of Sprengel's
        d.
    funnel d.
    fusiform d.

deformity—*Continued*
  gibbous d.
  Golding's d.
  gunstock d.
  hachet d.
  Haglund's d.
  Hill-Sachs d.
  hockey-stick d.
  hot cross bun d.
  Kirner's d.
  Klippel-Feil d.
  kyphotic d.
  lobster claw d.
  Madelung's d.
  Michel's d.
  napkin ring d.
  "parrot beak" d.
  "pencil-in-cup" d.
  "pencil-like" d.
  "penciling" d.
  pigeon breast d.
  poker d.
  "rat-tail" d.
  recurvatum d.
  saddle d.
  "shepherd's crook" d.
  spade d.
  Sprengel's d.
  swan-neck d.
  trefoil d.
  trigger finger d.
  ulnar drift d.
  valgus d.
  varus d.
  Velpeau's d.
  Volkmann's d.
degassing
degeneration
degenerative
  d. arthritis
  d. joint disease (DJD)
deglutition
  d. mechanism

degraded photon
dehiscence
  thoracic d.
Dehydroepiandrosterone
Deiter terminal fracture frame
Déjérine-Sottas syndrome
delayed
  d. operative
    cholangiogram
  d. operative
    cholangiography
  d. skeletal maturation
Delbet's
  D.'s classification
  D.'s fracture
Delclos applicator
DeLee catheter
deleterious
delimitation
delineation
Delphian node
delta
  d. mesoscapulae
  d. phalanx anomaly
  d. ray
  d. winding
deltoid
  d. ligament
  d. muscle
  d. tuberosity
deltoideopectoral node
deltoideus muscle
demagnification
  adiabatic d.
demarcation
  line of d.
  no line of d.
  shell-like d.
demifacet
demineralization
  d. bone matrix
demodulator
Demons-Meigs syndrome

Demuth hip screw
denatured
dendritic calculus
denervation
Denny-Brown syndrome
Denovilliers fascia
dens
    d. fracture
    d. view
dens, s.
    dentes, pl.
densitometer
densitometry
    dual photon d.
    Norland-Cameron photon d.
    quantitative d.
density
    background d.
    base d.
    calcific d.
    d. equalization filter
    d. latitude
    d. resolution
    film d.
    gradient d.
    hydrogen d.
    inherent d.
    ionization d.
    pulmonary d.
    radiographic d.
    spin d.
densogram
densography
dental
    d. abscess
    d. arch
    d. sac
dentate
    d. fascia
    d. fracture
    d. gyrus
    d. ligament
    d. line

    d. suture
dentes, pl.
    dens, s.
dentigerous cyst
dentoalveolar
    d. abscess
    d. joint
deossification
deoxyribonucleic acid (DNA)
Depage's position
DePalma hip prosthesis
dephasing
depilation
depressed fracture
depressor
    d. alae nasi muscle
    d. anguli oris muscle
    d. labii inferioris muscle
    d. septi muscle
    d. urethrae muscle
deprivation dwarfism
depth
    d. dose
    d. dose data
    d. dose distribution
    d. of focus
    d. perception
DePuy
    D. fracture frame
    D. plate
dequestration
dermatan sulfate
dermatoarthritis
    lipoid d.
dermatoglyphic
dermoid cyst
Desault dislocation
descending
    d. aorta
    d. artery
    d. colon
    d. myelopathy
    d. urography

Descot's fracture
Deseret catheter
desert fever
desferrioxamine
desiccated
Desilet catheter
Desilet-Hoffman introducer
desmoid tumor
desmoplastic fibroma
desquamation
desquamative interstitial
   pneumonitis
detached vitreous
detection
   beta d.
detector
   collimated scintillation
     d.
   crystalline phosphor d.
   d. aperture
   d. array
   d. channel
   d. collimator
   dielectric track d.
   Doppler blood flow d.
   radiation d.
   semiconductor d.
   tissue-equivalent d.
   x-ray d.
deteriorate
detoxify
detritus
detrusor sphincter dyssynergia
Deuel's halo sign
deuterium
deuteron
Deutschländer's disease
Deventer's diameter
device
   blade/plate d.
   compression d.
Devonshire catheter
dexamethasone
dextrad

dextran
dextroangiocardiogram
dextrocardia
dextrogram
dextrography
dextroposition
dextropositioned aorta
dextrorotation of the heart
dextrorotolevoscoliotic
dextroscoliosis
dextrosinistral
   d. plane
dextroversion of the heart
Deyerle
   D. apparatus
   D. pin
   D. plate
DFS (dynamic flow study)
DH (diaphragmatic hernia)
DI (diagnostic imaging)
diabetes mellitus
diabetic ulcer
diabrosis
diacondylar
   d. fracture
diaginol
Diagnorenol
diagnoses, pl.
   diagnosis, s.
diagnosis, s.
   diagnoses, pl.
Diagnost 120 (Philips, mfg.)
diagnostic
   d. capsules
   d. imaging (DI)
   d. impression
   d. pneumoperitoneum
   d. pneumothorax
   d.-related group (DRG)
   d. viewing console
diagonal conjugate
diagrammatic
   d. radiography
   d. radiology

dialogram
dialography
diamagnetic
    d. shift
diametaphyseal region
diaphanography
diaphragm
    Bucky's d.
    Potter-Bucky d.
diaphragma sellae
diaphragmatic
    d. cyst
    d. fascia
    d. flutter
    d. hernia (DH)
    d. "leaves"
    d. lymph n.
    d. pacemaker
    d. pinchcock
    d. pleura
    d. plexus
diaphyseal
    d. aclasis
    d. dysplasia
    d. sclerosis
    d. tuberculosis
diaphyses, pl.
    diaphysis, s.
diaphysis, s.
    diaphyses, pl.
diapositive
diarthric
diarthrodial
    d. cartilage
    d. joint
diasonics
Diasonics Cardiovue SectOR
  scanner
diasonogram
diasonography
diastasis
diastatic
    d. fracture
    d. skull fracture

diastematomyelia
diastole
diastolic
    d. murmur
    d. pressure
diastrophic
    d. dwarfism
    d. dysplasia
diathermy
diatomite fibrosis
Diatrast
diatrizoate
    d. meglumine
    d. methylglucamine
    d. sodium
    d. sodium solution
diatrizoic acid
Diaz' osteonecrosis
dicheiria
dichotomous ossification
Dickinson's syndrome
dicondylar
Dicopac
    D. kit
    D. test
dicrotic wave
didelphic
die plate
DIEDA (diethyl-iminodiacetic
  acid)
dielectric
    d. constant
    d. hysteresis
    d. insulator
    d. loss
    d. track detector
diencephalon
diethyl-iminodiacetic acid
  (DIEDA)
diethylenetriamine penta-
  acetic acid (DTPA)
Dietrich's syndrome
differential
    d. density sign

differential—*Continued*
  d. diagnosis
diffraction waves
diffuse
  d. abscess
  d. calcinosis
  d. esophageal spasm
  d. fibrosing alveolitis
  d. gastric polyadenoma
  d. goiter
  d. idiopathic skeletal
    hyperostosis (DISH)
  d. interstitial pulmonary
    fibrosis
  d. perichondritis
  d. spasm
diffusion
digastricus muscle
digestive tract
digital
  d. arteriography
  d. autofluoroscope
  d. compression
  d. fluoroscopy
  d. image
  d. isotope calibrator
  d. joint
  d. manipulation
  d. marking
  d. subtraction angiography
    (DSA)
  d. vascular imaging (DVI)
digital-to-analog converter (DAC)
digitofaciomental retardation
  syndrome
digitorum
digitoxin test set
Digitron DVI/DSA computer
digits
diglucuronide
digoxin
  d. I-125 imusay diagnostic
    kit

dihydroxycholecalciferol
  1,25-d.
  24,25-d.
diiodotyrosine (DIT)
diisofluorophosphate
diisopropyl flurophosphate
diisopropyl-iminodiacetic acid
  (DISIDA)
Dijodin
Dikol
dilatation
dilatator
  d. naris anterior muscle
  d. naris posterior muscle
dilated
  d. callosal sulcus sign
  d. common duct sign
dilation
dilator
  Amplatz d.
  Maloney d.
  Vance d.
dimelia
dimenhydrinate (Dramamine)
dimensional formulae
Dimer-X
dimercaptosuccinate (Tc 99m-
  DMSA)
dimerization
dimethylacetanilide
  iminodiacetic acid (HIDA)
dimethylnitrosamine (DMNA)
dimethylsuccinic acid (DMSA)
dimethylterephalate (DMT)
diminution
Dimitri-Sturge-Weber
  syndrome
dimple sign
Dinamap manometer
diode
diodine
diodone
Diodrast (iodopyracet)

Dionosil (propyliodone)
    D. aqueous
    D. oily
dioptric aberration
Diorast
diotyrosine
DIP (distal interphalangeal)
    joint
dip-coating autoradiography
Dipah
diphenhydramine
diphenylhydantoin, phenytoin
    (DPH)
diphenyloxazole
diphosphonate
diphtheritic myocarditis
diploë
diplogram
diploic
diploid
diploidy
dipolar
    d. coupling constant
    d. interaction
dipole, magnetic
diprotrizoate
dipyramidole
direct
    d. cardiac puncture
    d. current (d.c.)
    d. current generator
    d. display console (DDC)
    d. Fourier transformation
        imaging
    d. fracture
    d. mapping sequence
    d. measuring stereoscope
    d. percutaneous
        transhepatic
        cholangiogram
    d. puncture (DP)
    d. radiation
    d. reading caliper

dirty chest
disappearing bone disease
disarticulation
    hip d. (HD)
    knee d. (KD)
    shoulder d. (SD)
disc, see disk
discharge tube
discogenic
discogram
discography
discoidal atelectasis
discordant D-loop
discreet (means diminution)
discrete (means separate,
    distinct)
    d. Fourier transformation
    d. mass
    d. x-ray
discrimination
disease
    Addison's d.
    airflow obstructive d.
    air-space d.
    Alzheimer's d.
    Apert-Crouzon d.
    arc-welder's d.
    Arkin's d.
    Armenian d.
    arterial occlusive d.
    Ballingall's d.
    Barton's d.
    Basedow's d.
    bauxite worker's d.
    Bednar-Parrot d.
    Bekhterev's or
        Bechterew's d.
    Bekhterev-Strümpell-
        Marie d.
    Bergstrand's d.
    beriberi heart d.
    Bonfils' d.
    Bright's d.

disease—*Continued*
- Brinton's d.
- bronzed d.
- Buerger's d.
- Caffey's d.
- Caffey-Smyth d.
- Caisson d.
- Caroli's d.
- Castleman's d.
- celiac d.
- Chagas' d.
- Chandler's d.
- Charcot-Marie-Tooth d.
- Charcot's d.
- chronic granulomatous d. (CGD)
- chronic obstructive lung d. (COLD)
- chronic obstructive pulmonary d. (COPD)
- collagen d.
- collagen vascular d.
- coronary artery d. (CAD)
- Corvisart's d.
- Crohn's d.
- cytomegalic inclusion d. (CID)
- David's d.
- degenerative joint d. (DJD)
- Deutschländer's d.
- disappearing bone d.
- disc d.
- Dubin-Sprinz d.
- Durante's d.
- Ebstein's d.
- Ehrenfried's d.
- elastica d.
- English d.
- Evans' d.
- Fahr's d.
- Fairbank's d.
- Farber's d.
- fatal granulomatous d. of childhood
- Favre's d.
- fibrocystic d. of the breast
- focal d.
- Frieberg's d.
- Friedrich's d.
- Gaucher's d.
- Gee-Thaysen d.
- gestational trophoblastic d.
- Glisson's d.
- glycogen heart d.
- glycogen storage d. type I
- glycogen storage d. type II
- Graves' d.
- Greenfield's d.
- Haas' d.
- Hagner's d.
- Hand's d.
- Hand-Rowland d.
- Hand-Schüller-Christian d.
- heavy-chain d.
- Heine-Medin d. of the spine
- hemoglobin S d.
- Hippel-Lindau d.
- Hirschsprung's d.
- Hodgkin's d. (HD)
- Hodgson's d.
- homozygous hemoglobin S d.
- Hutchinson-Boeck d.
- Hutinel's d.
- hyaline membrane d. (HMD)
- hydroxyapatite deposition d. (HADD)
- I-cell d.
- idiopathic inflammatory bowel d.
- interstitial d.
- ischemic bowel d. (IBD)
- Jeune's d.

Jones' d.
Jüngling's d.
juvenile Paget's d.
Kahler's d.
Kahler-Bozzolo d.
Kartagener's d.
Kashin-Beck d.
Kienböck's d.
Kimmelstiel-Wilson d.
Klinger's d.
Klippel-Feil d.
Köhler's bone d.
Köhler's first d.
Köhler's second d.
Köhler-Mouchet d.
König's d.
Kugelberg-Welander d.
Kümmell's d.
Kümmell-Verneuil d.
Landing-Norman d.
Legg-Perthe's d.
Leroy's I-cell d.
Letterer-Siwe d.
Lindau's d.
Lindau-von Hippel d.
liver glycogen d.
Lobstein's d.
lückenschädel d.
Lyme d.
Malassez's d.
Marie-Sainton d.
Marie-Strümpell d.
Meige's d.
Meleda's d.
Ménétrier's d.
Mikulicz' d.
Milroy's d.
Möller-Barlow d.
Möller-Boeck d.
Morquio's d.
moyamoya d.
mushroom worker's d.
Myà's d.
Nielsen's d.

Nishimoto-Takeuchi-Kudo
d.
occupational lung d.
Odelberg's d.
old granulomatous d.
(OGD)
Ollier's d.
Osgood-Schlatter d.
Osler's d.
Otto's d.
Paget's d.
Paget's d. of the breast
Panner's d.
Parrot's d.
Patella's d.
Pel-Ebstein d.
Pelizaeus-Merzbacher d.
Pellegrini's d.
Pellegrini-Stieda d.
peptic ulcer d. (PUD)
Perthes-Jüngling d.
Peyronie's d.
Pick's d.
Pierre-Marie d.
pigeon breeder's d.
plantar perforating d.
Plummer's d.
Pompe's d.
Pott's d.
Preiser's d.
pulseless d.
Pyle's d.
Pyle-Cohn d.
Rathbun's d.
Reimann's periodic d.
Reiter's d.
Rokitansky's d.
Roske-de Toni-Caffey-
Smyth d.
Rustitskii's d.
Scheuermann's d.
Schmieden's d.
Schmitt's d.
Schüller's d.

disease—*Continued*
    Sever's d.
    silo-filler's d.
    Silverman's d.
    Sinding-Larsen d.
    Sternberg's d.
    Still's d.
    Strümpell's d.
    Tay-Sachs d.
    Terson's d.
    Thiemann's d.
    Thiemann-Fleischner d.
    thresher's d.
    Tokut-ze d.
    Trevor's d.
    triple vessel d.
    two-vessel d.
    Urov's d.
    van Buren's d.
    Van Neck's d.
    Vaquez-Osler d.
    Volkmann's d.
    von Gierke's d.
    von Hippel-Lindau d.
    von Recklinghausen's d.
    Wallgren's d.
    wet lung d.
DISH (diffuse iodopathic
  skeletal hyperostosis)
dish-pan fracture
DIIS (dorsiflexion intercalated
  instability) segment
DISIDA (diisopropyl-
  iminodiacetic acid)
DISIDA scan (formerly PIPIDA
  scan)
disintegration
    d. constant
    nuclear d.
    radioactive d.
disintegrations per second (dps)
disk or disc
    cervical d.
    choked d.

computed tomography
  (CT) d.
d. bulge
d. disease
d. herniation
d. interspace
d. margin
d. narrowing
d. space
floppy d.
intervertebral d. (IVD)
intra-articular d.
laser optical d.
lumbosacral d.
magnetic d.
Molnar retention d.
video d.
Winchester's d.
disk-shaped kidney
diskectomy
diskitis
diskogram
diskography
dislocation
    basketball foot d.
    carpal d.
    carpometacarpal d.
    coaches finger d.
    congenital hip d. (CHD)
    d. fracture
    d.-dissociation
    Desault d.
    dropped d.
    fracture-d.
    horseback rider's knee d.
    lunate d.
    Monteggia's d.
    Nélaton's d.
    nursemaid's elbow d.
    parachute jumper's d.
    perilunate d.
    scaphoid-capitate
      fracture- d.
    scaphoid-lunate d.

slice fracture-d.
subglenoid d.
transscaphoid perilunate
d.
vertebral d.
DISO (disofenin)
disofenin (DISO)
displaced
d. fat pad sign
d. fracture
display
A-mode d.
B-mode d.
d. matrix
d. monitor
d. status projection
d. system
M-mode d.
static image d.
displayed field of view
disposable catheter
dissecans
dissecting
d. aneurysm
d. hematoma
dissection
disseminated
d. condensing
osteopathy
d. intravascular
coagulation
d. lipogranulomatosis
d. lymphoma
dissipation
distal
d. convoluted tubule
d. humeral epiphysis
d. interphalangeal (DIP)
joint
d. myopathy
d. projection
distend
distensibility
distention

distinctor
distortion
geometric d.
pin-cushion d.
radiographic d.
distraction fracture
distribution
Boltzmann's d.
"butterfly" d.
d. transformer
depth dose d.
gaussian d.
maxwellian d.
Poisson's d.
spatial dose d.
disturbed motility pattern
DIT (diiodotyrosine)
Ditriokon
Ditrox
divergence
divergent
diverging collimator
diverticula, pl.
diverticulum, s.
diverticulitis
diverticulosis
diverticulum
acquired d.
bladder d.
bronchogenic d.
calyceal d.
esophageal d.
Hutch's d.
jejunal d.
laryngeal d.
Meckel's d.
pharyngeal d.
pharyngoesophageal d.
Rokitansky's d.
supradiaphragmatic d.
tracheal d.
Zenker's d.
diverticulum, s.
diverticula, pl.

DJD (degenerative joint
   disease)
dl (deciliter)
Dmax (maximum density) rads
DMNA (dimethylnitrosamine)
DMSA (dimethylsuccinic acid)
DMT (dimethylterephalate)
DNA (deoxyribonucleic acid)
Dobbhoff's tube
Docke murmur
Dockray's perirenal "P" sign
Dodd's solution
Dodge's principle
Doerner-Hoskins distribution
   law
dolichocephalic skull
dolichocephaly
dolichocolon
dolichoectasia
dolichostenomelia
dome
   d. fracture
   d. of the bladder
   d. of the urinary bladder
dome-shaped valve
Donohue's syndrome
donut configuration
Dooley-Caldwell-Glass method
Dooley hip nail
DOOR syndrome (deafness-
   onychodystrophy-
   osteodystrophy-retardation)
   syndrome
Doplette (mini Doppler)
Doppler
   D. blood flow detector
   D. effect
   D. technique
   D. ultrasound (U/S or US)
   pulse D.
Doptone
Dorello's canal
dormant
Dormia stone-basket catheter

dorsa, pl.
   dorsum, s.
dorsal
   d. bone
   d. cavity
   d. decubitus position
   d. elevated position
   d. inertia position
   d. kyphosis
   d. lithotomy position
   d. oblique position
   d. plate
   d. position
   d. recumbent position
   d. rigid position
   d. root entry zone (DREZ)
   d. vertebra
   d. view
dorsalis
dorsiflex
dorsiflexion intercalated
   segment instability (DISI)
dorsispinal
dorsoanterior
dorsocephalad
dorsodecubitus position
dorsointercostal
dorsolateral
dorsomedian
dorsonasal
dorsonuchal
dorsoplantar
   d. oblique position
   d. position
   d. projection
dorsoposterior
dorsoradial
dorsorecumbent position
dorsosacral position
dorsosupine position
dorsoventrad
dorsoventral
dorsum
   d. pedis

d. sellae
dorsum, s.
    dorsa, pl.
Dos Santos' needle
dose
    absorbed d.
    absorbed d. rate
    air d.
    allowable d.
    cumulative d.
    d. equivalent (DE)
    d. equivalent radiation
    d. estimate
    d. of focus
    d. rate
    d. reciprocity theorem
    d. rule
    depth d.
    depth d. data
    depth d. distribution
    doubling d.
    erythema d. (ED)
    exit d.
    exponential d.
    exponential d. rate
    exposure d.
    exposure d. rate
    fetal d.
    genetically significant d.
      (GSD)
    integral d.
    integrating d. meter
    LD_{50} (median lethal dose)
    lethal d. (LD)
    maximum permissible d.
      (MPD)
    mean d.
    mean gonad d.
    mean lethal d.
    mean marrow d. (MMD)
    measured d.
    midplane d.
    nominal single d. (NSD)
    oral fractionated d.

    organ d.
    organ tolerance d. (OTD)
    percent depth d.
    permissible d.
    radiation absorbed d.
      (rad)
    roentgen administered d.
      (RAD)
    skin d. (SD)
    threshold d.
    threshold erythema d.
      (TED)
    tissue d.
    tissue tolerance d. (TTD)
    tolerance d.
    tumor lethal d. (TLD)
dosimeter
    chemical d.
    d. FBX (ferrous sulfate-
      benzoic acid-xylenol
      orange)
    pencil d.
    pocket d.
    thermoluminescent d.
      (TLD)
    ultraviolet fluorescent d.
    Victoreen d.
dosimetric
dosimetrist
dosimetry
    estimation d.
    pion d.
    radiation d.
dot scan
    paper d. s.
    photo d. s.
Dotter
    D. balloon transluminal
      angioplasty catheter
    D. catheter
Dotter-Judkins technique
Dotter's tube
double
    d. ball sign

double—*Continued*
   d. coil intrauterine device
   d. exposure
   d. flexible-tipped guide
     wire
   d. focus tube
   d. fracture
   d. gastric fluid level
   d. lesion sign
   d. line of Sosman
   d. pneumonia
   d. suture line
   d. track sign
   "d. wall" sign
double-angle blade plate
"double-bubble"
   "d.-b." appearance
   "d.-b." sign
double-contrast
   d.-c. arthrogram
   d.-c. arthrography
   d.-c. barium enema
   d.-c. examination
   d.-c. study
   d.-c. upper GI series
   d.-c. visualization
double-current catheter
double-dose procedure
double-emulsion film
double-J
   d.-J catheter
   d.-J stent
   d.-J stent catheter
double-lumen catheter
double-outlet right ventricle
double-pole single throw (dpst)
double-step gait
doubling
   d. dose
   d. time
doughnut
   d. kidney
   d. lesion
   "d." sign

   d. transformer
Douglas'
   D.' abscess
Douglas, pouch of
Down's syndrome
doxorubicin HCL
DP (direct puncture)
DPA (dual photon
   absorptiometer)
DPH (diphenylhydantoin,
   phenytoin)
DPH reference serum
DPR (dynamic planar
   reconstructor)
dps (disintegrations per
   second)
dpst (double-pole single
   throw)
DPTA (diethyltriamine penta-
   acetic acid)
drag-to gait
drainage catheter
Dramamine (dimenhydrinate)
drape
   fenestrated d.
   Ioban d.
   Opraflex incise d.
   paper d.
   self-adhesive d.
   Steri-drape
   sterile d.
   textile d.
draping sign
drawer sign
Dressler's syndrome
Drew-Smythe catheter
Dreyfus' syndrome
DREZ (dorsal root entry zone)
DRG (diagnostic related group)
drip
   d. infusion pyelogram
   d. infusion pyelography
   d. infusion technique
   d. infusion urogram

d. infusion urography
dromedary
    d. hump
    d. left kidney
droop
    "Cooper's d."
drop
    d. finger
    d. heart
droplet
dropped
    d. dislocation
    d. finger
Drosophilia
"drowned newborn" syndrome
drugs used in radiology
    acacia
    amethocaine lozenge
    amphetamine sulfate
    Aquaphor (cholesterolized
      anhydrous petrolatum
      ointment)
    belladonna tincture
    Benadryl
      (diphenhydramine
      hydrochloride)
    castor oil
    chloral hydrate
    chloresium (chlorophyll)
    Dodd's solution
    Dramamine
      (dimenhydrinate)
    Dulcolax suppositories
      (bisacodyl)
    estradiol tablets
    Ex Tabac
    GoLYTELY (polyethylene
      glycol, sodium sulfate,
      sodium bicarbonate,
      sodium chloride,
      potassium chloride)
    liver extract
    methyl-bis-amine
      hydrochloride (B

      chloroethyl)
    Pontocaine (tetracaine)
    potassium permanganate
      powder
    propylthiouracil (PTU)
      tablets
    pyridoxine
    senna (compound)
      powder
    tannic acid
    testosterone propionate
    toluidine blue
    triethylenemelamine
    urethane (ethyl carbonate)
    zinc peroxide (medicinal)
drum crest
Drummond's marginal artery
drumstick appearance
drusen
Druy stents
dry
    d. abscess
    d. joint
dryer system
DSA (digital subtraction
   angiography)
DSR (dynamic spatial
   reconstructor)
D-tach needle
DTPA (diethylenetriamine
   penta-acetic acid)
dual
    d. photon absorptiometer
      (DPA)
    d. photon densitometry
    d. window
dual-contrast study
dual-energy
    d. computerized
      tomography (CT)
    d. scan
Dubin-Johnson syndrome
Dubin-Sprinz disease
Dubois' abscess

Dubovitz' syndrome
Duchenne's dystrophy
duck waddle test
duct
  alveolar d.
  Bartholin's d.
  bile d. (BD)
  common bile d. (CBD)
  common hepatic d.
  Cowper's d.
  cystic d.
  d. of Arantius
  d. of Botallo
  d. of Santorini
  d. of Vater
  d. of Wirsung
  endolymphatic d.
  extrahepatic biliary d.
  hepatic d.
  intrahepatic bile d.
  lacrimal d.
  mesonephric d.
  nasofrontal d.
  nasolacrimal d.
  omphalomesenteric d.
  pancreatic d.
  papillary ds.
  parotid d.
  Rivinus' d.
  Stensen's d.
  sublingual d.
  submandibular d.
  submaxillary d.
  thoracic d.
  thyroglossal d.
  Wharton's d.
  wolffian d.
ductal pattern
ductogram
ductography
  peroral retrograde
    pancreaticobiliary d.
ducts
  d. of Bellini
  lactiferous d.

  Müller's d.
  papillary d.
ductuli, pl.
  ductulus, s.
ductulus, s.
  ductuli, pl.
ductus
  d. bump
  d. choledochus
  d. sublingualis major
  d. venosus
Dudley-Klingenstein syndrome
Duhamel's operation
Dulcolax suppositories
  (bisacodyl)
dumping syndrome
Duncan's
    D.'s position
    D.'s ventricle
Duncan-Hoen method
Dunham's fan
Dunlap, Swanson and Penner
  method
duodenal
    d. atresia
    d. bulb
    d. C-loop
    d. loop
    d. papilla
    d. stasis syndrome
    d. sweep
    d. ulcer
duodenocholangeitis
duodenogastric bile reflux
duodenogram
duodenography
    hypotonic d.
duodenojejunal flexure
duodenum
Duografin
Duplay's bursitis
duplex
    d. Doppler
    d. kidney
duplication

d. cyst
esophageal d.
Dupuytren's
  D.'s contracture
  D.'s fracture
dura mater
  d. meninges
  d. sinus
dural
  d. sac
Durand-Zunin syndrome
Durante's disease
Dürck's node
Duroliopaque
Duroziez' sign or murmur
Dutt's view
Duverney's
  D.'s fracture
  D.'s gland
DVI (digital vascular imaging)
DVT (deep vein thrombosis)
DVTS (deep venous
  thromboscintigram)
dwarf kidney
dwarfism
  bird-headed d.
  camptomelic d.
  camptomicromelic d.
  diastrophic d.
  dyssegmental d.
  Laron's d.
  megaepiphyseal d.
  mesomelic d.
  metatrophic d.
  microcephalic d.
  osteoglophonic d.
  parastremmatic d.
  polydystrophic d.
  psychosocial d.
  short-limbed d.
  thanatophoric d.
  variable d.
DXR (deep x-ray)
d-xylose
dye

bengal d.
blue d.
brilliant d.
Cardio-Green d. (sterile
  indocyanine green)
d. column
d.-dilution method
halogenated
  phenolphthalein d.
rose bengal d.
Dyes' fracture
Dyggve-Melchior-Clausen
  syndrome
Dyke's
  D.'s blistering sign
  D.'s finger sign
  D.'s method
Dyke-Davidoff syndrome
dymelia
Dynamax
  D. 63
  D. 74
dynamic
  d. compression plate
  d. computerized
    tomography
  d. CT scan
  d. flow study (DFS)
  d. ileus
  d. magnetic field
  d. planar reconstructor
    (DPR)
  d. range
  d. scanning
  d. spatial reconstructor
    (DSR)
  d. volume imaging
dynamic-condenser
  electrometer
dynamo rule
dynamograph
DynaPak scanner
Dynapix
dyne
dysacromegaly

dysarthria
dyscephaly
    d., Saethre-Chotzen type
    François' d.
dyschondroplasia
dyschondrosteosis
dyscrasic fracture
dysencephalia
  splanchnocystica
dyserythropoiesis
dysesthesia
dysfunction
dysgerminoma
dysharmonic maturation
dyskinesis
dyslipotropism
dysmelia
dysmorphodystrophia
  mesodermalis congenita
dysosteosclerosis
dysostosis
    acrofacial d.
    cheirolumbar d.
    cleidocranial d.
    craniofacial d.
    Crouzon's d.
    d. cleidocranialis
    d. cleidocraniodigitalis
    d. cleidocraniopelvina
    d. cranio-orbitofacialis
    d. craniofacialis
      hereditaria
    d. enchondralis
      epiphysaria
    d. enchondralis
      metaphysaria
    d. mandibularis
    d. multiplex
    Kniest's d.
    mammary d.
    mandibulofacial d.
    metaphyseal d.
    orodigitofacial d.
    osteo-onycho d.

dysostotic idiocy
dysphagia lusoria
dysplasia
    acromesomelic d.
    acropectorovertebral d.
    camptomelic d.
    chondroectodermal d.
    cleidocranial d.
    craniocarpotarsal d.
    craniodiaphyseal d.
    cranioectodermal d.
    craniometaphyseal d.
    craniotelencephalic d.
    d. epiphysealis captis
      femoris
    d. epiphysealis
      hemimelica
    d. linguofacialis
    d. oculodentodigitalis
    d. oculovertebralis
    diaphyseal d.
    diastrophic d.
    ectodermal d.
    epiphyseal d. or epiphysial
      d.
    faciocardiomelic d.
    focal dermal d.
    frontometaphyseal d.
    frontonasal d.
    hip d.
    Kniest's d.
    mammary d.
    mandibulosacral d.
    metaphyseal d.
    metatropic d.
    monostotic fibrous d.
    oculoauriculovertebral d.
    oculodento-osseous d.
    onycho-osteoarthral d.
    otospondylomega-
      epiphyseal (OSMED) d.
    parastremmatic d.
    polyostotic fibrous d.
    pseudoachondroplastic d.

spondyloepiphyseal d.
spondylometaphyseal d.
ventriculoradial d.
dysplastic kidney
dyspnea
dysprosium
dysproteinemia
dysraphia
dyssegmental dwarfism
dyssynergia
dystelephalangy
dystonic gait

dystrophia
   d. brevicollis congenita
   d. mesodermalis congenita
   d. myotonica
dystrophic
dystrophy
   apical d.
   Duchenne's d.
   Fuchs' d.
   muscular d.
   reflex sympathetic d.
   thoracopelvophalangeal d.

Ee

E syndrome
E trisomy
EAC (external auditory canal)
Eagle's syndrome
EAM (external auditory
  meatus)
earth-eating syndrome
Easy catheter
Eaton's pneumonia
Eaton-Lambert syndrome
EBNA (Epstein-Barr nuclear
  antigen) test
Ebstein's
  E.'s anomaly
  E.'s disease
  E.'s malformation
eburnation
ECAT (emission computerized
  axial tomography)
eccentric
  e. pantomography
  e. projection
  e. target sign
eccentric-angle parieto-orbital
  projection
eccentro-
  osteochondrodysplasia
ECG (electrocardiogram)
ECG (electrocardiography)
echinococcal cyst
echo
  e. characteristic
  e. density
  echinococcus cyst e.
  e. pattern
  e. planar imaging
  e. texture
  e. time (ET)
  endometrial e.

  spin e. (SE)
ECHO (echocardiogram)
echo-containing mass
echo-dense structure
echo-planar image
echo-ranging
echocardiogram (ECHO)
  2-dimensional e.
  M-mode e.
  cross-sectional e.
echocardiography
echodense
echoencephalogram
echoencephalography
echogenicity
echogram
echography
echolaminogram
echolaminography
ECMO (extracorporeal
  membrane oxygenation)
ECT (emission computed
  tomography)
ectasia
ectatic aneurysm
ectethmoid
ectocondyle
ectocuneiform
ectoderm
ectodermal dysplasia
ectoentad
ectopic
  e. calcification
  e. infusion
  e. kidney
  e. myelopoiesis
  e. ossification
  "e. pinealomas"
  e. pregnancy

ectopic—*Continued*
    e. thyroid
    e. ureter
ectrodactyly
ectrodactyly-ectodermal
   dysplasia-clefting (EEC)
   syndrome
ectromelia-ichthyosis
   syndrome
ED (end diastole)
ED (erythema dose)
Eddowes' syndrome
eddy current
Edebohl's position
edentulous
edge
    Compton e.
    e. enhancement
    e. gradient
    e. gradient artifact
    e. packing
    e. response function
edge-enhancing kernel
EDH (epidural hematoma or
   hemorrhage)
E-dial calibration
Edison
    E. effect
    E. fluoroscopy
Edmondson Grading System
EDR (effective direct radiation)
EDTA (ethylenediamine tetra-
   acetic acid)
EDTMP (ethylenediamine
   tetramethylene phosphoric
   acid)
Edwards catheter
Edwards'
    E.' node
    E.' syndrome
EEC syndrome (ectrodactyly-
   ectodermal dysplasia-
   clefting) syndrome
EEG (electroencephalogram)
EEG (electroencephalography)

EF (ejection fraction)
EF (erythroblastosis fetalis)
effaced
effacement
effacing
effect
    Auger e.
    Compton's e.
    Doppler's e.
    Edison e.
    isotope e.
    Overhauser e.
    photoelectric e.
    piezoelectric e.
    radiographic e.
    Volta e.
    Warburg e.
    "washboard" e.
effective
    e. atomic number
    e. current
    e. detector aperture
    e. direct radiation (EDR)
    e. focal spot
    e. foramen of magnum
    e. half-life
    e. mass attenuation
      coefficient
    e. renal plasma flow
      (ERPF)
    e. value
    e. voltage
effector
efferent (conducting
   outward)
effort thrombosis
effusion
    extraperitoneal e.
    interlobar e.
    intraperitoneal e.
    joint e.
    pericardial e.
    pleural e.
EG (esophagogastric)
Egan's technique

EGBPS (equilibrium gated blood pool study)
"egg-in-the-cup" deformity
egg-shaped heart
egg-shell deposits
Eggers
    E. contact splint
    E. plate
    E. screw
EGJ (esophagogastric junction)
EHDP (ethane-1-hydroxy-1, 1-diphosphonate)
Ehlers-Danlos syndrome
Ehrenfried's disease
Eindhoven magnet
Einstein's law
einsteinium
Einthoven galvanometer
Eisenmenger
    E. complex
Eisenmenger's
    E.'s reaction
ejection
    e. fraction (EF)
    e. murmur
Ekman-Lobstein syndrome
elastic
    e. collision
    e. scattering
elastica disease
elastosis dystrophica
elbow joint
elbowed catheter
electric
    e. field intensity
    e. flux
    e. lines of force
electrical
    e. artifact
    e. capacitor
    e. energy
    e. field
    e. force
    e. ring

    e. ripple
    e. sensitivity
    e. temperature
Electrical and Musical Industries (EMI) (scanner)
electrification
electrobiological
electrocardiogram (ECG)
electrocardiography
electrochemical equivalent
electrode
    e. placement
    focusing e.
electrodynamic
electrodynamometer
electroencephalogram (EEG)
electroencephalography (EEG)
electrokymogram
electrokymography
electroluminescent sensitometer
electrolysis
electrolyte studies
electromagnet
    e. video tape
    iron-core e.
electromagnetic
    e. energy
    e. field
    e. flowmeter (emf)
    e. induction
    e. radiation
    e. spectrum
    e. unit
    e. wave
electrometer
    dynamic-condenser e.
    vibrating-reed e.
electromotive force
electromyography (EMG)
electron
    Auger e.
    bound e.
    Compton e.

electron—*Continued*
 e. beam
 e. beam tube
 e. capture
 e. cloud
 e. energy
 e. flow
 e. gun
 e. linear accelerator
 e. multiplier tube
 e. neutrino
 e. orbit
 e. paramagnetic resonance
  (EPR)
 e. radiography
 e. recoil
 e. spin resonance (ESR)
 e. stream
 e. theory
 e. transmission system
 e. tube
 e. valence
 e. volt (eV)
 free e.
 negative e.
 orbital e.
 oscillating e.
 secondary e.
electron-positron pair
electronic
 e. circuit
 e. device
 e. grid
 e. linear accelerator
 e. noise
 e. subtraction
 e. timer
electro-oculogram (EOG)
electrophoresis
electrophysiology studies (EPS)
electroretinogram (ERG)
electroscope
electrostatic
 e. force

 e. generator
 e. imaging
 e. induction
 e. law
 e. method
 e. repulsion
 e. unit (esu)
element
 chemical e.
 daughter e.
 parent e.
 radioactive e.
elementary particle
elements
elevation of diaphragm
ELF (extremely low frequency)
Elliot's position
Elliott plate
ellipse sign
ellipsoid lesion
ellipsoidal
 e. cast
 e. joint
elliptical motion
Ellis' line
Ellis-van Creveld syndrome
Elon
elongation
 e. of aorta
Elscint Excel 905 scanner
elusive ulcer
elution technique
elutriation
emanate
Embden-Meyerhof glycolytic
  pathway
embedded
embolectomy catheter
emboli, pl.
 embolus, s.
embolic
 e. aneurysm
 e. phenomenon
 e. pneumonia

embolism
embolization
embolomycotic aneurysm
embolus, s.
    emboli, pl.
embryo
embryoblast
embryology
embryonal
    e. adenosarcoma
    e. carcinosarcoma
    e. cell carcinoma
    e. nephroma
    e. nephrotomography
    e. sarcoma
embryonic
    e. sac
embryopathy
    fetal anticoagulant e.
    fetal warfarin e.
emesis
emf (electromagnetic
    flowmeter)
EMG (electromyography)
EMI (Electric and Muscial
    Industries)
    EMI 7070 scanner
    EMI CT 500 scanner
    EMI unit
eminence
    thenar e.
eminentia arcuata
emissary
    e. foramen
    e. vein
emission
    beta e.
    e. computed tomography
      (ECT)
    e. computerized axial
      tomography (ECAT)
    e. spectrum x-ray
    e. tomography
    filament e.

negative e.
negatron e.
photoelectric e.
secondary e.
thermionic e.
emitter
emphysema
    alveolar e.
    bullous e.
    centrilobular e.
    compensatory e.
    gangrenous e.
    glass-blower's e.
    idiopathic unilobar e.
    interlobular e.
    interstitial e.
    lobar e.
    panacinar e.
    panlobular e.
    paracicatricial e.
    paraseptal e.
    pulmonary interstitial e. (PIE)
    senile e.
emphysematous
    e. bleb
    e. bulla
    e. cholecystitis
    e. cystitis
    e. gastritides
    e. gastritis
    e. pyelonephritis
    e. vaginitis
emprosthotonos position
empty
    e. intestine
    e. sella turcica
empty-sella syndrome
empyema
    pneumococcal e.
    postpneumonectomy
      tuberculous e.
    streptococcal e.
    subdural e.
    "technical" e.

emulsion
    nuclear e.
en bloc (French: "as a whole")
en face
    e. field
    e. projection
en plaque meningioma
enamel niche
enameloma
enantiomeric
enarthritis
enarthrodial joint
encapsulated
    e. empyema
    e. pleural fluid
encephalogram
encephalography
encephalolith
encephaloma
encephalomeningitis
encephalometry
encephalomyelitis
    e. disseminata
encephalon
encephalopathy
encephalotrigeminal
    angiomatosis
enchondroma
enchrondromatosis
encroachment
encysted
end
    e. diastole (ED)
    e. systole (ES)
end-plate sclerosis
end-to-side (E-S)
endaortitis
endarteritis
    e. calcificans cerebri
    e. obliterans
    e. proliferans
endaural

endemic goiter
endergic reaction
Enders
    E. nail
    E. rod
Endobile
endocardial
    e. dysplasia
    e. fibroelastosis
endocardium
endocervical canal
endocervix
endochondral ossification
endocrine
    e. fracture
    e. gland
    e. osteoporosis
endoderm
endodiascope
endoergic reaction
endogenous
Endografin
endolymphatic
    e. duct
    e. labyrinth
    e. sac
endometrial
    e. carcinoma
    e. echo
endometriosis
endometrium
endomyocardial fibrosis
endoprosthesis
endoscopic
    e. duodenal biopsy
    e. retrograde
        cholangiogram
    e. retrograde
        cholangiography
    e. retrograde
        cholangiopancreatogram
        (ERCP)
    e. retrograde

cholangiopancrea-
tography (ERCP)
e. ultrasonography
endoscopy
endosteal
e. sclerosis
endosternum
endosteum
endostoma
endothelial myeloma
endothelioma
endothelium
endothermic
endothoracic fascia
endotracheal (ET) tube
endouterine
enema
air contrast barium e.
barium e. (BE or BaE)
cleansing e.
double-contrast barium e.
opaque e.
single-contrast barium e.
energy
atomic e.
binding e.
chemical e.
e. fluence
e. frequency
e. resolution
e. spectrum
e. wavelength
electrical e.
electromagnetic e.
electron e.
excitation e.
gravitational potential e.
heat e.
kinetic e.
nuclear e.
photon e.
potential e.
quantum e.

radiant e.
radiation e.
thermal e.
x-ray e.
Engel-Lysholm maneuver
Engel–von Recklinghausen
syndrome
Engelmann's syndrome
English
E. disease
E. position
engorgement
enhanced scan
enophthalmos
enostosis
ensiform process
enteric lymphadenitis
enteritis
Crohn's granulomatous e.
eosinophilic e.
enterobiliary fistula
enterochromaffin
enterocolitis
bacterial e.
infectious e.
necrotizing e. (NEC)
pseudomembranous e.
enterocutaneous
enterocystocele
enterocystoma
enteroepiplocele
enterogenous cyst
enterohydrocele
enteroinvasive
enteron
enteropathic arthritis
enteropathogenic *Escherichia
coli* (EPEC)
enteropathy
exudative e.
enteroptosis
enterostenosis
enterovesical

enthesis
enthesitis
entoderm
entodermal
    e. canal
entrance wound
entry catheter
enucleation
environmental density artifact
enzyme
EOA (erosive osteoarthritis)
EOG (electro-oculogram)
eosinophil
eosinophilic
    e. enteritis
    e. gastritis
    e. gastroduodenum
    e. granuloma
    e. granulomatosis
    e. meningoencephalitis
    e. pneumonia
eparterial bronchus
epaxial
EPEC (enteropathogenic
   Escherichia coli)
ependyma
ependymal cyst
ependymoma
Epi-testosterone
epiarticular osteochondromata
epibronchial right pulmonary
   artery syndrome
epicardia, pl.
   epicardium, s.
epicardium, s.
   epicardia, pl.
epicerebral space
epicolic lymph node
epicondyle
epicondylic ridge
epicranial aponeurosis
epicranius muscle
epidermis
epidermoid

epidermoidoma
epidermolysis bullosa
   dystrophica
epididymides, pl.
   epididymis, s.
epididymis, s.
   epididymides, pl.
epididymogram
epididymography
epididymo-orchitis
epididymovesiculogram
epididymovesiculography
epidural
    e. abscess
    e. cyst
    e. fat
    e. hematoma
    e. space
    e. venography
epidurography
epigastric
    e. lymph node
    e. zone
epigastrium
epiglottiditis
epiglottis
epiglottitis
epilation
epileptiform
    e. seizure
epiloia
epiphyseal or epiphysial
    e. coxa magna
    e. coxa plana
    e. coxa valga
    e. coxa vara
    e. dysplasia
    e. fracture
    e. plate
    e. plate line
    e. staple
epiphyses, pl.
   epiphysis, s.
epiphysiolysis

epiphysis
    capital e.
    cone e.
    distal humeral e.
    femoral e.
    ivory e.
    slipped capital femoral e.
    stippled e.
epiphysis, s.
    epiphyses, pl.
epiphysitis
epiplocele
epiploenterocele
epiploic
    e. abscess
    e. foramen
    e. sac
epipyramis
episcleral space
epispadias
epispinal space
epistaxis
epistropheus axis
epithelial
    e. tumor
epithelium
    Barrett's e.
    columnar e.
epithermal neutron
epitransverse process
epitympanic
    e. recess (EPR)
    e. space
Eppendorf catheter
EPR (electron paramagnetic resonance)
EPR (epitympanic recess)
EPS (electrophysiology studies)
epsilon sign
Epstein-Barr nuclear antigen (EBNA) test
Epstein's malformation
Eq. (equilibrium)

equally loaded opposed lateral portals
equation
    Bloch's e.
    Bohr's e.
    Bragg's e.
    Fick's e.
    hamiltonian e.
    Larmor's e.
    Schrödinger's e.
    Stewart-Hamilton e.
    transformer e.
equator
equilibratory ataxia
equilibrium (Eq.)
    e.-gated blood pool study (EGBPS)
    e.-gated format
    e. study
    e. thickness
    radioactive e.
    secular e.
    transient e.
equinovalgus
equinovarus
equinus
equivalence
    mass energy e.
equivalent
    e. resistence
    e. roentgen
    electrochemical e.
equivocal
Eraso's method
Erb's
    E.'s point
    E.'s paralysis
erbium (Er)
ERCP (endoscopic retrograde cholangiographic pancreatography)
ERCP (endoscopic retrograde cholangiopancreatogram or cholangiopancreatography)

Erdheim's syndrome
erect
  e. anteroposterior projection
  e. fluoro spot projection
  e. oblique projection
  e. position
erector
  e. clitoridis muscle
  e. penis muscle
  e. spinae muscle
erg (a centimeter-gram-second) (CGS)
ERG (electroretinogram)
ergocalciferol
ergometer
  Cybex e.
ergonovine maleate
ergot
Erlacher-Blount syndrome
Erlenmeyer's
  E.'s "flask-like" appearance
  E.'s "flask-like" deformity
Ernst radium applicator
erosion arthritis
erosive
  e. gastritis
  e. osteoarthritis (EOA)
ERPF (effective renal plasma flow)
erroneous projection
erythema
  brisk e.
  e. dose (ED)
  e. doubling
  e. fugax
  e. multiforme
  e. nodosum
erythematous
erythroblastic anemia
erythroblastosis fetalis
erythrocyte
Erythroflex catheter
erythroid

erythrokinetic study
erythropoietin
  e. assay
  e. bioassay
ES (end systole)
E-S (end-to-side)
Escudero-Nemenov sign
ESD (esophagus, stomach and duodenum)
esophageal
  e. atresia
  e. carcinoma
  e. dilatation
  e. diverticulum
  e. duplication
  e. dysmotility
  e. hiatus
  e. lip
  e. lung
  e. motility
  e. obstruction
  e. reflux
  e. rupture
  e. sclerosis
  e. spasm
  e. stricture
  e. transit time (ETT)
  e. ulcer
  e. varices
  e. vestibule
  e. web
esophagectasia
esophagitis
esophagogastric (EG)
  e. junction
esophagogastroduodenoscopy
esophagogram
esophagography
esophagomalacia
esophagopleural fistula
esophagoscopic (EG)
  e. catheter
  e. junction (EGJ)
esophagoscopy

esophagostomal hernia
esophagram
    Besey e.
esophagraphy
esophagus
    abdominal e.
    Barrett's e.
    corkscrew e.
    e. stomach and duodenum
      (ESD)
Esophotrast (barium sulfate)
esosinophilic
    e. granuloma
ESR (electron spin resonance)
essential
    e. brown induration of the
      lung
    e. lipoid histocytosis
    e. pulmonary
      hemosiderosis
Essex-Lopresti fracture
esthesioneuroblastoma
estimation dosimetry
estradiol
    e. RIA antiserum
    e. tablets
estriol
estrogen
estrone
esu (electrostatic unit)
ESWL (extracorporeal shock
  wave lithotripsy)
ET (echo time)
ET (endotracheal) tube
état mammelonné
ethane-1-hydroxyl-1, 1
  diphosphonate (EHDP)
Ethiodane
ethiodized oil
Ethiodol (ethiodized oil)
ethmoid
    e. antrum
    e. bulla
    e. canal

ethmoidal
    e. air cell
    e. concha
    e. infundibulum
    e. labyrinth
    e. notch
    e. sinus
ethmoidomaxillary suture
ethmovomerine plate
ethyl
    e. diiodo stearate
    e. triiodo stearate
ethylene
    e. glycol
ethylenediamine tetra-acetic
  acid (EDTA)
ethylenediamine
  tetramethylene phosphoric
  acid (EDTMP)
ethyl iodophenylundecylate
  (Myodil)
etiology
etoposide (Vepesid)
ETT (esophageal transit time)
ETT (exercise tolerance test)
Etter's line
EU (excretory urogram or
  urography)
Euler's number
eunuchoidism
europium
eustachian
    e. canal
    e. catheter
    e. tube
euthyroid
eutonic stomach
eV (electron volt)
Evac-Q-Kwik
evagination
Evans-Lloyd-Thomas syndrome
Evans blue (T-1824)
Evans'
    E.' disease

Evans'—*Continued*
  E.' method
evaporation of filament
Evart's method
eventration
  e. treatment
Evermed catheter
eversion
  e. fracture
  e. position
evert
every night (q.n.)
Ewart's sign
Ewing's
  E.'s sarcoma
  E.'s tumor
Ex Tabac
exaggerated Waters' position
examination
  dark-field e.
  double-contrast e.
exchange
  e. coupling
  e. narrowing
excitation
  e. energy
excited
  e. atom
  e. electron
  e. state
excrescence
excretion
excretory
  e. cystogram (XC)
  e. cystography (XC)
  e. nephrourogram
  e. nephrourography
  e. urethrogram
  e. urogram or urography (XU)
exenteration
exercise tolerance test (ETT)
exergic reaction
exfoliation
exfoliative gastritis

exhalation
exit
  e. dose
  e. wound
exocrine gland
exoergic reaction
exomphalos-macroglossia-
  gigantism syndrome
exophthalmos
exophytic
  e. lesion
exostosis
  cartilaginous e.
  e. luxurians
  e. multiplex cartilaginea
  subungual e.
  "turret" e.
exostotic dysplasia
exothermic
expel
expiration
  e. view
expiratory film
exponential
  e. decay
  e. dose rate
exposure
  double e.
  e. angle
  e. dose
  e. dose rate
  e. meter
  e. rate
  e. time
  overcouch e.
  radiation e.
expressed skull fracture
expression
  e. cystourethrogram
  e. cystourethrography
extensibility
extension
  e. contracture
  e. position

extensor
- e. carpi radialis brevis muscle
- e. carpi radialis longus muscle
- e. carpi ulnaris muscle
- e. digiti minimi muscle
- e. digiti quinti proprius muscle
- e. digitorum brevis muscle
- e. digitorum communis muscle
- e. digitorum longus muscle
- e. hallucis brevis muscle
- e. hallucis longus muscle
- e. indicis muscle
- e. ossis metacarpi pollicis muscle
- e. pollicis brevis muscle
- e. pollicis longus muscle
- e. primi internodii pollicis muscle
- e. proprius hallucis muscle
- e. secundi internodii pollicis muscle
- e. tendon

external
- e. abdominal oblique muscle
- e. auditory canal (EAC)
- e. auditory meatus (EAM)
- e. beam
- e. capsule
- e. carotid artery
- e. conjugate
- e. fixation
- e. oblique aponeurosis
- e. occipital protuberance
- e. radiation

extirpation
extra-articular fracture
extracalyceal extravasation
extracapsular fracture
extracardiac shunt

extracellular
extracorporeal
- e. lithotripsy
- e. membrane oxygenation (ECMO)
- e. shock wave lithotripsy (ESWL)

extracorticospinal tract
extradural
- e. abscess
- e. defect
- e. space

extrahepatic biliary duct
extraluminal gas
extramedullary myelopoiesis
extraoral projection
extraperitoneal
- e. air
- e. effusion
- e. fat
- e. fluid

extrapleural
- e. air
- e. defect
- e. hematoma
- e. sign
- e. space

extrapolate
extrapolation ionization chamber
extrapyramidal tract
extrarenal fat
extratracheal
extrauterine
extravasation gas
extravascular
extremely low frequency (ELF)
extremity osteochondrodystrophy syndrome
extrinsic
extrophy
exuberant callus
exudation

exudative
- e. angina
- e. arthritis
- e. ascites
- e. enteropathy

eye
- e. bolt
- e. studies
- Sweet's e.

eye-ear plane

E-Z-CAT

E-Z-Em disposable barium enema

E-zero offset

E-Z-Gas

E-Z-H-D barium sulfate

E-Z-Paque

Ff

F (form of
 acropectorovertebral
 dysplasia)
f (frequency)
F. R. Thompson prosthesis
F syndrome
FA (femoral artery)
FA (fetal age)
fabella sign
fabella, s.
 fabellae, pl.
fabellae, pl.
 fabella, s.
Fabry-Anderson syndrome
Fabry's syndrome
face-down position
face-on
facet joint
faceted
faceting
facial
 f. fracture appliance
 f. hemiatrophy
 f. hemihypertrophy
 f. lymph node
 f. profile
 f. trophoneurosis
facial-digital-genital syndrome
facies, s. and pl.
faciocardiomelic
 f. dysplasia
faciodigitogenital syndrome
FACR (Fellow of the American
 College of Radiology)
factitious clinodactyly
factor
 Boltzmann's distribution f.
 Boltzmann's f.

F. III multimer assay
filling f.
geometry f.
intensification f.
intrinsic f.
magnification f.
power f.
rheumatoid f.
slice f.
Fahr's disease
failing lung sign
Fairbank's disease
falces, pl.
 falx, s.
falciform
 f. aponeurosis
 f. ligament
falcine meningioma
fallacious finding
fallopian
 f. aqueduct
 f. arch
 f. artery
 f. catheter
 f. ligament
 f. tube
Fallot's
 F.'s pentalogy
 F.'s tetrad
 F.'s tetralogy
 F.'s trilogy
false
 f. aneurysm
 f. double sellar floor
 f. joint
 f. rib
false-negative report
false-positive report

falx
- f. cerebelli
- f. cerebri

falx, s.
- falces, pl.

familial
- f. acrocephalosyndactyly
- f. acropathia ulceromutilans
- f. adenomatosis coli
- f. amaurotic idiocy
- f. asphyxiant thoracic dystrophy
- f. cardiomegaly
- f. carpal necrosis
- f. chromaffinomatosis
- f. dominant acro-osteolysis
- f. dysautonomia
- f. dysplastic osteopathy
- f. fibrous dysplasia of the jaw
- f. form of Sprengel's deformity
- f. hemorrhagic telangiectasia
- f. idiopathic osteoarthropathy
- f. juvenile nephrophthisis
- f. lumbosacral syringomyelia
- f. Mediterranian fever
- f. metaphyseal dysplasia
- f. multiple exostosis
- f. neurovascular dystrophy
- f. neurovisceral lipidosis
- f. osseous dystrophy
- f. osteoclasia with macrocranium
- f. osteoectasia
- f. paroxysmal polyserositis
- f. perforating ulcers of the foot
- f. progressive cerebral sclerosis
- f. recurring polypositis
- f. splenic anemia

Fanconi's
- F.'s anemia
- F.'s pancytopenia
- F.'s panmyelopathy
- F.'s syndrome

Fanconi-Albertini-Zellweger syndrome

Fanconi-de Toni-Debré syndrome

Fanconi-Hegglin syndrome

far
- f. field
- f. ultraviolet
- f. wall echo

farad

faraday

Faraday's
- F.'s cage
- F.'s constant
- F.'s dark space
- F.'s law
- F.'s shield

faradic electrical stimulation

Farber's disease

Farber-Uzman syndrome

farmer's lung

fascia
- Abernethy's f.
- anal f.
- Buck's f.
- bulbar f.
- cervical, deep f.
- cervical, superficial f.
- Cloquet's f.
- Colles' f.
- cribriform f.
- Denonvillier's f.
- dentate f.
- diaphragmatic f.
- endothoracic f.
- f. lata
- f. of Laimer

fascia—*Continued*
  Gerota's f.
  iliac f.
  infundibuliform f.
  intercolumnar f.
  lateroconal f.
  lumbodorsal f.
  pectineal f.
  pelvic f.
  perirenal f.
  psoas f.
  quadratus lumborum f.
  renal f.
  Taldt fusion f.
  Tenon's f.
  thyrolaryngeal f.
  transversalis f.
  Zuckerkandl's f.
fascia, s.
  fasciae or fascias, pl.
fasciae or fascias, pl.
  fascia, s.
fasciagram
fasciagraphy
fascias or fasciae, pl.
  fascia, s.
fascicle
fascicular lymphosarcoma
fasciculation
fasciitis
  Gerota's f.
fasciolar gyrus
fast
  f. Fourier transformation
    (FFT)
  f. neutron
  f. single slice method
FasTENS
fat
  epidural f.
  extraperitoneal f.
  extrarenal f.
  f. absorption breath test
  f. embolism

  f. pad sign
  orbital f.
  pararenal f.
  peribiliary f.
  perirenal f.
  preperitoneal f. line
  properitoneal f. stripe
fat-absorption test
fat-free meal
fatal granulomatous disease of
    childhood
fatigue fracture
fatty
  f. acid resonance
  f. infiltration
  f. meal
fauces, pl.
  faux, s.
faucial
  f. catheter
  f. eustachian catheter
  f. tonsil
faux, s.
  fauces, pl.
Favre's disease
FBX dosimeter (ferrous
    sulfate-benzoic acid-xylenol
    orange)
FB (foreign body)
FCC (fracture, compound,
    complex)
Fe (iron)
feather analysis
feathered
feathery
  f. margin of calyces
  f. mucosal pattern
fecal
  f. abscess
  f. material
fecalith
feeding tube
  f. t. tip
Fein antrum trocar needle

Feist's method
Feist-Mankin
    F.-M. method
    F.-M. position
Fellow of American College of
    Radiology (FACR)
felon
Felty's syndrome
female pseudo-Turner's
    syndrome
femora or femurs, pl.
    femur, s.
femoral
    f. aortic flush
    f. aortic flush catheter
    f. arteriography
    f. artery (FA)
    f. canal
    f. condylar plate
    f. condyle
    f. epiphysis
    f. fracture
    f. head
    f. length
    f. neck
    f. neck fracture
    f. shaft
    f. shaft fracture
    f. sheath
    f. torsion
    f. triangle
    f. visceral renal curve
        catheter
femorocele
femorocerebral angiography
femoroiliac
femoropatellar joint
femorotibial
femtoliter (fL)
femur-fibula-ulna (FFU)
    syndrome
femur length (FL)
femur, s.
    femurs or femora, pl.

femurs or femora, pl.
    femur, s.
fencing position
fender fracture
fenestra
    f. choledocha
    f. cochleae
    f. rotunda
    f. vestibuli
fenestra, s.
    fenestrae, pl.
fenestrae, pl.
    fenestra, s.
fenestral otosclerosis
fenestrated
    f. catheter
    f. drape
Ferguson's
    F.'s angle
    F.'s fracture
    F.'s measurement
    F.'s method
Fermi's theory
fermium
Ferrein, ligament of
ferrite contrast medium
ferrite rings
ferritin
ferrokinetic data
ferromagnetic relaxation
ferrous
    f. ascorbate
    f. citrate
ferrutope-Fe-59
fertilization
festinating gait
fetal
    f. achondroplasia
    f. age (FA)
    f. alcohol syndrome
    f. aminopterin
    f. anticoagulant
        embryopathy
    f. cephalometry

fetal—*Continued*
  f. demise
  f. Dilantin syndrome
  f. dose
  f. endocarditis
  f. fibroelastosis
  f. folic acid antagonist
    syndrome
  f. growth
  f. growth retardation
    (FGR)
  f. height
  f. hydantoin syndrome
  f. length
  f. lobulation
  f. methotrexate
  f. movement
  f. osteoporosis
  f. position
  f. retardation
  f. thalidomide
  f. warfarin embryopathy
fetid
fetogram
fetography
fetometry
fetopathy
Fett navicular balls
fetus papyraceous
fetus, s.
  fetuses, pl.
fetuses, pl.
  fetus, s.
FEV (forced expiratory volume)
FFD (focal film distance)
FFT (fast Fourier
  transformation)
FFU (femur-fibula-ulna)
  syndrome
fibercolonoscope
fibergastroscope
fiberglass cast
fiber-illuminated

fiberoptic
  f. bronchoscopy
  f. esophagogastric
    duodenoscopy
  f. probe
  f. scope
fiberscope
fibril
fibrin ball
fibrinogen
fibrinous
fibro-osseous
  f.-o. otitis media
  f.-o. tumor
fibro-osteoma
fibroadenoma
fibroangiomatous polyp
fibroatrophy
fibroblast
fibroblastoma
fibrocalcareous
fibrocalcific
fibrocarcinoma
fibrocartilage
fibrocartilaginous joint
fibrocaseous
fibrocavitary tuberculosis
fibrocellular
fibrochondroma
fibrocollagenous
fibrocyst
fibrocystic disease of the
  breast
fibrocystoma
fibrodysplasia
  f. elastica generalisata
  f. ossificans
  f. ossificans progressiva
fibroepithelioma
fibroflocculent
fibrogenesis
  f. imperfecta ossium
fibroglandular opacity

fibroglioma
fibrolipoma
fibrolipomatosis
fibroma
    ameloblastic f.
    cementifying f.
    chondromyxoid f.
    desmoplastic f.
    nonossifying f.
    nonosteogenic f.
    ossifying f.
fibroma, s.
    fibromas or fibromata, pl.
fibromas or fibromata, pl.
    fibroma, s.
fibromatoid
fibromatosis
    juvenile hyaline f.
    Stout's f.
fibromyalgia
fibromyeloid medullary
  reticulosis
fibromyitis
fibromyoma
    f. uteri
fibromyositis
fibromyxoma
    odontogenic f.
fibromyxosarcoma
fibropapilloma
fibroplasia
    retrolental f.
fibropurulent
fibrosarcoma
fibroserous
fibrosis
    cartilaginous anulus f.
    congenital hepatic f.
    cystic f.
    diatomite f.
    endomyocardial f.
    f. uteri
    graphite f.

    idiopathic pulmonary f.
    idiopathic retroperitoneal
      f.
    interstitial f.
    mediastinal f.
    neoplastic f.
    nodular subepidermal f.
    panmural f.
    perianeurysmal f.
    periureteric f.
    postfibrinous f.
    progressive portal f.
    proliferative f.
    pulmonary f.
    replacement f.
    retroperitoneal f.
    root sleeve f.
    submucosal f.
fibrositis
    capsular f.
    f. ossificans
fibrothorax
fibrous
    f. band
    f. cavernitis
    f. cortical defect
    f. dysplasia
    f. goiter
    f. histiocytoma
    f. joint
    f. long-spacing FLS
      (collagen)
    f. myocarditis
    f. obliteration
    f. osteoma
    f. pneumonia
    f. replacement
    f. sclerosis of the penis
    f. streaking
    f. tissue
    f. xanthoma
fibrovascular
fibroxanthoma

fibula, s.
    fibulae or fibulas, pl.
fibulae or fibulas, pl.
    fibula, s.
fibular
    f. malleolus
    f. notch
    f. shaft fracture
fibulas or fibulae, pl.
    fibula, s.
fibulocalcaneal
Fick's
    F.'s equation
    F.'s law
    F.'s method
    F.'s position
    F.'s principle
fictitious polyps
FID (free induction decay)
FID (free induction delay)
Fiedler's myocarditis
field
    absolute f.
    alternating f.
    dynamic magnetic f.
    electrical f.
    electromagnetic f.
    f. coil
    f. emission x-ray system
    f. focusing nuclear
        magnetic resonance
    f. frequency
    f. gradient
    f. intensity
    f. line
    f. lock
    f. magnet
    f. of force
    f. of view (FOV)
    f. size
    f. strength
    helmet f.
    magnetic f.
    pulsed radiofrequency f.

static magnetic f.
    wedge-shaped f.
Fielding's classification
Fiessinger-Leroy syndrome
fifth
    f. finger
    f. or O-shell
    f. ventricle
figure "8"
    f. "8" heart
    f. "8" optic canal
fila, pl.
    filum, s.
filament
    ammeter f.
    evaporation of f.
    f. circuit
    f. current
    f. emission
    f. saturation
    f. stabilizer
    f. transformer
    f. voltage
    thorinated tungsten f.
filariasis
filiform
    f. and followers
    f. catheter
filiform-tipped catheter
filling
    f. defect
    f. factor
film
    acetate f.
    cine f.
    comparison f.
    copy f.
    double-emulsion f.
    expiratory f.
    f. acetate
    f. badge
    f. base
    f. bin
    f. changer

f. contrast
f. corner cutter
f. defect
f. density
f. density calibration
f. dispenser
f. emulsion
f. exposure
f. field collimator
f. graininess
f. hangers
f. plate
f. ring
f. screen contact test tool
f. screen technique
　mammogram
f. sensitivity
f. speed
f. subtraction
flat f.
gamma f.
grid f.
high-contrast f.
lateral decubitus f.
overhead f.
overpenetrated f.
plain f.
port f.
postevacuation f.
postreduction f.
preliminary f.
rapid processing f.
scout f.
screen type f.
screen-f.
semierect f.
sequential f.
serial f.
single-emulsion f.
soft-tissue f.
split-f.
spot f.
streaky f.
stress f.

strip f.
subtraction f.
wet f.
film changer
　Sanchez-Perez automatic f. c.
　Schonander f. c.
　Schonander rapid biplane
　　f. c.
film-stripping autoradiography
film-tube distance
filmy adhesion
filter
　alpha f.
　beam-flattening f.
　bow-tie f.
　compensating f.
　density equalization f.
　f. radiography
　f. safelight
　f. therapy
　GBX f.
　Greenfield's f.
　high-pass f.
　inherent f.
　low-pass f.
　Mobin-Uddin vena caval f.
　primary f.
　radiography f.
　secondary f.
　spatial f.
　Thoraeus' f.
　Wedge's f.
　Wratten's 6B f.
filtered-back projection
filtration
　f. fraction
　glomerular f.
　inherent f.
filum
　f. terminale
filum, s.
　fila, pl.
fimbria, s.
　fimbriae, pl.

fimbriae, pl.
    fimbria, s.
fimbriate
fine needle
    f. n. aspiration (FNA)
    f. n. aspiration biopsy(FNAB)
    f. n. biopsy
fine-grain
finger
    baseball f.
    claw-like f.
    coach's f.
    dropped f.
    f. pads
    f. plate
    fifth f.
    mallet f.
    trigger f.
    webbed f.
    webbed trigger f.
Finnish-type nephrosis
Finsen's treatment
first
    f. arch syndrome
    f. dorsal segment
    f. generation
    f. metacarpal
    f. metatarsal
    f. or K-shell
    f. rib
first-order
    f.-o. beam hardening
      correction
    f.-o. subtraction
first-pass
    f.-p. isotope angiography
    f.-p. radionuclide
      angiocardiography
    f.-p. view
Fischgold's
    F.'s bimastoid line
    F.'s biventer line
    F.'s digastric line
"fish" vertebrae
fish-scale gallbladder

Fisher numbering
Fiske's method
FISP (MRI sequences)
fission
    f. products
    f. yield
    nuclear f.
fissula, s.
    fissulae, pl.
fissulae, pl.
    fissula, s.
fissura
    f. calcarina
    f. hippocampi
fissura, s.
    fissurae, pl.
fissurae, pl.
    fissura, s.
fissural
fissure
    anal f.
    azygos lobe f.
    calcarine f.
    f. fracture
    f. of Rolando
    f. of Sylvius
    glaserian f.
    interhemispheric f. (IHF)
    interlobar hepatic f.
    intersegmental hepatic f.
    intrapulmonary f.
    longitudinal f.
    orbital f.
    parieto-occipital f.
    petrosquamous f.
    petrotympanic f.
    pulmonary f.
    sylvian f.
    transverse f.
fissured
    f. fracture
    f. pelvis
fistula
    aortoduodenal f.
    arteriovenous f. (AVF)

bronchopleural f.
cholecystocolic f.
cholecystoenteric f.
colovesical f.
enterobiliary f.
esophagopleural f.
gastrocolic f.
Gross' tracheoesophageal
    f., type E
sigmoid-vesical f.
thyroglossal f.
tracheoesophageal f.
    (TEF)
tracheoinnominate f.
fistula, s.
    fistulas or fistulae, pl.
fistulae or fistulas, pl.
    fistula, s.
fistulogram
fistulography
fistulous
    f. tract
    f. ulcer
Fitz' syndrome
five T group
fixation
    external f.
    flexible rod f.
    internal f.
fixation nail
fixed
    f. angle method
    f. defect
fixed-field therapy
fixing
    f. bath
    f. time
fL (femtoliter)
FL (femur length)
flaccid
Flack's node
flail
    f. chest
    f. joint
    f. valve

flair valve
flange
flank
    f. shadow
    "f. stripe"
    "f. stripe" sign
flap fracture
FLASH (MRI sequences)
flask-like
flask-shaped heart
flat
    f. film
    f. plate
    f. roentgenogram
    f. waist sign
flatfoot
flatulence
flatus
flaval ligament
fleck
    f. formation
    f. sign
Fleischner's
    F.'s atelectasis
    F.'s line
    F.'s method
    F.'s pointed ileum sign
    F.'s position
    F.'s spearhead sign
Fleming's rule
Fletcher's
    F.'s ovoid system for
        afterloading
    F.'s projection
        (cervicothoracic)
Fletcher-Suit applicator
Fletcher-Suit-Delclos (FSD)
    applicator
flex-i-tip
flexible
    f. bronchoscopy
    f. catheter
    f. guide wire
    f. metal catheter
    f. rod fixation

flexible—*Continued*
    f. sigmoidoscopy
flexion
    acute f.
    f. contracture
    f. extension projection
    f. fracture
    f. position
    partial f.
    Towne's f.
flexor (muscle)
    f. accessorius muscle
    f. brevis minimi digiti
        muscle
    f. carpi radialis muscle
    f. carpi radialis tendon
    f. carpi ulnaris muscle
    f. digiti quinti brevis muscle
    f. digitorum brevis muscle
    f. digitorum longus muscle
    f. digitorum profundus
        muscle
    f. digitorum profundus
        tendon
    f. digitorum sublimis
        muscle
    f. digitorum superficialis
        muscle
    f. hallucis brevis muscle
    f. hallucis longus muscle
    f. pollicis brevis muscle
    f. pollicis longus muscle
    f. tunnel
flexura coli sinistra
flexure (a bend)
    colic f.
    duodenojejunal f.
    hepatic f.
    splenic f.
flicker-free image
flip angle
flip-flop phenomenon
floating
    f. catheter

f. elbow
f. gallstones
f. kidney
f. knee
"f. mine" sign
f. patella (knee cap)
f. rib
f. spleen
f. table top
"f. tooth" sign
flocculation
flocculent
flocculonodular
    f. lobe
Flocks' technique
flood source
floor plate
floppy
    f. atrial septum
    f. disk
    f. valve syndrome
florid
    f. pulmonary edema
    f. reactive periostitis
flow
    blood f. measurement
    cerebral blood f.
    collateral f.
    effective renal plasma f.
        (ERPF)
    electron f.
    f. graph
    f. imaging
    f. potential
    f. study
    pulmonary f.
flow-directed catheter
flower pattern
flowing hyperostosis
flowmeter
    electromagnetic f. (emf)
    Gould electromagnetic f.
    Statham electromagnetic
        f.

FLS (fibrous long-spacing)
   collagen
fluctuating muscular rigidity
fluence and intensity
fluffy margins
fluid
   bland f.
   cerebrospinal f.
   extraperitoneal f.
   free peritoneal f.
   intraperitoneal f.
   mediastinal f.
   pleural f.
   synovial f.
   toxic f.
fluid-filled structure
fluid-fluid level
fluorescein
   f. angiogram
   f. angiography
   f. uptake
fluorescence
fluorescent
   f. ray
   f. scan
   f. screen
   f. yield
Fluorex
Fluoricon
fluoride
fluoride therapy
fluorine 18 (18F)
fluorine-fluoride
fluorochloride
fluorometer
fluorometry
fluoronephelometer
fluororoentgenography
fluoroscopic
   f. contrast
   f. evaluation
   f. examination
   f. guidance
   f. image

f. image intensifier
f. localization
f. timer
fluoroscopist
fluoroscopy
   C-arm f.
   cine f. foot
   computerized f.
   digital f.
   image-amplified f.
fluorosis
flush
   f. aortogram
   f. syndrome
flushing technique
flutter
   atrial f.
   auricular f.
   diaphragmatic f.
   mediastinal f.
   ventricular f.
flutter-fibrillation
flux
   electric f.
   f. jumping
   f. line
   magnetic f.
   photon f.
FNA (fine needle aspiration)
FNAB (fine needle aspiration
   biopsy)
focal
   f. dermal dysplasia
   f. dermal hypoplasia
   f. disease
   f. film distance (FFD)
   f. finding
   f. length
   f. myelopathy
   f. neurologic deficit
   f. neuropathy
   f. plane level
   f. plane tomography
   f. pyelonephritis

focal—*Continued*
    f. skin distance (FSD)
    f. spot
    f. thyroiditis
    f. zone (FZ)
foci, pl.
    focus, s.
focus
    conjugate f.
    f. film distance
    f. grid
    f. object distance (FOD)
    f. size
    line f.
    linear f.
    virtual f.
focus, s.
    foci, pl.
focus-skin distance
focused
    f. collimator
    f. grid
    f. nuclear magnetic
        resonance (FONMR)
focusing
    f. collimator
    f. cup
    f. electrode
FOD (focus-object distance)
fog
Fogarty
    F. artery embolectomy
        catheter
    F. balloon biliary catheter
    F. catheter
folate
fold
    aryepiglottic f.
    axillary f.
    bulboventricular f.
    gastric f.
    lacrimal f.
    medullary f.
    pharyngoepiglottic f.
    rugal f.

semilunar f.
    vestibular f.
folds
    Kerckring's f.s
Foley
    F. catheter
Foley-Alcock catheter
follicle
follicular
    f. adenoma
    f. atresia
    f. gastritis
    f. lymphadenopathy with
        splenomegaly
    f. lymphoma
    f. lymphoreticuloma
    f. reticulosis
    f. ulcer
folliculi, pl.
    folliculus, s.
folliculoma
    f. lipidique
folliculus, s.
    folliculi, pl.
Fölling's syndrome
Foltz catheter
Fong's
    F.'s lesion
    F.'s syndrome
FONMR (focused nuclear
    magnetic resonance)
fontanel (also fontanelle)
fontanelle (also fontanel)
foot
    f. plate
    Madura f.
    rocker-bottom f.
foot-candle
foot-lambert
foot-pound
foot-poundal
"football" sign
foramen
    anterior sacral f.
    basal f.

effective f. of magnum
emissary f.
epiploic f.
f. caecum
f. intervertebral
f. lacerum
f. lacerum posterius
f. magnum
f. magnum line
f. of Bochdalek
f. of Botallo
f. of Hyrtl
f. of Luschka
f. of Magendie
f. of Monro
f. of Morgagni
f. of Vesalius
f. of Winslow
f. ovale
f. ovale septi atriorum
f. rotundum
f. spinosum
f. transversarium
hypoglossal f.
infraorbital f.
interventricular f.
intervertebral f.
jugular f.
mandibular f.
mental f.
neural f.
nutrient f.
obturator f.
olfactory f.
optic f.
palatine f.
parietal f.
pseudo-optic f.
sacral f.
stylomastoid f.
supraorbital f.
transverse f.
vascular f.
venous f.
vertebral f.

zygomaticofacial f.
foramen, s.
foramina, pl.
foramina of Luschka
foramina, pl.
foramen, s.
foraminal
f. node
f. stenosis
foraminous spiral tract
force
centripetal f.
Coulomb's f.
electric lines of f.
electrical f.
field of f.
gravitational f.
Lorentz's f.
molecular f.
nuclear f.
forced expiratory volume
(FEV)
forearm
forebrain
forefoot
f. valgus
foreign body (FB)
aspirated f.
f. granuloma
metallic f. (MFB)
penetrating f.
radiopaque f.
retained f.
swallowed f.
foreshortened
Forestier and Rotés-Querol
syndrome
forked
f. rib
f. ureter
format camera
formation
bone f.
"ruffled border"
bone f.

formation—*Continued*
  "ruffled border" f.
formatter
forme fruste of Hurler's
  syndrome
formula
  autotransformer f.
  power f.
  projection f.
forniceal invasion
fornices, pl.
  fornix, s.
fornix, s.
  fornices, pl.
Forssell's sinuses
fortuitous
forty-inch Bucky
forward-biased voltage
FOS (full of stool)
fossa
  cerebral f.
  condyloid f.
  coronoid f.
  cubital f.
  f. of Rosenmüller
  f. ovalis
  gallbladder f.
  glenoid f.
  Gruber's f.
  hepatorenal f.
  hypophyseal f.
  iliac f.
  infraspinatus f.
  intercondylar f.
  intercondyloid f.
  interpeduncular f.
  Jobert's f.
  jugular f.
  malleolar f.
  mandibular f.
  nasal f.
  olecranon f.
  paraduodenal f.
  paravesical f.

  parietal f.
  patellar f.
  pituitary f.
  popliteal f.
  posterior f.
  pterygoid f.
  pterygopalatine f.
  radial f.
  renal f.
  semilunar f.
  supraclavicular f.
  supraspinatus f.
  temporal f.
  temporomandibular f.
  tibiofemoral f.
  trochanteric f.
  ulnar f.
  zygomatic f.
fossa, s.
  fossae, pl.
fossae, pl.
  fossa, s.
Foster fracture frame
Foster-Kennedy syndrome
four-cavities position
four days technique of Salzman
four-field box
four-flanged pin
four-hole side plate
four-point gait
four-valve-tube rectification
four-vessel
  f.-v. angiography
  f.-v. study
four-view chest x-ray
four-way stopcock
four-wing Malecot retention
  catheter
fourchette
Fourier
    F. direct transformation
      energy
    F. direct transformation
      imaging

F. discrete transformation
F. multislice KWE direct
    imaging
F. multislice modified
F. transform (FT)
F. transformation
    reconstruction
F. transformation
    zeugmatography
F. two-dimensional
    imaging
F. two-dimensional
    projection
    reconstruction
fourth
    f. generation
    f. or N-shell
    f. ventricle
FOV (field of view)
fovea centralis
fovea, s.
    foveae, pl.
foveae, pl.
    fovea, s.
foveola
Fowler's
    F.'s position
    F.'s segment
Fr. (French)
fraction
    absorbed f.
    branching f.
    ejection f. (EF)
    packing f.
    penetration f.
    scatter f.
fractional
fractionation
fracture (fx)
    acetabular f.
    acromial f.
    acute f.
    agenetic f.
    anterior malleolus f.

apophyseal or apophysial f.
articular f.
atrophic f.
aviator's astragulus f.
avulsion f.
backfire f.
Bado's f.
Bankart's f.
Barton's f.
basal neck f.
basal skull f.
bending f.
Bennett's f.
Bennett's reverse f.
bent f.
bimalleolar f.
blow-in f.
blow-out f.
boot-top f.
Bosworth's f.
boxer's f.
Boyd f.
bucket-handle f.
buckle f.
bumper f.
bunkbed f.
bursting f.
butterfly f.
buttonhole f.
calcaneal f.
capillary f.
carpal f.
carpometacarpal f.
cementum f.
central f.
Chance's f.
Chauffeur's f.
chip f.
chisel f.
chondral f.
Chopart's f.
circumferential f.
clavicular f.
"clay-shoveler's" f.

fracture (fx)—*Continued*
    cleavage f.
    closed f.
    Colles' f.
    Colles' reverse f.
    comminuted f.
    complete f.
    complex f.
    complex simple f.
    complicated f.
    composite f.
    compound f.
    compression f.
    condylar f.
    congenital f.
    convulsive f.
    coracoid process f.
    cortical buckle f.
    Cotton's f.
    cough f.
    dashboard f.
    de Quervain's f.
    deferred f.
    Delbet's f.
    dens f.
    dentate f.
    depressed f.
    Descot's f.
    diacondylar f.
    diastatic f.
    diastatic skull f.
    direct f.
    dish-pan f.
    dislocation f.
    displaced f.
    distraction f.
    dome f.
    double f.
    Dupuytren's f.
    Duverney's f.
    Dyes' f.
    dyscrasic f.
    endocrine f.
    epiphyseal or epiphysial f.

    Essex-Lopresti f.
    eversion f.
    extra-articular f.
    extracapsular f.
    f. alignment
    f. by contrecoup
    f. clamp
    f. *en coin* (French)
    f. *en rave* (French)
    f. fragment
    f. frame
    f. line
    f. nail
    f. of contrecoup
    f. plate
    f. rod
    f. splint
    f. table
    f., compound, complex
      (FCC)
    fatigue f.
    femoral f.
    femoral neck f.
    femoral shaft f.
    fender f.
    Ferguson's f.
    fibular shaft f.
    fissure f.
    flap f.
    flexion f.
    Frykman's f.
    Galeazzi's f.
    "gamekeeper's" thumb f.
    Garden f.
    golfer's f. of the ribs
    Gosselin's f.
    greenstick f.
    grenade-thrower f.
    "growing" f.
    Guérin's f.
    gutter f.
    hairline f.
    hangman's f.
    head-splitting f.

Henderson's f.
Heydenreich's f.
hickory-stick f.
hip pointer f.
Hoffa f.
Holstein-Lewis f.
horizontal f.
horizontal maxillary f.
humeral condyle f.
Hutchinson's f.
iliopubic ramus f.
impacted f.
implosion f.
impression f.
incomplete f.
indirect f.
inflammatory f.
insufficiency f.
intercondylar f.
internal f.
interperiosteal f.
intertrochanteric f.
intra-articular f.
intracapsular f.
intraperiosteal f.
intrauterine f.
inversion f.
ischial f.
Jefferson's f.
joint f.
Jones' f.
jumper's f.
Kocher's f.
Kohler's f.
lap-type seat belt f.
Laugier's f.
Le Fort's f.
Le Fort's I f.
Le Fort's II f.
Le Fort's III f.
lead pipe f.
linear f.
Lisfranc's f.
long bone f.

longitudinal f.
loose f.
lorry driver f.
lumbar f.
Maisonneuve's f.
malar f.
Malgaigne's f.
malleolus f.
malunited f.
march f.
mechanical bull thumb f.
metacarpal f.
metacarpal head f.
metacarpal neck f.
metaphyseal corner f.
metatarsal f.
midnight f.
Monteggia's "reverse" f.
Monteggia's f.
Montercaux's f.
Moore's f.
Mouchet's f.
multiple f.
Myer-McKeever f.
navicular f.
Neer's I f.
Neer's II f.
neoplastic f.
neurogenic f.
nightstick f.
nonarticular f.
oblique f.
occult f.
olecranon f.
open f.
osteochondral f.
paratrooper's f.
parry f.
patellar f.
pathologic f.
Pauwels' f.
pelvic ring f.
perforating f.
periarticular f.

fracture (fx)—*Continued*
   pertrochanteric f.
   phalangeal f.
   Piedmont f.
   pillion f.
   ping-pong f.
   plafond f.
   pond f.
   Posada's f.
   Pott's f.
   Pouteau's f.
   pressure f.
   pubic rami f.
   pyramidal f.
   Quervain's f.
   resecting f.
   ring f.
   Rolando's f.
   root puller's f.
   Salter's f.
   Salter-Harris f.
   scaphoid f.
   screwlike f.
   seat-belt f.
   secondary f.
   segmental f.
   Segond's f.
   Shepherd's f.
   sideswipe f.
   silver-fork f.
   simple f.
   simple skull f.
   ski boot f.
   ski pole f.
   Skillern's f.
   skull f.
   Smith-Goyrand f.
   Smith's f.
   spinous process f.
   spiral f.
   splintered f.
   spontaneous f.
   sprain f.
   sprinter's f.
   stellate f.
   Stieda's f.
   straddle f.
   strain f.
   stress f.
   subcutaneous f.
   subperiosteal f.
   supracondylar f.
   T-f.
   T-shaped f.
   teardrop f.
   thoracolumbar f.
   Thurston-Holland f.
   tibial condylar f.
   tibial plafond f.
   tibial shaft f.
   Tillaux-Kleiger's f.
   Tillaux's f.
   toddler's f.
   tongue f.
   torsion f.
   torus f.
   transcervical f.
   transcondylar f.
   transverse f.
   transverse facial f.
   transverse maxillary f.
   trimalleolar f.
   triplane f.
   trophic f.
   "tripod" f.
   tuft f.
   TV f.
   ulnar styloid f.
   uncinate process f.
   ununited f.
   volar plate f.
   wagonwheel f.
   Wagstaffe's f.
   Walther's f.
   willow f.
   Wilson's f.
   Y-f.
fracture appliance
   Cameron f. a.
   craniofacial f. a.

facial f. a.
Roger Anderson facial f. a.
fracture frame
  Balkan f. f.
  Böhler f. f.
  Bradford f. f.
  Cole f. f.
  Deiter terminal f. f.
  Depuy f. f.
  Foster f. f.
  Goldthwait f. f.
  head f. f.
  Hibbs f. f.
  hyperextension f. f.
  laminectomy f. f.
  occluding f. f.
  overhead f. f.
  quadriplegic standing f. f.
  rainbow f. f.
  reading f. f.
  reducing f. f.
  Stryker f. f.
  Thomson f. f.
  trial f. f.
  turning f. f.
  Whitman f. f.
fracture-dislocation
fractured kidney
Fraenkel, white line of
fragilitas ossium
  congenita
fragmentation
  f. myocarditis
  f. sign
Fraley's syndrome
Franceschetti's syndrome
francium
François'
  F.' dyscephaly
  F.' syndrome
François-Haustrate
  syndrome
Fränkel's sign
Frankfort's
  F.'s line

F.'s plane
Franseen
  F. lung biopsy needles
  F. needle
Fraunhofer zone
Fray's
  F.'s cranial angle method
  F.'s proportional method
"frayed string" appearance
fraying
free
  f. air
  f. air ionization chamber
  f. electron
  f. induction decay (FID)
  f. isolated spin
  f. ligand
  f. peritoneal air
  f. peritoneal fluid
  f. thyroxin index (FTI)
  f. tissue water
free-air chamber
free-floating cradle table
free-flowing
free-induction decay
free-induction sign
freely movable joint
Freeman-Sheldon
  syndrome
Freeman–Swanson
  prosthesis
Frei's test
Freiberg's
  F.'s disease
  F.'s infarction
  F.'s infraction
fremitus
French (Fr)
  F. catheter
  F. Foley catheter
  F. fundus (bas-fond)
  F. Mani
  F. pigtail
  F. polyethylene catheter
  F. Robinson catheter

frenula, pl.
  frenulum, s.
frenulum, s.
  frenula, pl.
frequency
  angular f.
  energy f.
  f. encoding
  f. modulation
  f. pattern
  f. waves
  Larmor's f.
  Larmor's precession f.
frequency (f)
Fresnel zone plate
Freund's adjuvant
friction marks
Friedländer's
  F.'s bacillus
  F.'s pneumobacillus
  F.'s pneumonia
Friedman's
  F.'s method
  F.'s position
Friedrich's
  F.'s disease
  F.'s necrosis
  F.'s syndrome
Friend catheter
frilling
fringe joint
Fritsch catheter
frog-leg
  f.-l. position
  f.-l. view
frog-like position
Fröhlich's obesity syndrome
frons
frontad
frontal
  f. abscess
  f. anterior position
  f. antrum

f. bone
f. dura mater
f. fundus
f. gyrus
f. horn
f. lobe
f. lobe sulcus
f. plane
f. posterior position
f. process
f. projection
f. region
f. sinus
f. star
f. suture
f. transverse position
f. view
frontalis muscle
frontipetal
frontoanterior position
frontodigital
frontoethmoidal
  f. suture
frontolacrimal
frontomalar
  f. suture
frontomaxillary
  f. suture
frontometaphyseal
  f. dysplasia
frontonasal
  f. dysplasia
  f. suture
fronto-occipital position
frontoparietal
  f. suture
frontopolar sign
frontopontine
  f. tract
frontoposterior position
frontosphenoid
  f. suture
frontotemporal

frontotransverse position
frontozygomatic
    f. suture
Frostberg's
    F.'s epsilon sign
    F.'s sign
Frykman's
    F. classification
    F. fracture
FSD (Fletcher-Suit-Delclos)
    applicator
FSD (focal skin distance)
FT (Fourier transform)
FT line
FTI (free thyroxin index)
Fuchs'
    F.' anteroposterior
      position
    F.' dystrophy
    F.' method
    F.' oblique position
    F.' position
fucose
FUDR (fluorodeoxyuridine)
fuel rod
fulcrum
full
    f. scan
full-column barium enema
full-line scan
full-size
full-wave
    f.-w. rectification
    f.-w. rectifier
full-width
    f.-w. at half maximum
      (FWHM)
Fuller-Albright syndrome
function
    line spread f.
    modulation transfer f.
      (MTF)
    point spread f.

    Shepp-Logan filter f.
    Zeeman's hamiltonian f.
fundamental unit
fundi, pl.
    fundus, s.
fundiform
fundoplication
    Nissen's f.
fundus
    uterine f.
fundus uteri
fundus, s.
    fundi, pl.
funduscopy
fungal
    f. abscess
    f. osteomyelitis
fungus ball in the bladder
funicular
    f. myelopathy
funiculi, pl.
    funiculus, s.
funiculoepididymitis
funiculus, s.
    funiculi, pl.
funnel
    f. breast
    f. chest
    f. deformity
    mitral f.
    pial f.
    vascular f.
funnel-shaped pelvis
funnelization
Furniss' catheter
furosemide
Furst-Ostrum syndrome
fused
    f. kidney
fusiform
    f. aneurysm
    f. deformity
    f. gyrus

fusion
  atlantoaxial f.
  capitate-hamate f.
  capitate-trapezoid f.
  f. fascia
  lunate-scaphoid f.
  lunate-triquetrum f.
  nuclear f.
  pisiform-hamate f.
  scaphoid-trapezium f.
  sutural f.
  trapezium-trapezoid f.
  triquetrum-hamate f.
  triquetrum-lunate f.
  vertebral f.
FWHM (full-width at half-maximum)
fx (fracture)
FZ (focal zone)

Gg

G (gauss)
G syndrome
Ga (gallium)
Ga-67 citrate
gadolinium (Gd)
    g. 159 hydroxycitrate
    g. DTPA
    g. oxysulfide
gadopentetate dimeglumine
Gaenslen acetabulum cup
gag reflex
gain
    g. compensation time
    g. correction
gait
    antalgic g.
    ataxic g.
    athetotic g.
    cerebellar g.
    Charcot's g.
    choreic g.
    cogwheel g.
    double-step g.
    drag-to g.
    dystonic g.
    festinating g.
    four-point g.
    glue-footed g.
    gluteus medius g.
    heel-toe g.
    helicopod g.
    hemiplegic g.
    listing g.
    Oppenheim's g.
    reeling g.
    scissors g.
    shuffling g.
    spastic g.

    steppage g.
    swing-to g.
    tabetic g.
    three-point g.
    Trendelenburg's g.
    two-point g.
galactocele
galactose
galea aponeurotica
Galeazzi's fracture
Galen
    G., great vein of
Galen's
    G.'s vein aneurysm
    G.'s venous system
    G.'s ventricle
Galisol
gallbladder (GB)
    Courvoisier's g.
    fish-scale g.
    g. calculi
    g. fossa
    g. scan
    g. series
    g. study
    "porcelain" g.
    sandpaper g.
    stasis g.
    wandering g.
gallium (Ga)
    g. citrate (Ga 67)
    g. scanning
    g. uptake
    radioactive g. (Ga 67)
gallstone ileus
galvanoionization
galvanometer
    Einthoven's g.

string g.
thread g.
galvanotherapy
galvanotropism
Gambro catheter
gamekeeper's thumb
gamma
  g. aminobutyrate
  g. camera
  g. cascade
  g. counter
  g. emitter
  g. film
  g. globulin
  g. heating
  g. knife
  g. level indicator
  g. photo
  g. photon
  g. radiation
  g. radiography
  g. reference source sets
  g. scanning
  g. scintillation camera
  g. spectrometer
  g. well counter
gamma ray
gamma-ray
  g.-r. capture
  g.-r. counter
  g.-r. level indicator
  g.-r. spectra
Gamma/COR RCG cardiac
  probe
gammagram
gammagraphic
ganglia or ganglions, pl.
  ganglion, s.
ganglioglioma
ganglion
  gasserian g.
  Gasser's g.
ganglion, s.
  ganglia or ganglions, pl.

ganglioneuroblastoma
ganglioneuroma
ganglioneuromatosis
ganglions or ganglia, pl.
  ganglion, s.
gangrenous
  g. abscess
  g. emphysema
gantry
  g. angulation
  g. aperture
gap
  air-bone g.
  ausculatory g.
  Bochdalek's g.
  g. in anatomy
  g. technique
Garceau catheter
Garden fracture
Gardner-Bosch syndrome
Gardner's syndrome
gargoyle syndrome
gargoylism
  Pfaundler-Hurler g.
Garland-Thomas method
Garn's method
Garré's
  G.'s osteomyelitis
  G.'s sclerosing osteomyelitis
Gartner's duct cyst
gas
  alveolar g.
  extraluminal g.
  extravasation g.
  g. abscess
  g. amplification
  g. chromatograph
  g.-containing
  g. density line
  g. in nucleus pulposus
  g. in soft tissues
  g. in the portal venous
    system
  g. infarction

gas—*Continued*
  g. myelography
  g. outlet
  g. pattern
  g. phenomenon
  g. tube
  intraluminal g.
  intramural g.
  intraperitoneal g.
  retroperitoneal g.
  ventilator-induced g.
gas-capped niche
gas-filled
gas-flow counter
gas-obstructed visualization
gas-tight needle
gaseous distention
Gaskell's bridge
Gasser's ganglion
gasserian ganglion
gastrectomy
gastric
  g. air-trapping sign
  g. antrum
  g. artery
  g. atrophy
  g. bezoar
  g. bubble
  g. carcinoma
  g. cardia
  g. corpus
  g. crescent-shaped opacity
  g. crises
  g. duplication
  g. emptying
  g. emptying half-time (GET 1/2)
  g. emptying time (GET)
  g. fold
  g. fundus
  g. inlet jet
  g. lung
  g. lymph n.
  g. mucosa

g. mucosal pattern
g. myiasis
g. outlet
g. parietography
g. perforation
g. pouch
g. pull-through segment
g. regurgitation
g. remnant snydrome
g. resection
g. residual
g. rugae
g. ulcer
gastric cancer
  g. c. type I
  g. c. type II
  g. c. type II-a
  g. c. type II-b
  g. c. type II-c
  g. c. type III
Gastriloid
Gastrin immutope kit
gastrinoma
gastritides, pl.
  gastritis, s.
gastritis
  antral g.
  atrophic g.
  catarrhal g.
  cirrhotic g.
  corrosive g.
  cystic g.
  emphysematous g.
  eosinophilic g.
  erosive g.
  exfoliative g.
  follicular g.
  hemorrhagic g.
  hypertrophic g.
  phlegmonous g.
  polypous g.
  pseudomembranous g.
  radiation g.

toxic g.
zonal g.
gastritis, s.
  gastritides, pl.
Gastro-Conray
gastro-omental lymph node
gastrocamera
gastrocardiac syndrome
gastrocele
gastrocnemial ridge
gastrocnemius muscle
gastrocolic
  g. artery
  g. fistula
  g. omentum
gastroduodenal junction
gastroduodenoscopy
gastroenteritis
  eosinophilic g.
  g. typhosa
gastroenterocolitis
gastroenteroptosis
gastroenterostomy
  catheter
gastroepiploic
  g. gland
  g. lymph node
gastroesophageal
  g. (GE)
  g. reflux
gastrogenic cyst
Gastrografin (diatrizoate
  methyl-glucamine and
  sodium diatrizoate)
gastrograph
gastrohepatic
gastrointestinal (GI)
  g. blood loss test
  g. hemorrhage
  g. motility studies
  g. protein loss test
  g. series
  g. studies
  g. tract (GIT)

g. tract studies
g. bleeding scan
gastrojejunostomy
gastrolith
Gastropaque
gastroparesis
gastrophthisis
gastropyloric
gastroradiculitis
gastrosplenic omentum
Gastroview
gated
  g. blood pool imaging
  g. blood pool study
    (GBPS)
  g. CT scanner
  g. image
gating
  cardiac g.
Gaucher's disease
Gaucher-Schlagenhaufer
  syndrome
gauss (G)
gaussian
  g. curve
  g. distribution
  g. line saturation
  g. mode profile laser beam
gavage
Gaynor-Hart
  G.-H. method
  G.-H. position
GB study (gallbladder study)
GBD tablets
GBPS (gated blood pool
  study)
GBX filter
Gd (gadolinium)
Gd-DTPA radioiostope
GE (gastroesophageal)
Ge (germanium)
Gee-Herter-Heubner
  syndrome
Gee-Thaysen disease

gegenhalten
Geiger
    G. counter
    G. region
    G. threshold
Geiger-Müller (G-M)
    G.-M. counter
    G.-M. tubes
Gelobarin
gemellus
    g. inferior muscle
    g. superior muscle
General Electric
    (manufacturer)
    G. E. 8800 scanner
    G. E. CT/T 8800 scan
    G. E. CT/T7 800 scanner
generator
    6-pulse, 3-phase g.
    12-pulse, 3-phase g.
    direct current g.
    electrostatic g.
    Minitec g.
    molybdenum-technetium
        g.
    polyphase g.
    pulse g.
    resonance g.
    six-pulse, three-phase g.
    supervoltage g.
    technetium-99m g.
    three-phase g.
    Triphasix g.
    Ultra-Technekow FM g.
    Van de Graaff's g.
    x-ray g.
genesistasis
genetic effect of radiation
genetically significant dose
    (GSD)
genial apophysis
genicula, pl.
    geniculum, s.
geniculate (branches)

g. bodies
g. ganglion
geniculocalcarine tract
geniculotemporal tract
geniculum, s.
    genicula, pl.
genioglossal
genioglossus muscle
geniohyoglossus muscle
geniohyoid
geniohyoideus muscle
genital dwarfism
genitocrural
genitofemoral nerve
genitography
genitourinary (GU) tract
Gensini arterial percutaneous
    catheter
gentamicin (I-125)
    radioimmunoassay kit
genu
    g. corpus collosum
    g. equivalgum
    g. impressum
    g. internal capsule
    g. recurvatum
    g. valgum
    g. varum
genu, s.
    genua, pl.
genua, pl.
    genu, s.
genucubital position
genufacial position
genupectoral position
geographic
geometric
    g. artifact
    g. distortion
geometrical
    g. efficiency
    g. projection
geometry
    g. factor

Golay g.
geophagia-dwarfism-
    hypogonadism syndrome
Gerdy's tubercle
Gerlach's tendon
German horizontal plane
germanium (Ge)
germicidal
germinal disc
germinoma
    pineal g.
Gerota's
    G.'s capsule
    G.'s fascia
    G.'s fasciitis
    G.'s layer
    G.'s method
Gesco catheter
gestational
    g. sac
    g. trophoblastic disease
GET (gastric emptying time)
GET 1/2 (gastric emptying half-
    time)
GeV (giga electron volt)
GFR (glomerular filtration rate)
GHA (glucoheptanoic acid or
    glucoheptonate)
Ghantus, tables of
Ghon complex
Ghon's
    G.'s focus
    G.'s primary lesion
    G.'s tubercle
ghost reflection
GI (gastrointestinal)
giant
    g. blue nevus
    g. fibroadenoma
    g. follicle lymphosarcoma
    g. follicular
        lymphoblastoma
    g. follicular lymphoma
    g. hairy nevus

    g. lymph node hyperplasia
    g. osteoid osteoma
    g. rugal hypertrophy
giant cell
    g. c. arteritis
    g. c. chondrodysplasia
    g. c. granuloma
    g. c. myeloma
    g. c. myocarditis
    g. c. pneumonitis
    g. c. tumor
    g. c. xanthoma
Gianturco coil
Giardia
    G. intestinalis
    G. lamblia
giardiasis
gibbous deformity
gibbus (noun)
Gibson's
    G.'s groove
    G.'s valve
    G.'s vestibule
Giedion's syndrome
giga electron volt (GeV)
giggle incontinence
Gilbert's catheter
Gill's method
gill-arch skeleton
Gillespie's syndrome
Gimbernat's ligament
gingiva, s.
    gingivae, pl.
gingivae, pl.
    gingiva, s.
gingival abscess
ginglymoarthrodial
ginglymoid joint
ginglymus
Giordano's sphincter
Girdany-Golden method
girdle
    pectoral g.
    pelvic g.

girdle—*Continued*
    shoulder g.
Girout's method
GI (gastrointestinal) series
    lower GI s.
    upper GI s.
GIT (gastrointestinal tract)
glabella
glabelloalveolar line
glabellomeatal line
glabrous
glacial acetic acid
gladiolus
gladiomanubrial
gland
    accessory g.
    adrenal g.
    454Bartholin's g.
    Brunner's g.
    bulbocavernous g.
    bulbourethral g.
    carotid g.
    Duverney's g.
    endocrine g.
    exocrine g.
    g. of Tyson
    g. of Zeis
    gastroepiploic g.
    gustatory g.
    Henle's g.
    lacrimal g.
    mammary g.
    meibomian g.
    merocrine g.
    mesenteric g.
    mucous g.
    nabothian g.
    parathyroid g.
    parotid g.
    pineal g.
    pituitary g.
    preputial g.
    prostate g.
    Rosenmüller's g.
    salivary g.

    sublingual g.
    submandibular g.
    submaxillary g.
    suprarenal g.
    synovial g.
    Theile's g.
    thymus g.
    thyroid g. uptake
    Virchow's g.
glandulography
Glanzmann-Riniker
    syndrome
glaserian fissure
glass
    crown g.
    g. envelope
    g. jaw
    g. ray
    hepatic test of g.
    lithium g.
    quartz g.
glass-blower's emphysema
glaukomflecken
Glenn's procedure
glenohumeral
    g. joint
    g. ligament
glenoid
    g. cavity
    g. fossa
    g. ligament
    g. process
glia
glial tumor
gliding
    g. dorsiflexion
    g. joint
glioblastoma
    g. multiforme
glioma
    brainstem g.
    optic chiasm g.
    pontine g.
Glisson's
    G.'s capsule

G.'s disease
global
    g. ischemia
    g. renal infarction
globi, pl.
    globus, s.
globoid
globose
globular
globulin
globus
    g. pallidus
globus, s.
    globi, pl.
glomangioma
glomera, pl.
    glomus, s.
glomerular filtration rate
   (GFR)
glomeruli, pl.
    glomerulus, s.
glomerulonephritis
glomerulonephropathy
glomerulopathy
glomerulosclerosis
glomerulose
glomerulus, s.
    glomeruli, pl.
glomus
    g. jugulare tumor
    g. tympanicum tumor
glomus, s.
    glomera, pl.
glossa
glossoepiglottic
glossopalatine
glossopalatinus muscle
glossopharyngeal
glottic atresia
glottides or glottises, pl.
    glottis, s.
glottis, s.
    glottides or glottises, pl.
glottises or glottides, pl.
    glottis, s.

glow modular tube
glucagon
glucagonoma
glucocerebrosidase deficiency
glucocorticoid
glucoheptanoic acid
   (GHA)
glucoheptonate (GHA)
gluconeogenesis
glucosaminidase
glucose-6-phosphatase
   dehydrogenase deficiency
glue-footed gait
glutamate
glutaraldehyde
gluteal
    g. fold
    g. line
    g. lymph node
gluten-induced enteropathy
gluteofemoral
gluteoinguinal
gluteus
    g. maximus muscle
    g. medius muscle
    g. minimus muscle
glutitis
glycemia
glycerine
glycerolphosphorylcholine
   (GPC)
glycogen
    g. heart disease
    g. storage disease, type I
    g. storage disease, type II
glycolipid lipidosis
glycosaminoglycan
gm (gram)
GM1 gangliosidosis
GM2 gangliosidosis
goblet sign
Goeckerman's treatment
Goetz needle
goiter
    aberrant g.

goiter—*Continued*
   adenomatous g.
   Basedow's g.
   colloid g.
   congenital g.
   diffuse g.
   endemic g.
   fibrous g.
   intrathoracic g.
   mediastinal g.
   multinodular g. (MNG)
   nontoxic g.
   retrosternal g.
   retrovascular g.
   substernal g.
Golay
   G. coil
   G. geometry
gold (Au)
   g. (Au 198)
   g. colloid
Goldblatt's kidney
Golden's
   G.'s "S" sign
   G.'s disturbed motility
      pattern
Golden-Kantor syndrome
Goldenhar's syndrome
Golding's deformity
Goldschneider's syndrome
Goldstein's ray
Goldthwait fracture frame
golfer's fracture of the ribs
Golgi
   G. apparatus
   G. complex
Goll's tract
Goltz-Gorlin syndrome
GoLYTELY (polyethylene
   glycol, sodium sulfate,
   sodium bicarbonate, sodium
   chloride, potassium chloride)
Gombault's neuritis
gompholic joint

gonad
   mean g. dose
gonadal
   g. agenesis
   g. dysgenesis syndrome
   g. shield
gonadoblastoma
gonia, pl.
   gonion, s.
gonion, s.
   gonia, pl.
gonitis
gonocampsis
gonococcal arthritis
gonycampsis
gonyoncus
Goodale-Lubin catheter
Goodpasture's syndrome
Goodsell line
Gorham's syndrome
Gorlin-Chaudhry-Moss
   syndrome
Gorlin-Goltz syndrome
Gorlin-Psaume syndrome
Gosselin's fracture
gothic palate
Gotmori-Takamatsu procedure
Gott-Daggett valve
Gougerot-Houwer-Sjögren
   syndrome
Gould electromagnetic
   flowmeter
Gouley catheter
gouty node
Goutz catheter
Gowers' tract
GPC
   (glycerolphosphorylcholine)
G.P. prep emulsion
graafian
   g. follicle
   g. vesicle
gracilis muscle
graded MUGA

Gradenigo's syndrome
gradient
    edge g.
    field g.
    g. coil
    g. density
    g. echo sequence
    g. magnetic field
    g. power amplifier
    g. system
    g. waveform generation
    potential g.
graft
    aortocoronary artery
      bypass g.
    aortoiliac g.
    coronary artery bypass g.
    intra-abdominal g.
    saphenous vein
      aortocoronary bypass g.
Graham's test
Graham-Steell syndrome
graininess
grainy
gram (gm)
gram-calorie
gram-rad (grd)
gram-roentgen
grand mal
Grandy's method
Granger's
    G.'s 107 degrees position
    G.'s 17 degrees position
    G.'s 23 degrees position
    G.'s line
    G.'s method
    G.'s position
granular cell tumor
granulation tissue
granulocytes
granuloma
    calcified g.
    caseating g.
    eosinophilic g.

    foreign body g.
    g. annulare
    g. faciale
    g. gangraenescens
    g. inguinale
    g. venereum
    midline g.
    optic g.
    periapical g.
    plasma cell g.
    pulmonary g.
    pyogenic g.
    Wegener's g.
granulomatosis
    eosinophilic g.
    g. benigna
    lymphomatoid g.
    Wegener's g.
granulomatous
    g. arteritis
    g. colitis
    g. inflammation
    g. lymphoma
    g. pneumonitis
graphite fibrosis
Grashey's
    G.'s aphasia
    G.'s method
    G.'s position
Graves'
    G.' disease
    G.' scapula
gravid
gravida
Gravigards intrauterine device
gravitation abscess
gravitational
    g. force
    g. potential energy
gravity abscess
Grawitz's tumor
gray
    g. matter
    g. ramus

gray (Gy)
    g. bar
    g. scale
gray-scale
    g.-s. imaging
    g.-s. ultrasonography
grd (gram-rad)
great
    g. anastomotic vein
    g. anterior medullary
      artery
    g. anterior radicular artery
    g. toe
    g. vein of Galen
greater
    g. auricular nerve
    g. multangular bone
    g. omentum
    g. sac of peritoneum
    g. superficial petrosal
      nerve
    g. trochanter
    g. trochanter muscle
    g. tuberosity
Grebe's
    G.'s chondrodysplasia
    G.'s syndrome
Greene
    G. biopsy needle
    G. needle
Greenfield
    G. filter
Greenfield's
    G.'s disease
greenstick fracture
Greig's
    G.'s cephalopolydactyly
    G.'s syndrome
grenade-thrower fracture
grenz ray
Greulich and Pyle (bone age)
    G. and P. atlas
Gribbs phenomenon
grid
    Bucky g.

    crosshatch g.
    electronic g.
    focus g.
    focused g.
    g. cassette (or oscillating
      g.)
    g. controlled x-ray
    g. film
    g. focus
    g. index
    g. line
    g. or sieve therapy
    g. radius
    g. ratio
    linear g.
    Lysholm g.
    moving g.
    oscillating g.
    parallel g.
    Potter-Bucky g.
    radiographic g.
    radius g.
    ratio g.
    reciprocating g.
    rhombic g.
    stationary g.
Griffith's point
Grignolo's syndrome
Grisel's syndrome
Grob's dysplasia linguofacialis
Groedel index
groin
Groll catheter
Grollman
    G. pigtail catheter
    G. pulmonary pigtail
      catheter
    short-arm G.
Grönblad-Strandberg
  syndrome
Grönblad-Strandberg-Touraine
  syndrome
groove
    bicipital g.
    costal g.

Gibson's g.
interosseous g.
medullary g.
mylohyoid g.
obturator g.
occipital g.
optic g.
radial g.
sagittal g.
subclavian g.
subcostal g.
supraorbital g.
trigeminal g.
ulnar g.
vascular g.
Groshong catheter
Gross'
 G.' esophageal atresia,
  type A
 G.' esophageal atresia,
  type B
 G.' esophageal atresia,
  type C
 G.' esophageal atresia,
  type D
 G.' tracheoesophageal
  fistula, type E
Grossman's principle
ground
 g. state
 g. wire
growth plate
Gruber's fossa
Gruentzig or Grüntzig catheter
grumous
Grüntzig or Gruentzig catheter
Grynfelt-Lesgaft triangle
Grynfelt's hernia
gryposis
GSD (genetically significant
 dose)
GU (genitourinary tract)
gubernaculum
 g. chorda
 g. testis

Hunter's g.
Gudden's tract
Guérin's fracture
Guérin-Stern syndrome
guide wire
 Amplatz stiff g. w.
 "basket" g. w.
 Bentson cerebral curved
  safe-T-J g. w.
 Bentson cerebral straight
  g. w.
 catheter exchange curved
  safe-T-J g. w.
 catheter exchange straight
  g. w.
 Coons interventional g. w.
 Cope mandrel or mandril
  g. w.
 double flexible tipped g. w.
 Hanafee cerebral straight
  g. w.
 J-tipped g. w.
 Lunderquist exchange g. w.
 Lunderquist-Ring torque
  g. w.
 Newton g. w.
 pig-tailed g. w.
 straight g. w.
guides
 Hawkins g.
 Moses g.
 Newton g.
 Ring IV torque g.
 Rosen g.
 Torq-Flex g.
Guidi's canal
Guillain-Barré syndrome
gull-wing sign
gumma, s.
 gummata, pl.
gummata, pl.
 gumma, s.
Gumprecht's shadow
Gunson's
 G.'s method

Gunson's—*Continued*
    G.'s position
gunstock deformity
Gunther's classification
gustatory gland
gutter
    g. fracture
    pelvic g.
    pericolonic g.
Guyon's canal
Gy (gray)
gynecography
gynecoid
gynecomastia-
    aspermatogenesis syndrome
gyri
    g. breves insulae
gyri, pl.
    gyrus, s.
gyromagnetic
    g. field
    g. ratio
gyromagnetic ratio

gyrus
    angular g.
    Broca's g.
    callosal g.
    callosomarginal g.
    cingulate g.
    dentate g.
    fasciolar g.
    frontal g.
    fusiform g.
    g. rectus
    hippocampal g.
    intralimbic g.
    lingual g.
    occipitotemporal g.
    olfactory g.
    orbital g.
    parahippocampal g.
    supracallosal g.
    temporal g.
gyrus, s.
    gyri, pl.

Hh

H-1-H (headhunter) catheter
H (henry)
H (Hounsfield units)
H (hydrogen)
H (magnetic field)
H reflex study
H space
H tritiated water
H type of horseshoe kidney
"H" vertebrae
HA (hepatic artery)
Haab magnet
Haaga biopsy needle
Haas'
    H.' disease
    H.' method
    H.' position
    H.' prone position
    H.' view
habenular commissure
habitus
    asthenic h.
    body h.
    hypersthenic h.
    hyposthenic h.
    sthenic h.
hachet deformity
HADD (hydroxyapatite
    deposition disease)
Hadlock's method (OB/US)
Haferkamp's syndrome
hafnium (Hf)
Hagie pin
Haglund plate
Haglund's
    H.'s deformity
    H.'s osteonecrosis
Haglund-Läwen-Frund
    syndrome

Hagner catheter
Hagner's disease
hairline fracture
hairspray artifact
Hakim valve
    system
Hakion catheter
halation
half scan
half-axial
    h.-a. position
    h.-a. projection
half-cycle
half-life
    biological h.-l.
    effective h.-l.
    physical h.-l.
half-moon pattern
half-shadow
half-thickness
half-time of exchange
half-value layer (HVL)
half-wave rectification
Hallermann-Streiff-François
    syndrome
Halliday's hyperostosis
halluces, pl.
    hallux, s.
hallux
    h. dolorosa
    h. flexus
    h. malleus
    h. rigidus
    h. valgus
    h. varus
hallux, s.
    halluces, pl.
halo
    h. sign

h. traction
halogenated phenolphthalein
    dye
halopelvic traction
halter traction
HAM (human albumin
    microspheres)
hamartoblastoma
hamartoma
        chondromatous h.
hamartomatous cystic kidney
hamate
hamatometacarpal ligament
hamatum metacarpus
hamiltonian
        h. equation
        Zeeman's h. function
Hamman-Rich syndrome
Hamman's sign
hammer toe
Hampton's
        H.'s aortic line
        H.'s gastric line
        H.'s hump
        H.'s view
hamstring tendon
hamulus process
HAN (hyperplastic alveolar
    nodules)
Hanafee
        H. catheter
        H. cerebral straight guide
            wire
hand
        Myobock artificial h.
        "rosebud" h.
        "windswept" h.
Hand's disease
hand-foot syndrome
hand-foot-genital syndrome
hand-foot-uterus syndrome
Hand-Rowland disease
Hand-Schüller-Christian
        H.-S.-C. disease

H.-S.-C. syndrome
hanging-head position
hangman's
        h.'s fracture
        h.'s sign
Hanhart's syndrome
Hansen-Street
        H.-S. diamond-shaped nail
        H.-S. pin
        H.-S. plate
haploid
haploidy
"happy puppet" syndrome
hard
        h. burr type of vesical
            calculus
        h. copy
        h. disk
        h. palate
        h. palate sign
        h. x-ray
Hare's syndrome
Harkavy's syndrome
Harrington's
        H.'s hernia, type I
        H.'s hernia, type II
Harrison-Stubbs method
Hartley's ball sign
Hartmann catheter
Hartmann's
        H.'s pouch
        H.'s procedure
Harwood-Nash catheter
Hashimoto's
        H.'s struma
        H.'s thyroiditis
Hasner, valve of
hat sign
Hatch catheter
Hatcher pin
Hatt's method
Haudeck's
        H.'s niche
        H.'s sign

Hauder's pelvis
haustra, pl.
   haustrum, s.
haustral
   h. churning
   h. fold
   h. pattern
   h. sacculations
haustration
haustrum, s.
   haustra, pl.
Haven's syndrome
haversian
   h. canal
   h. glands
   h. lamella
   h. space
   h. systems
   h. typical system
Hawkins
   H. accordion catheter
      drainage set
   H. catheter
   H. coaxial wire guides
   H. exchange tip deflecting
      wire guides
   H. guide
Hawkins'
   H.' classification
   H.' sign
Haygarth's node
hazard
HCS (hydroxycorticosteroid)
HD (hip disarticulation)
HD (Hodgkin's disease)
H and D curve (Hurter and
   Driffield photographic curve)
HDP (hydroxydiphosphonate)
He (helium)
He-Ne (helium-neon) beam
head
   h. fracture frame
   h. scan
head-dependent position

head-low position
head-splitting fracture
headhunter catheter (H-1-H)
heart
   crisscross h.
   "snowman" h.
heat
   h. dissipation
   h. effect
   h. energy
   h. exchanger
   h. quantity
   h. unit (HU)
heavy
   h. duty straight safety wire
      guides
   h. ion imaging
   h. ion irradiation
   h. particle therapy
   h. water
heavy-chain disease
Heberden's node
Hector's tendon
Hedinger's syndrome
Hedspa
heel-pad thickness sign
heel-toe gait
Hefke-Turner sign
Hegar dilator
Heiland galvanometer
Heine-Medin disease of the
   spine
Heiner's syndrome
Heinz bodies
Heister's
   H.'s diverticulum
   H.'s fold
   H.'s valve
helicis
   h. major muscle
   h. minor muscle
helicopod gait
helium (He)
   h. atom

helium-neon (He-Ne) beam
helix
Hellmer's sign
helmet field
Helmholtz
   H. coil
   H. pair
Helmholtz-Harrington
   syndrome
helminthic abscess
hemal node
hemangiectatic
   h. hypertrophy
hemangioblastoma
hemangioma
   orbital h.
   subglottic h.
   vertebral h.
hemangiomata
hemangiomatosis
   intraosseous h.
hemangiopericytoma
hemangiosarcoma
Hemaquet catheter
hemarthrosis
hematencephalon
hematobilia
hematocolpos
hematocrit
   mean circulatory h.
hematogenous
hematologic osteomyelitis
hematolymphangioma
hematoma
   cerebral h.
   epidural h.
   extrapleural h.
   hepatic h.
   iliacus h.
   intracapsular h.
   intracerebral h.
   intracranial h.
   intramural h.
   intrarenal h.

intrasplenic h.
paraspinal h.
perianal h.
perinephric h.
pulmonary h.
retrouterine h.
splenic h.
subcapsular h.
subdural h.
subungual h.
hematomyelia
hematopoiesis
hematuria
Hemed catheter
hemianopia or hemianopsia
hemiataxia
hemiatrophy
hemiazygos
hemicentrum
hemicranium
hemidiaphragm
hemigigantism
hemimelia
hemiparesis
hemiplegic gait
hemiscrotum
hemisphere
hemispherization
hemithorax
hemivertebra
hemobilia
hemochromatosis
hemocoelom
hemocytoblastoma
hemodynamic
hemoglobin S disease
hemolysis
hemolytic
   h. anemia
   h. icterus
hemolytic-uremic syndrome
hemopericardium
hemoperitoneum
hemophilic joint

hemorrhage
   cerebellar h.
   gastrointestinal h.
   intracerebral h.
   intracranial h. (ICH)
   intraperitoneal h.
   mediastinal h.
   parenchymal h.
   perirenal h.
   pulmonary h.
   retroperitoneal h.
   subarachnoid h.
   subdural h.
   tracheobronchial h.
   variceal h.
hemorrhagic
   h. cyst
   h. gastritis
   h. jaundice
   h. myelopathy
   h. shock
hemorrhoid
hemorrhoidal zone
hemostasis
hemostat
hemostatic catheter
hemothorax
Henderson-Jones syndrome
Henderson's fracture
Henle's
   H.'s gland
   H.'s loop
Henoch-Schönlein purpura
Henoch's purpura
henry (H)
Henschen's
   H.'s method
   H.'s position
   H.'s view
Henschen, Schüller, and
   Lysholm method
Hensen's
   H.'s node
   H.'s plane

Hepacon catheter
hepar
heparitinuria
hepatic
   h. abscess
   h. angiography
   h. angle
   h. arteriography
   h. artery (HA)
   h. cord
   h. duct
   h. flexure
   h. hematoma
   h. laceration
   h. lobe
   h. lymph node
   h. metastasis
   h. parenchymal cells
   h. sphincter
   h. test of Glass
   h. uptake
   h. vein catheterization
hepato-iminodiacetic acid
   (HIDA) scan
hepatobiliary
   h. scan
hepatoblastoma
hepatocellular carcinoma
hepatocholangitis
hepatocirrhosis
hepatocolic
hepatodiaphragmatic
   interposition
hepatoenteric
hepatogastric
hepatogram
hepatography
hepatojugular reflux (HJR)
hepatolenticular degeneration
hepatolienal fibrosis
hepatolienogram
hepatolienography
hepatomegaly
hepatophlebography

hepatoptosis
hepatorenal
    h. fossa
    h. glycogenosis
hepatosplenomegaly
Hepler's concept
hereditary
    h. adenomatosis
    h. cutaneomandibular
      polyoncosis
    h. deforming
      chondrodysplasia
    h. extremity malformation
      syndrome
    h. gerodermia
      osteoblastica
    h. goiter and deafness
    h. hematuria-nephropathy-
      deafness syndrome
    h. multiple ankylosing
      arthropathy
    h. multiple diaphyseal
      sclerosis
    h. ocular hypertelorism
    h. osteo-onychodysplasia
    h. osteochondrodystrophy
    h. polyposis and
      osteomatosis
    h. sensory radicular
      neuropathy
    h. thymic dysplasia
    h. trophedema
Hering's canal
hernia
    Bochdalek's h.
    diaphragmatic h.
    esophagostomal h.
    hiatal h. (HH)
    inguinal h.
    intercostal
    Morgagni's h.
    omental h.
    paraesophageal h.
    pericardial h.

    spigelian h.
    umbilical h.
hernial
    h. aneurysm
    h. sac
herniated
    h. nucleus pulposus (HNP)
    h. vertebra
herniation
herniogram
herniography
Herrick's syndrome
Herter's infantilism
Hertwig's sheath
Hertwig-Weyers syndrome
hertz (Hz)
hertzian wave
Heschl's gyrus
hesitation marks
Hesselbach's triangle
heterogeneous radiation
heterotopic
    h. calcification
    h. ossification (HO)
Heublein's method
Heubner-Herter syndrome
Heubner's artery
Hexabrix
hexamethonium
hexamethylmelamine (HMM)
Heydenreich's fracture
Heyman's capsules
Hf (hafnium)
Hg meralluride
Hg-chlormerodrin
HGA (homogentisic acid)
HH (hiatal hernia)
hiatal hernia (HH)
hiatus
Hibbs fracture frame
Hickey's
    H.'s position for the femur
    H.'s position for the
      mastoid process

Hickey's—*Continued*
    H.'s view
Hickman catheter
hickory-stick fracture
Hicks radius plate
Hicks' syndrome
HIDA (hepato-iminodiacetic
    acid) scan
hide-bound small bowel
Higgins catheter
high
    h. cecum
    h. convergence sign
    h. count rates
    h. definition intensifying
        screens
    h. efficiency particulate
        arrestance
    h. energy collimator
    h. field strength scanner
    h. overlay sign
    h. placental position
    h. speed intensifying
        screens
    h. vacuum
    h. voltage transformer
high-contrast area
high-contrast film
high-detail technique
high-energy collimator
high-frequency
high-lying patella
high-pass
    h.-p. filter
    h.-p. spatial filtering
high-powered liquid
    chromatography
    (HPLC)
high-resolution collimator
high-resolution image
high-sensitivity collimator
high-velocity particle
high-voltage
    h.-v. roentgen therapy
    h.-v. transformer

highlights
Highmore, antrum of
hila, pl.
    hilum, s.
Hilal
    H. aortogram catheter
    H. catheter
    H. coaxial embolization set
        and component
    H. modified headhunter
        cerebral catheter
Hilal-Grossman
    H.-G. curved safe-T-J wire
        guide
    H.-G. straight safety wire
        guide
hilar
    h. adenoma
    h. adenopathy
    h. angle
    h. clouding
    h. dance
    h. infiltration
    h. lymph node
    h. lymphadenopathy
    h. nodule
    h. silhouette
    h. vascular shadow
Hilgenreiner line
hili, pl.
    hilus, s.
Hill's procedure
Hill-Sachs
    H.-S. defect
    H.-S. deformity
    H.-S. lesion
Hilton's sac
hilum
    h. convergence sign
    h. overlay sign
hilum, s.
    hila, pl.
hilus of the meningioma
hilus, s.
    hili, pl.

Hinck
    H. headhunter cerebral
      catheter
    H. myelography
    H. myelography needle
    H. spinal needle with
      depth guide
hindbrain
hindfoot valgus
hinge
    h. joint
    h. position
hip
    h. disarticulation (HD)
    h. dysplasia
    h. joint
    h. pointer fracture
    h. spica cast
Hippel-Czermack
  syndrome
Hippel-Lindau disease
hippocampal gyrus
hippocratic fingers
Hippodin
Hippuran I-131 injection
Hipputope I-125 [radio-
  iodinated sodium
  iodohippuruate (^{131}I)]
Hirsch's
    H.'s sphincter
    H.'s syndrome
Hirschsprung's disease
Hirtz'
    H.' method
    H.' position
    H.' projection
    H.' view
HIS (hospital information
  system)
His, angle of
histiocytic lymphoma
histiocytosis
histogram mode
histology
histopathologic

histoplasmic lymphadenitis
histoplasmoma
histoplasmosis
historadiography
hitchhiker's thumb
Hittorf's tube
Hitzenberger's sniff test
HIV (human immunodeficiency
  virus)
HJR (hepatojugular reflex)
HMD (hyaline membrane
  disease)
HMDP (hydroxymethylene
  diphosphonate)
HMM (hexamethylmelamine)
HNP (herniated nucleus
  pulposus)
HO (heterotopic
  ossification)
Ho (holmium)
HO (hypertrophic
  osteoarthropathy)
Hobbin's method (OB
  ultrasound)
hobnail liver
Hoboken's valve
hockey-stick
    h.-s. deformity
    h.-s. ureter
Hodge's plane
Hodgkin's
    H.'s disease (HD)
    H.'s lymphoma
Hodgson's disease
Hoen
    H. plate
    H. ventricular needle
Hoffa's
    H.'s fracture
    H.'s method
Hoffa-Kastert syndrome
Hofmeister's
    H.'s defect
    H.'s operation
holarthritis

hold-back carrier
hold-up
hole of the doughnut
hole-pair limiting resolution
hollow
Holly's method
Holmblad's
    H.'s method
    H.'s position
holmium (Ho)
hologram
holography
holosystolic prolapse
holotelencephaly
Holstein-Lewis fracture
Holt-Oram syndrome
Holter valve system
Holtermüller-Wiedemann
  syndrome
Holzknecht's
    H.'s space
    H.'s stomach
    H.'s unit
homeostasis
homogeneity
homogeneous radiation
homogentisic acid (HGA)
homologous
homotypical cortex
homozygous hemoglobin S
  disease
honeycomb
    h. lung
HOOD (hereditary onycho-
  osteodysplasia) syndrome
hooded anode
hook
    h. sign
    Mikaelsson h.
    Shepherd h.
Hook visceral catheter
horizontal
    h. fracture
    h. heart
    h. maxillary fracture

    h. plane
    h. position
    h. ray method
horizontal-beam study
horn
    anterior h.
    frontal h.
    inferior h.
    occipital h.
    temporal h.
Horner's
    H.'s sign
    H.'s syndrome
hornpipe position
horseback rider's knee
  dislocation
horseshoe
    h. configuration
    h. kidney
hospital information system
  (HIS)
hot
    h. abscess
    h. cathode
    h. cathode x-ray tube
    h. cross bun deformity
    h. cross bun skull
    h. lesion
    h. nodule
    h. spot
    h. wire
Hough's method
Houndsfield unit (Hu)
Hounsfield's
    H.'s number
    H.'s scale
hourglass
    h. bladder
    h. chest
    h. stomach
    h. tumor
hourglass-shaped sella
Houston's valve
Howship's lacuna
Hozay's syndrome

HPA-23 (antimonium
  tungstate)
HPLC (high powered liquid
  chromatography)
HPO (hypertrophic pulmonary
  osteoarthropathy)
Hryntschak catheter
HSA (human serum albumin)
HSG (hysterosalpingogram)
HSG (hysterosalpingography)
Hsieh's
  H.'s method
  H.'s position
HU (heat unit)
HU (Hounsfield unit)
Hubbard plate
Hudson brace
Hufnagel's operation
Hughes-Stovin syndrome
Hughston's
  H.'s method
  H.'s view
Huldshinsky radiation
Hultkrantz syndrome
human
  h. albumin microspheres
    (HAM)
  h. immunodeficiency virus
    (HIV)
  h. serum albumin (HSA)
humeral condyle fracture
humeri, pl.
  humerus, s.
humeroradial joint
humeroulnar joint
humerus, s.
  humeri, pl.
humped left kidney
hundredth-normal solution
Hünermann's syndrome
Hunner's ulcer
Hunt needle
Hunter-Hurler syndrome
Hunter's
  H.'s canal

  H.'s gubernaculum
  H.'s syndrome
Hurler's syndrome
Hurler-Scheie compound
Hurter and Driffield
  photographic curve (H and D
  curve)
Hutch's
  H.'s diverticulum
  H.'s theory
Hutchinson's fracture
Hutchinson-Boeck
  H.-B. disease
  H.-B. granulomatosis
Hutchinson-Gilford syndrome
Hutchinson-Weber-Peutz
  syndrome
Hutinel-Pick syndrome
Hutinel's disease
HVL (half-value layer)
hyaline
  h. arteriosclerosis
  h. cartilage
  h. cast
  h. membrane disease
    (HMD)
hyalinosis cutis et mucosae
hyaloid canal
hybrid
hydantoin syndrome
hydatid
  h. cyst
  h. resonance
hydatidiform mole
hydramnios
hydranencephaly
hydrarthrosis
hydrated
  h. pyelogram
  h. pyelography
hydrocephalus
  adult h.
  atrophic h.
  communicating h.
  h. internus

hydrocephalus—*Continued*
   h. occlusus
   intermediate h.
   noncommunicating h.
   obstructive h.
hydrochloric acid
hydrocolpos
hydrocystadenoma
hydrogen (H)
   h. atom
   h. density
   h. in concentrate (pH)
hydrogen [tritium] (^{3}H)
Hydrombrine
hydrometer
hydrometrocolpos polydactyly
   syndrome
hydromyelia
hydronephrosis
hydrophilic nonflocculating
   barium
hydropneumothorax
hydrops
   h. fetalis
   h. folliculi
hydroquinone
hydrosalpinx
hydrothorax
hydroxyapatite deposition
   disease (HADD)
hydroxycitrate
hydroxycorticosteroid (HCS)
   17-hydroxycorticosteroid
hydroxydiphosphonate
   (HDP)
hydroxymethylene
   diphosphonate (HMDP)
hygroma
hymen
hyoglossus muscle
hyoid
hyoidal
hyoidean
hyopharyngeus muscle

Hypaque (diatrizoate
   meglumine, diatrizoate
   sodium, iodine)
   H. 25%
   H. 30%
   H. 76 (diatrizoate)
Hypaque-Cysto
Hypaque-DIU 30%
Hypaque-meglumine 60%
Hypaque-meglumine 75%
Hypaque-meglumine 90%
hyparterial bronchus
hypaxial
hyperaeration
hyperbaric
hypercallosis
hypercorticism
hypercortisolism
hypercycloidal
   tomography
hyperechoic (US)
hyperesthesia
hyperextension
   h. fracture frame
   h. position
hyperfractionation
hypergastric
hypergastrium
hyperlucency
hyperlucent lung syndrome
hypernephroid tumor
hypernephroma
   h. halo sign
hyperostoses, pl.
   hyperostosis, s.
hyperostosis
   cortical h.
   diffuse idiopathic skeletal h.
   h. corticalis generalisata
   h. corticalis infantilis
   h. cranii
   h. frontalis interna
   h. generalisata with
      striations

h. palmaris et plantaris
infantile cortical h.
van Buchem's endosteal h.
hyperostosis, s.
hyperostoses, pl.
hyperparathyroid
h. osteoporosis
hyperphosphatasemia tarda
hyperpigmentation
hyperplasia
h. fascialis ossificans
h. fascialis progressiva
hyperplastic
h. alveolar nodules (HAN)
h. osteoarthritis
h. periostosis
hypersthenic habitus
hypertensive
h. arteriosclerosis
h. urography
hyperthecosis of the ovary
hyperthermal
hyperthermia
hypertonic
h. solution
hypertrophic
h. arthritis
h. cardiomyopathy
h. gastritis
h. interstitial neuritis
h. marginal spurring
h. osteoarthropathy (HO)
h. prostate
h. pulmonary
osteoarthropathy (HPO)
h. spurring
hypertrophy
ventricular h.
hypervolemia
hypoaeration
hypocalcemic convulsions-
dwarfism syndrome
hypochondriac region
hypochondrium

hypochondroplasia
hypocomplementemic
hypocycloidal
h. motion
h. movement
h. tomography
hypoechoic
hypogastric zone
hypogastrium
hypoglossal
h. canal
h. foramen
hypohyperparathyroidism
hypokinesis
hypomotility
hypoparathyroid cretinism
hypoparathyroidism
hypophosphatasia
hypophysial or hypophyseal
h. duct tumor
h. fossa
h. syndrome
hypophysiothalamic syndrome
hypopituitarism syndrome
hypoplasia
camptomelic h.
central h.
focal dermal h.
spondylohumerofemoral h.
hypoplastic thrombocytopenia
hypospadias
hypostatic abscess
hyposthenic habitus
hyposulfite of sodium
hypotension
hypothalamic
h. hamartoblastoma
syndrome
h. tegmentum
hypothalamicohypophyseal
tract
hypothenar hammer syndrome
hypothesis
hypothyroid myopathy

hypotonic
    h. duodenography
    h. stomach
hypovolemia
hypoxia
Hyrtl, foramen of
Hyrtl's sphincter
hysterectomy
hysteresis loss

hysteria
hysteric joint
hysterogram
hysterography
hysterosalpingogram (HSG)
hysterosalpingography (HSG)
hysterotubogram
Hytrast
Hz (hertz)

I 131 thyroidal accumulation
I (iodine)
I-123
I-125
I-131
IAC (internal auditory canal)
IACB (intra-aortic counterpulsation balloon)
IACR (The InterAmerican College of Radiology)
IADSA (intra-arterial digital subtraction angiography)
IAM (internal auditory meatus)
iatrogenic
 i. afferent loop syndrome
 i. osteoporosis
IBC (iron-binding capacity)
IBD (ischemic bowel disease)
ICA (internal carotid artery)
"iceberg"
 "i." configuration
 "i." sign
iced intestine
I-cell disease
ICH (intracranial hemorrhage)
ichthyosis palmaris et plantaris
ICP catheter
ICR (International Congress of Radiology)
ICRU (International Commission on Radiation Units and Measurements)
icteric-hepatic pigmentation syndrome
ID (inside diameter)
IDA (iminodiacetic acid)
idiopathic
 i. capsulitis

i. chronic lymphedema
i. cortical sclerosis
i. curve
i. familial acro-osteolysis
i. hereditary lymphedema
i. hypercalcemia
i. hypertrophic osteoarthropathy (IHO)
i. hypertrophic subaortic stenosis (IHSS)
i. inflammatory bowel disease
i. interstitial fibrosis
i. juvenile osteoporosis
i. megacolon
i. megatrachea
i. myocarditis
i. osteoarthropathy
i. pulmonary atrophy
i. pulmonary fibrosis
i. pulmonary hemosiderosis
i. renal acidosis
i. retroperitoneal fibrosis
i. scoliosis
i. steatorrhea
i. unilobar emphysema
idiopathy
IDIS (intraoperative digital subtraction angiography)
IDK (internal derangement of the knee)
IDS (incremented dynamic scanning)
iduronidase
I/E (inspiratory/expiratory) ratio
IHA (infusion hepatic arteriography)

IHF (interhemispheric fissure)
IHO (idiopathic hypertrophic osteoarthropathy)
IHSS (idiopathic hypertrophic subaortic stenosis)
ileac also ileal
ileal also ileac
ileitis
ileocecal
    i. junction
    i. valve
ileocolic lymph node
ileostogram (loopogram)
ileum (small intestine)
ileus
    adynamic i.
    colonic i.
    dynamic i.
    gallstone i.
    mechanical i.
    meconium i.
    paralytic i.
    spastic i.
ili(o) (pelvic)
ilia, pl. (hip bone)
    ilium, s.
iliac
    i. angle
    i. circumflex lymph node
    i. colon
    i. crest
    i. crest apophysis
    i. fascia
    i. fossa
    i. horns
    i. index
    i. lymph node
    i. osteomyelitis
    i. region
    i. spine
    i. spur
    sign of i. artery
iliaci, pl.
    iliacus, s.

iliacus
    i. hematoma
    i. muscle
iliacus, s.
    iliaci, pl.
iliococcygeal muscle
iliocostal space
iliocostalis
    i. cervicis muscle
    i. dorsi muscle
    i. lumborum muscle
    i. thoracis muscle
iliofemoral ligament
ilioischial column
iliolumbar ligament
iliolumbocostoabdominal
iliopectineal line
iliopelvic
iliopsoas
    i. abscess
    i. bursitis
    i. muscle
    i. sign
iliopubic
    i. column
    i. ramus fracture
    i. tract
iliosacral
iliotibial tract
iliotrochanteric ligament
ilium, s. (hip bone)
    ilia, pl.
illumination
illuminator
IMA (inferior mesenteric artery)
image
    alias-free i.
    amplifier i.
    bone-negative i.
    calculated i.
    contrast enhanced i.
    echo-planar i.
    flicker-free i.

image—*Continued*
  fluoroscopic i.
  gated blood pool i.
  gated i.
  high-resolution i.
  i. acquisition time
  i. aliasing
  i. amplifier
  i. analysis
  i. chains
  i. contrast
  i. converter
  i. flip feature
  i. intensification
  i. intensifier
  i. intensifier system
  i. intensifier tube
  i. modification
  i. modulation
  i. noise
  i. orthicon tube
  i. quality
  i. receptor
  i. reconstruction
  i. reformation
  i. resolution
  i. sharpness
  i. slice thickness
  i. storage
  indirect volume i.
    reconstruction
  insert i.
  inversion recovery i.
  laser-generated i.
  latent i.
  localized i.
  multiecho coronal i.
  nuclear magnetic resonance i.
  object-to-i. receptor
    distance (OIRD)
  phantom i.
  "pruned-tree" i.
  radiographic i.
  reference i.
  saturation recovery i.
  scout i.
  soft tissue-negative i.
  spin-echo i.
  static i. display
  static renal i.
  suboptimal i.
  T1-weighted coronal i.
  tomographic i.
  x-ray i.
  zoomed i.
image-amplified fluoroscopy
image-forming system
imaging
  adrenal i.
  blood pool i.
  cardiac blood pool i.
  coded-aperture i.
  correlative i.
  diagnostic i. (DI)
  digital vascular i. (DVI)
  direct Fourier
    transformation i.
  dynamic volume i.
  echo-planar i.
  electrostatic i.
  flow i.
  Fourier multislice KWE
    direct i.
  Fourier two-dimensional i.
  gated blood pool i.
  gray-scale i.
  heavy ion i.
  infarct-avid i.
  isotope colloid i.
  isotope hepatobiliary i.
  line i.
  longitudinal section i.
  lymph node i.
  magnetic resonance i.
    (MRI)
  multigated i.
  multiplanar i.
  multiple-gated blood pool
    i.
  multiple line-scan i.

multiple plane i.
multiple spin echo total
    volume i.
multislice modified KWE
    direct Fourier i.
myocardial infarct i.
myocardial perfusion i.
nuclear i.
nuclear magnetic
    resonance (NMR) i.
phase i.
pinpoint i.
planar i.
planar-spin i.
point i.
projection reconstruction
    i.
Purkinje's i.
pyrophosphate (PYP) i.
quantitative brain i.
radionuclide i.
reconstructive i.
reticuloendothelial i.
rotating frame i.
selective excitation
    projection
    reconstruction i.
sensitive plane projection
    reconstruction i.
sequential first-pass i.
sequential plane i.
sequential point i.
simultaneous volume i.
single-slice modified KWE
    direct Fourier i.
spin-warp i.
thallium-201 i.
three-dimensional echo
    planar i.
three-dimensional Fourier
    i.
three-dimensional i.
three-dimensional KWE
    direct Fourier i.
three-dimensional

projection
    reconstruction i.
transverse section i.
two-dimensional Fourier i.
two-dimensional Fourier
    transformation i.
two-dimensional KWE
    direct Fourier i.
two-dimensional modified
    KWE direct Fourier i.
ultrasound i.
ventilation-perfusion i.
volume i.
Imatron scanner
imbecilitas phenylpyruvica
imbricate
IMC (internal mammary chain)
imidodiphosphonate
iminodiacetic acid (IDA)
immersion
    i. coupling
    i. scanning
    i. technique
imminent
immobilization device
    Pigg-O-Stat i. d.
immovable joint
immune serum globulin (ISG)
immunoadsorbent
immunoassay
immunoblastic
    lymphadenopathy
immunoelectrophoresis
immunofiltration
immunofluorescence
immunogenetics
immunoglobulin
immunoradiometric assay
    (IRMA)
immunosuppression
immunosuppressive therapy
impacted fracture
impaction
impaired
impalpable

impedance
 i. plethysmography (IPG)
impediment
imperforate anus
IMPH (1-iodomercuri-2-
 hydroxypropane)
impinge
impingement
implant
 augmentation
  mammoplasty i.
 cochlear i.
 Syed i.
 therapeutic radiology i.
implantation
implied solidity
implosion fracture
impression
 basilar i.
impulse
 apical i.
 i. timer
IMV (inferior mesenteric
 vein)
In (indium)
in plastic (IP)
in situ
in utero
in vitro
in vivo
In-111-bleomycin
In-111-DTPA
In-111-labeled WBCs
inadequate
incandescence
incarcerate
incidentally
incipient
incisor
incisura
 i. angularis
 i. cardiaca
incisura or incisure, s.
 incisurae or incisures, pl.

incisurae or incisures, pl.
 incisura or incisure, s.
incisure or incisura, s.
 incisurae or incisures, pl.
incisures or incisurae, pl.
 incisura or incisure, s.
incoherent scattering
incomplete
 i. fracture
 i. mandibulofacial
  dysostosis
incontinence
 giggle i.
 overflow i.
 paradoxical i.
 stress i.
 urge i.
increased attenuation
incremented
 i. dynamic scanning (IDS)
 i. scan
incudes, pl.
 incus, s.
incudomalleal joint
incudostapedial
 i. articulation
 i. joint
incus, s.
 incudes, pl.
indentation
 "ring-like" i.
 "wasp-waist" i.
in-depth
indeterminate diagnosis
index
 Cronqvist's cranial i.
 sesamoid i.
index, s.
 indices, pl.
Indian Club needle
indices, pl.
 index, s.
indirect
 i. fracture

i. volume image
reconstruction
indium
    i. 111
    i. 111 chloride
    i. 111 leukocyte scanning
    i. 111 leukocytoscan
    i. 111 oxine
    i. 113m
indocyanine green dye
indolent myeloma
induced radioactivity
inductance
induction
    electromagnetic i.
    electrostatic i.
    i. coil
    i. motor
inductive reactance (XL)
inductogram
induration
industrial
    i. monitoring
    i. radiography
indwelling
    i. catheter
    i. Foley
    i. T-tube
inelastic
    i. scattering
inert
inertia
infant
    i. catheter
    i. female catheter
    i. male catheter
infantile
    i. acromegaloid gigantism
    i. cortical hyperostosis
    i. hemorrhagic diathesis
    i. hereditary
        chondrodysplasia
    i. metachromatic
        leukodystrophy

i. myxedema-muscular
    hypertrophy
i. pseudospondylitis
i. pulmonary
    reticuloendotheliosis
i. scurvy
i. sponge kidney
i. stomach
i. thoracic dystrophy
infarct-avid imaging
infarct scan
infarction
    anteroseptal i.
    atrial i.
    bone i.
    cerebral i.
    Freiberg's i.
    gas i.
    global renal i.
    lacunar i.
    mesenteric i.
    myocardial i. (MI)
    renal i.
    splenic i.
    subendocardial i.
    thrombotic i.
    transmural i.
    watershed i.
infected aneurysm
infectious
    i. colitis
    i. disease
    i. enterocolitis
    i. jaundice
    i. mononucleosis
infective
    i. endocarditis
inferior
    i. accessory fissure
    i. accessory lobe
    i. articular process
    i. caval
    i. horn
    i. mesenteric artery (IMA)

inferior—*Continued*
   i. mesenteric vein (IMV)
   i. olive
   i. point of the pubic bone
     (IPP)
   i. radioulnar joint
   i. ramus
   i. tibiofibular joint
   i. vena cava
   i. venacavogram (IVC)
   i. venacavography (IVC)
inferior-superior projection
inferior-superior tangential
  projection
inferoapical
inferoposterior
inferosuperior
   i. axial projection
   i. projection
infiltrate
infiltration
inflammatory
   i. fracture
   i. process
inflation
influenzal pneumonia
infraclavicular
infracostales
   i. externus muscle
   i. internus muscle
infraction
   Freiberg's i.
infradiaphragmatic
inframammary crease
inframesocolic
infraoral projection
infraorbital
   i. canal
   i. foramen
   i. line
   i. margin
   i. suture
infraorbitomeatal line (IOML)
infraperitoneal

infrared radiation
infraroentgen ray
infrasellar
infrasound
infraspinatus
   i. fossa
   i. muscle
infrasylvian region
infratentorial lesions
infratragal notch
infundibula, pl.
   infundibulum, s.
infundibular
   i. subaortic stenosis
   i. systolic/diastolic ratio
infundibular/bulb ratio
infundibuliform fascia
infundibuloventricular line
infundibulum
   ethmoidal i.
   i. of hypothalamus
   i. of the gallbladder
   i. of uterine tube
infundibulum, s.
   infundibula, pl.
Infuse-a-port
infused
infusion
   i. hepatic arteriography (IHA)
   i. nephrotomography
infusion-type scan
Ingram trocar catheter
inguinal
   i. canal
   i. hernia
   i. inion
   i. ligament
   i. lymph node
   i. region
   i. sphincter
inhalation
   i. bronchography
inhalation/perfusion lung scan
inhale

inherent
  i. density
  i. filter
  i. filtration
  i. resistance
inhibition
inhomogeneity
in-house film distribution
  network
inion
initis
injection
  cisternal i.
  contrast i.
  i. urethrogram
  opaque i.
  perinephric air i.
  radionuclide i.
  transduodenal fiberscopic
    duct i.
injury
  i. monitor
  i. physics
  i. therapy
  i. warning symbol
  i. window
inlet
  i. position
  pelvic i.
  thoracic i.
inner tunnel
innocent murmur
innominate
  i. aneurysm
  i. artery
  i. bone (hip)
  i. cartilage
  i. vein
inorganic
inosculation
inotropic
in-phase
insert image
in-service

inside diameter (ID)
insoluble
insonatic (ultrasound curves)
inspiration
inspiratory collapse
inspissated milk syndrome
instability
instep
instillation
insufficiency fracture
insufflation
  perirenal i.
  retroperitoneal gas i.
insulation
insulin
insulinase
insulinoma
INT (internal)
integral
  i. dose
  i. timer
integrating
  i. circuit
  i. dose meter
  i. ionization chamber
  i. timer
integumentary
integumentum
intensification factor
intensifier
intensifying
  i. factor
  i. screen
intensity
  i. magnetization
intentional transoperative
  hemodilution
interaction
interarticular
  i. joint
  i. ridge
interarytenoid space
interatrial septum
intercalary ossicle

intercarpal joint
intercartilaginous rim
intercavitary radiation
interchondral joint
interclavicular notch
intercolumnar fascia
intercompartmental
intercondylar
   i. eminences
   i. fossa
   i. fracture
   i. notch
   i. process
intercondyle
intercondyloid fossa
intercostal
   i. catheter
   i. hernia
   i. lymph node
   i. margin
   i. space
intercostohumeral
intercristal space
intercrural space
intercuneiform joint
interdependence
interdigital
interendognathic suture
interface
interfacet
interfascial space of Tenon
interference phenomenon
interfragmentary screw
interhemispheric
   i. cistern
   i. fissure (IHF)
interiliac lymph node
interior
interlace
interleaved images
interleaving ray data samples
  technique
interlobar
   i. effusion
   i. hepatic fissure

interlobular
   i. emphysema
interlock
interlocking IM
  (intramedullary) nail
intermalleolar line
intermaxillary suture
intermediate
   i. cuneiform
   i. hydrocephalus
   i. neutron
intermetacarpal joint
intermetatarsal joint
intermittent venous
  claudication
internal (INT)
   i. auditory canal (IAC)
   i. auditory meatus
    (IAM)
   i. capsule
   i. carotid artery (ICA)
   i. conversion
   i. derangement of the knee
    (IDK)
   i. fixation
   i. fracture
   i. granuloma
   i. mammary chain (IMC)
   i. radiation hazard
   i. resistance
internally deposited
  radionuclides
internasal suture
International
   I. 10-20 system
   I. Commission on
    Radiation Units and
    Measurements (ICRU)
   I. Congress of Radiology
    (ICR)
   I. System (SI)
interorbital line
interossei
   i. dorsales manus muscle
   i. palmares muscle

i. volares muscle
interosseous
    i. cartilage
    i. dorsalis pedis muscle
    i. groove
    i. plantaris muscle
    i. ridge
    i. space
interparietal
    i. plane
    i. suture
interpectoral lymph node
interpediculate
interpeduncular
    i. cistern (IPC)
    i. fossa
interperiosteal fracture
interphalangeal (IP)
    i. joint (IPJ)
interphase
interpolation
interpulse time
interpupillary line
interrenal
interscan delay
intersegmental hepatic fissure
interseptal space
interspace
interspinales, pl.
    interspinalis, s.
interspinalis, s.
    interspinales, pl.
interspinous
intersternal joint
intersternebral joint
interstice
interstitial
    i. amyloidosis
    i. calcification
    i. calcinosis
    i. cystitis
    i. disease
    i. edema
    i. emphysema
    i. fibrosis

i. infiltrates
    i. irradiation
    i. markings
    i. myelopathy
    i. myocarditis
    i. myositis
    i. pneumonitis
    i. radiation
    i. radiotherapy
    i. therapy
interstitium
intertarsal joint
interthalamic
intertrabecular space
intertransversarii muscle
intertrochanteric
    i. crest
    i. fracture
    i. ridge
intertuberal line
intertubercular plane
interureteric ridge
interval
interventional
    i. angiography
    i. radiobiology
interventricular
    i. foramen
    i. septum
intervertebral
    i. cartilage
    i. disc or disk (IVD)
    i. foramen
    i. joint
    i. notch
    i. osteoarthritis
    i. space
intervillous space
intestina, pl.
    intestinum, s.
intestinal
    i. atresia
    i. carcinoid syndrome
    i. duplication
    i. gas pattern

intestinal—*Continued*
  i. infantilism
  i. knot syndrome
  i. malrotation
  i. obstruction
  i. sand
  i. string sign
  i. tract
intestine
  blind i.
  empty i.
  iced i.
  jejunoileal i.
  mesenterial i.
  segmented i.
  straight i.
intestinum, s.
  intestina, pl.
intra-abdominal
  i.-a. abscess
  i.-a. graft
intra-alveolar
intra-aortic counterpulsation
  balloon (IACB)
intra-arterial
  i.-a. digital subraction
    angiography (IADSA)
  i.-a. infusion
intra-articular
  i.-a. disk or disc
  i.-a. fracture
intrabronchial
intracapsular
  i. fracture
  i. hematoma
intracardiac
  i. catheter
  i. shunt
  i. thrombus
intracartilaginous ossification
Intracath (catheter)
intracavitary
  i. radiotherapy
  i. radium insertion
  i. therapy

intracavity
intracellular
intracerebral
  i. hematoma
  i. hemorrhage
intracoronary
intracranial
  i. abscess
  i. aneurysm
  i. bleed
  i. calcification
  i. cyst
  i. exostosis
  i. hematoma
  i. hemorrhage (ICH)
intraductal obstruction
intradural abscess
intrahepatic
  i. abscess
  i. bile duct
  i. biliary drainage
intralimbic gyrus
intraluminal
  i. catheter
  i. gas
  i. mass
intramammary abscess
intramastoid abscess
intramedullary
  i. cyst
  i. nail
  i. rod
intramembranous ossification
intramural
  i. gas
  i. hematoma
  i. jejunal calcification in
    meconium
intranodal
intraoccipital
intraoperative
  i. cholangiogram (IOC)
  i. cholangiography (IOC)
  i. digital subtraction
    angiography (IDIS)

i. electron beam therapy (IOEBT)
i. radiation therapy (IORT)
intraoral
intraorbital
intraosseous
    i. ganglia
    i. hemangiomatosis
    i. venogram
intrapericardial cyst
intraperiosteal
    i. catheter
    i. fracture
intraperitoneal
    i. abscess
    i. air
    i. catheter
    i. effusion
    i. fluid
    i. gas
    i. hemorrhage
intrapleural air
intrapulmonary
    i. fissure
    i. foci
intrarenal
    i. abscess
    i. hematoma
    i. reflux
intrasellar
intrasplenic
    i. hematoma
    i. lymphangioma
intrathecal
intrathoracic goiter
intrauterine
    i. catheter
    i. device (IUD)
    i. fetal growth retardation (IUFGR)
    i. fracture
    i. growth retardation (IUGR)
    i. pregnancy

intrauterine device (IUD)
    copper T i. d.
    copper-7 i. d.
    Dalkon shield i. d.
    double coil i. d.
    Gravigards i. d.
    Lippes' loop i. d.
    Progestasert i. d.
    Saf-T coils i. d.
intravaginal irradiation
intravascular fetal air sign
intravenous (IV)
    i. angiocardiography (ACG)
    i. catheter
    i. cholangiogram (IVC)
    i. cholecystogram (IVC)
    i. digital subtraction angiography (IVDSA)
    i. hyperalimentation
    i. pyelogram (IVP)
    i. pyelography (IVP)
    i. urogram (IVU)
    i. urography (IVU)
intraventricular hemorrhage (IVH)
intrinsic
    i. factor
    i. motion
introducer
    aortic assist balloon i.
    Bentson i.
    Check-Flo i.
    Desilets-Hoffman i.
    peel-away i.
    Schwartz i.
    Tuohy-Bost i.
introitus
Intron
Intropaque (barium sulfate)
intubate
intubation
intussuscepting polyp
intussusception

invasive
inverse
    "i. comma" appearance
    i. voltage
inverse-square law
inversion
    i. fracture
    i. position
    i. recovery (IR)
    i. recovery image
    i. recovery sequence
    i. time (TI)
invert
inverted
    "i. 3" sign
    i. goblet sign
    i. horseshoe kidney
    i. jackknife position
    i. Marfan's syndrome
    i. transposition
    "i. V" sign
    i. ventricles
invisible spectrum
involucrum
involuntary
    i. guarding
    i. motion
    i. muscle
    i. spasm
Ioban drape
iobenzamic acid
iobutoic acid
IOC (intraoperative
    cholangiogram)
IOC (intraoperative
    cholangiography)
iocarmate meglumine
iocarmic acid
iocetamate
iocetamic acid
Iod-Cholegnostyl
iodamic acid
iodamide
iodatol
iodecol

Iodeikon
iodide
    potassium i.
    silver i.
    sodium i.
iodinated
    i. I-125 fibrinogen
    i. I-125 serum albumin
    i. I-131 aggregated albumin
        (human)
    i. I-131 serum albumin
        (human)
iodination
iodine (I)
    I 123
    I 125
    I 131
    I 132
    i. chelate
    radioactive i.
iodine-based
iodipamic acid
iodipamide meglumine
    injection
iodized
    i. oil
    i. oil study
iodoalphionic acid
Iodocaps I-125 or I-131
Iodochlorol
iodocholesterol
Iodognost
iodohippurate
iodomethamate
iodomethyl-19-norcholes-5-
    (10)-en-3B-ol (NP-59)
iodophen
iodophendylate
iodophor
iodophthalein
iodopyracet
Iodosol
Iodotope (sodium iodide-I-
    131)
iodoventriculography

iodoxamate
iodoxamic acid
iodoxyl
Ioduron
IOEBT (intraoperative electron
  beam therapy)
ioglicate
ioglicic acid
ioglucol
ioglucomide
ioglunide
ioglycamic acid
ioglycamide
iohexol
iomide
IOML (infraorbitomeatal line)
ion
    amphoteric dipolar i.
    i. exchange
    i. pair
ionic
    i. charge
    i. intravascular
    i. polar valence
    i. solution
    i. strength
ionium (thorium)
ionization
    avalanche i.
    i. chamber
    i. constant
    i. current
    i. density
    i. instrument
    i. interferene
    i. potential
    specific i.
ionizing
    i. energy
    i. event
    i. particle
    i. radiation
ionograph
ionography
ionophore

iopamidol
Iopan
iopanoate
iopanoic acid
iopanoic tablets
Iopax
iophendylate
iophenoxic acid
ioprocemic acid
iopromide
iopronic acid
iopydol
iopydone
Iopyracil
IORT (intraoperative radiation
  therapy)
iosefamate
iosefamic acid
iosefamide
ioseric acid
iosulamic acid
iosulamide
iosumetic acid
iotasul
iotetric acid
iothalamate
iothalamic acid
iotrol
iotroxamide
iotroxic acid
ioxaglate
ioxaglic acid
ioxithalamate
ioxithalamic acid
iozomic acid
IP (in plastic)
IP (interphalangeal)
IPC (interpeduncular cistern)
IPG (impedance
  plethysmography)
IPJ (interphalangeal joint)
ipodate
    i. calcium
    i. sodium
ipodic acid

IPP (inferior point of the pubic bone)
ipsilateral ramus
ipsilateral, also ipsolateral
ipsolateral, also ipsilateral
192IR (iridium)
IR (inversion recovery)
IRA-400 resin
iridium (Ir-192)
IRMA (immunoradiometric assay)
iron (Fe)
    i. 55 (Fe55)
    i. 59 (Fe59)
    i. hydroxide
    radioactive i.
iron-binding capacity (IBC)
iron-core
    i. electromagnet
    i. transformer
Irosorb-59 diagnostic kit
irradiate
irradiation
    heavy ion i.
    i. change
    i. damage
    i. procedure
    i. therapy
    i. time
    interstitial i.
    whole-body i.
irregular
irrigating catheter
irritability
irritable joint
irritative radiation
ischemia
    global i.
    i. retinae
    mesenteric i.
    myocardial i.
    renal i.
    silent i.
    transient myocardial i.

ischemic
    i. bowel disease (IBD)
    i. colitis
ischia, pl.
    ischium, s.
ischial
    i. bursa
    i. fracture
    i. ramus
    i. tuberosity
    i. varus sign
ischioacetabular
ischioanal
ischiobulbar
ischiocapsular
ischiocavernosus muscle
ischiocele
ischiococcygeal
ischiococcygeus muscle
ischiofibular
ischiopubic junction
ischiorectal
    i. abscess
    i. space
ischium, s.
    ischia, pl.
Iselin's osteonecrosis
ISG (immune serum globulin)
Isherwood's
    I.'s method
    I.'s position
Ishihara plate
island of Reil
islands (or islets) of Langerhans
islet cell carcinoma
iso-osmotic
ISO/Meridrin Hg 197, 203
Iso-rodeikon
isobar
isobaric transition
isocentric mounting
Isocon camera
isocount curves
isodense

isodose
    i. charts
    i. curve
isoechoic
isoelectric
    i. focusing
    i. point
isolated ventricular inversion
isolation
isomer
isomeric
    i. decay
    i. transition (IT)
Isopaque
    I. 280
    I. 370
    I. 440
    I. B
isopropyl alcohol
isoresponse curve
isosthenuria
isosulfan blue (Lymphazurin)
isotope
    i. bone scan
    i. colloid imaging
    i. dilution mass
        spectrometry
    i. effect
    i. hepatobiliary imaging
    i. placentography
    i. separation
    i. study
    i. venogram
    i. voiding
        cystourethrogram
        (IVCU)
    i. voiding
        cystourethrography
        (IVCU)
    radioactive i.
    stable i.

isotopic
    i. tracer
    i. track
Isovue (iopamidol with
    tromethamine and edetate
    calcium disodium)
    I.-M
isthmus
IT (isomeric transition)
Itard catheter
IUD (intrauterine device)
IUFGR (intrauterine fetal
    growth retardation)
IUGR (intrauterine growth
    retardation)
IV (intravenous)
IV catheter
IVC (inferior venacavogram)
IVC (inferior venacavography)
IVC (intravenous
    cholangiogram)
IVC (intravenous
    cholangiography)
IVCU (isotope voiding
    cystourethrography)
IVD (intervertebral disk)
IVDSA (intravenous digital
    subtraction angiogram)
IVDSA (intravenous digital
    subtraction angiography)
Ivemark's syndrome
IVH (intraventricular
    hemorrhage)
ivory
    i. bones
    i. epiphysis
    i. phalanx
IVP (intravenous pyelogram or
    pyelography)
IVU (intravenous urogram)
IVU (intravenous urography)

Jj

J (joule)
Jaccoud's
    J.'s arthritis
    J.'s arthropathy
jackknife
    j. position
    j. view
Jackson-Huber nomenclature
Jackson-Pratt catheter
Jackson's membrane
jackstone type of vesical
    calculus
Jaeger plate
Jaeger-Whiteley catheter
Jaffe-Lichtenstein syndrome
Jaffe-Lichtenstein-Uehlinger
    syndrome
Jahnke's syndrome
Jamshidi needle
Jannetta's procedure
Jansen's metaphyseal
    dysostosis
Janus' syndrome
Japanese classification
jaundice
    cholestatic j.
    hemorrhagic j.
    infectious j.
    leptospiral j.
    obstructive j.
    spirochetal j.
Javid catheter
JB1 catheter
JB3 catheter
JCAHO (Joint Commission on
    Accreditation of Healthcare
    Organizations)

Jefferson's
    J.'s fracture
    J.'s syndrome
jej (jejunum)
jejunal
    j. carcinoma
    j. diverticulum
    j. intussusception
    j. neoplasm
    j. syndrome
    j. ulcer
jejunocolic anastomosis
jejunoileal
    j. bypass
    j. intestine
jejunoileostomy
jejunojejunostomy
jejunostomy
jejunum (jej)
Jelco catheter
jelly-like
Jelm catheter
jet
    j. aneurysm
    j. sign
Jeune's disease
Jewett
    J. brace
    J. nail
    J. plate
Jewett-Marshall system
Jobert's fossa
jockey-style
Jodafen
Jodairal
Jodobilan
Jodosol

Jodtetragnost
Joduron
Johannson lag screw
Johanson's vein
Johnie McL's syndrome
Johnson and Dutt view
Johnson's
    J.'s method
    J.'s position
joint
    acromioclavicular j. (ACJ)
    amphidiarthrodial j.
    ankle j.
    antecubital j.
    anterior cervical j.
    anterior intraoccipital j.
    apophyseal j.
    arthrodial j.
    atlanto-occipital j.
    atlantoaxial j.
    atlantoepistropheal j.
    ball-and-socket j.
    biaxial j.
    bicondylar j.
    bilocular j.
    bleeders' j.
    Brodie's j.
    Budin's j.
    calcaneocuboid j.
    capitular j.
    carpal j.
    carpometacarpal j. (CMJ)
    cartilaginous j.
    Charcot's j.
    chondrocostal j.
    Chopart's j.
    Clutton's j.
    coccygeal j.
    cochlear j.
    coffin j.
    collateral j.
    composite j.
    compound j.
    condylar j.

condyloid j.
costochondral j.
costotransverse j.
costovertebral j.
cotyloid j.
cricoarytenoid j.
cricothyroid j.
Cruveilhier's j.
cubital j.
cuboideonavicular j.
cuneocuboid j.
cuneometatarsal j.
cuneonavicular j.
dentoalveolar j.
diarthrodial j.
digital j.
DIP (distal
    interphalangeal) j.
dry j.
elbow j.
ellipsoidal j.
enarthrodial j.
facet j.
false j.
femoropatellar j.
fibrocartilaginous j.
fibrous j.
flail j.
freely movable j.
fringe j.
ginglymoid j.
glenohumeral j.
gliding j.
gompholic j.
hemophilic j.
hinge j.
hip j.
humeroradial j.
humeroulnar j.
hysteric j.
immovable j.
incudomalleal j.
incudostapedial j.
inferior radioulnar j.

inferior tibiofibular j.
interarticular j.
intercarpal j.
interchondral j.
intercuneiform j.
intermetacarpal j.
intermetatarsal j.
interphalangeal j. (IPJ)
intersternal j.
intertarsal j.
intervertebral j.
irritable j.
j. calcification
j. capsule
j. contracture
j. effusion
j. fracture
j. instability
j. line
j. mice
j. of Luschka
j. spurring
j. stability
jaw j.
knee j.
lateral atlantoaxial j.
lateral atlantoepistrophic j.
ligamentous j.
Lisfranc's j.
lumbosacral j.
Luschka's j.
mandibular j.
manubriosternal j.
median atlantoaxial j.
metacarpal-carpal (MCC) j.
metacarpophalangeal
    (MCP) j.
metatarsocuneiform j.
metatarsophalangeal j.
    (MTPJ)
midcarpal j.
midtarsal j.
mixed j.
mortise j.

movable j.
multiaxial j.
navicular j.
neurocentral j.
neuropathic j.
open j.
peg-and-socket j.
petro-occipital j.
phalangeal j.
PIP (proximal
    interphalangeal) j.
pisotriquetral j.
pivot j.
plane j.
polyaxial j.
posterior intraoccipital j.
proximal interphalangeal
    (PIP) j.
radiocarpal j.
radioulnar j.
rotary j.
sacrococcygeal j.
sacroiliac j.
saddle j.
scapuloclavicular j.
schindyletic j.
screw j.
sellar j.
shoulder j.
simple j.
socket j.
spheno-occipital j.
spheroidal j.
spiral j.
sternal j.
sternoclavicular j.
sternocleidomastoid j.
sternocostal j.
stifle j.
Street finger j.
subtalar j.
subtaloid j.
superior radioulnar j.
suture j.

joint—*Continued*
  synarthrodial j.
  synchondrodial j.
  syndesmodial j.
  synovial j.
  talocalcaneal j.
  talocalcaneonavicular j.
  talofibular j.
  talonavicular j.
  talotibial j.
  tarsal j.
  tarsometatarsal j.
  temporomandibular (TMJ) j.
  thigh j.
  Thompson finger j.
  through j.
  tibiofibular j.
  trochoid j.
  uncovertebral j.
  uniaxial j.
  unilocular j.
  von Gies' j.
  wedge-and-groove j.
  wrist j.
  xiphisternal j.
  zygapophyseal j.
Joint Commission on
  Accreditation of Healthcare
  Organizations (JCAHO)
Jones'
  J.' disease
  J.' fracture
  J.' position
Jonnson's maneuver
joule (J)
JRA (juvenile rheumatoid
  arthritis)
J-shaped stomach
J-tipped guide wire
Judd's
  J.'s method
  J.'s position
Judet
  J. acrylic prosthesis

Judet's view
Judkins
  J. coronary artery straight
    safety wire guide
  J. left coronary catheter
  J. pigtail catheter
  J. right coronary catheter
Judkins' technique
juga cerebralia, pl.
  jugum cerebralia, s.
jugal (zygoma, malar, or
  cheek)
  j. suture
jugular
  j. foramen
  j. foramen syndrome
  j. fossa
  j. lymph node
  j. lymph sac
  j. notch
  j. reflux
  j. vein (JV)
  j. venous catheter
jugulo-omohyoid lymph node
jugulodigastric lymph node
jugum cerebralia, s.
  juga cerebralia, pl.
jugum sphenoidale
Julien Marie's syndrome
jumper's fracture
junction
  bulbomedullary j.
  cervico-occipital j.
  corticomedullary j.
  craniovertebral j.
  esophagogastric j.
  gastroduodenal j.
  ileocecal j.
  ischiopubic j.
  myoneural j.
  rectosigmoid j.
  sclerocorneal j.
  ureteropelvic j.
  ureterovesical j. (UVJ)

junctura, s.
    juncturae, pl.
juncturae, pl.
    junctura, s.
Jung's muscle
Junghans'
    J.' pseudospondylolisthesis
Jüngling's
    J.'s disease
    J.'s polycystic osteitis
juvenile
    j. angiofibroma
    j. arrhythmia
    j. chronic polyarthropathy
    j. hyaline fibromatosis
    j. idiopathic osteoporosis
    j. kyphosis dorsalis
    j. Paget's disease
    j. pilocytic astrocytoma
    j. rheumatoid arthritis
      (JRA)
    j. tertiary syphilis
juxta-articular osteoporosis
juxtacortical chondroma
juxtaintestinal node
juxtamedullary
juxtangina
juxtaphrenic
juxtaposition
juxtapyloric
juxtavertebral
JV (jugular vein)

K42 (potassium)
K (kelvin)
K (potassium)
K or Kohm (kilohm)
K radiation
Kaes' line
Kahler-Bozzolo disease
Kahler's disease
Kahn
    K. needle
    K. tenaculum
kalemia
Kalischer's syndrome
Kandel's method
Kantor's sign
Kapandjy's sphincter
Kaplan-Meier survival curves
Kaposi's
    K.'s sarcoma (KS)
    K.'s varicelliform eruption
Kapp-Beck serration
Karnofsky
    K. scale
    K. status
Karplus relationship
Kartagener's
    K.'s disease
    K.'s syndrome
    K.'s triad
Kasabach's
    K.'s method
    K.'s view
Kashin-Beck
    K.-B. disease
    K.-B. syndrome
Kast's syndrome
Kawasaki syndrome
Kaye catheter

Kaznelson's syndrome
kc (kilocycle)
Kcal or kcal (kilogram-calorie)
K-capture
kCi (kilocurie)
KD (knee disarticulation)
Kearns-Sayre syndrome
Keith's node
Keith-Wagener classification
K-electron capture
Kelman phacoemulsification
keloid
kelvin (K)
Kemp Harper's method
Ken
    K. nail
    K. plate
Kenney-Caffey syndrome
Kenotron tube
Kent bundle
Keraphren
kerasin
keratan sulfate
keratinization
keratoacanthoma
    subungual k.
keratosulfaturia
Kerber
    K. catheter
    K. cerebral catheter
Kerckring's
    K.'s center
    K.'s folds
    K.'s ossicle
    K.'s valve
Kerlan-Ring catheter
Kerley
    K. A line

Kerley—*Continued*
  K. B line
  K. C line
kerma
kernel
kernicterus
Kernig's sign
Kernohan notch
Kessel plate
ketamine
ketone bodies
keV or kev [kilo (thousand)
  electron volts]
kHz (kilohertz)
kidney
  abdominal k.
  arteriosclerotic k.
  atrophic k.
  cicatricial k.
  contracted k.
  cyanotic k.
  cystic k.
  "doughnut" k.
  duplex k.
  dysplastic k.
  ectopic k.
  floating k.
  fused k.
  horseshoe k.
  k. abscess
  k. biopsy
  k. failure
  k. internal splint/stent (KISS)
  k. position
  k. shutdown
  k. studies
  k. transplant
  k. wash-out
  lardaceous k.
  medullary sponge k.
  multicystic k.
  myelin k.
  Page's k.
  parenchymal k.

  pelvic k.
  polycystic k.
  pyelonephritic k.
  sacciform k.
  sigmoid k.
  sponge k.
  supernumerary k.
  thoracic k.
  wandering k.
kidneys, ureters, bladder
  (KUB)
Kiel classification
Kienböck's
  K.'s atrophy
  K.'s disease
  K.'s unit (X)
Kiernan's space
Kiesselbach's space
Kilian's pelvis
kilo (thousand) electron volts
  (keV or kev)
kilocalorie
kilocurie (kCi)
kilocycle (kc)
kilogram-calorie (Kcal or kcal)
kilohertz (kHz)
kilohm (K or Kohm)
kilomegacycle (kMc)
kilometer (km)
kilopascal (kPa)
kilosecond
kilovolt (kV)
  k. constant potential
    (kVcp)
  k. peak (kVp)
  k.-ampere (kVA)
kilovoltage (kV)
  k. peak (kVp)
kilovoltmeter
kilowatt (kw)
Kimball catheter
Kimberlin's method
Kimmelstiel-Wilson disease
Kimmerle's anomaly

Kim-Ray Greenfield filter
   insertion
kineradiogram
kineradiography
kinescope radiography
kinetic energy
Kinevac (sincalide)
King-Armstrong unit
kinking of the aorta
"kinky hair" syndrome
Kirchhoff's law
Kirdani's method
Kirklin's meniscus complex
Kirner's deformity
Kirschner wire (K-wire)
KISS (kidney internal splint/
   stent)
KISS catheter
"kissing" spine
Kistner tracheal "button"
Kite's method
Klatskin needle
Klatzkin's tumor
Klebsiella
   K. oxytoca
   K. pneumoniae
kleeblattschädel syndrome
Klein-Nishina Formula
Klein's technique
Klein-Waardenburg syndrome
Klinefelter-Reifenstein-Albright
   syndrome
Klinefelter's syndrome
Klinger's disease
Klippel-Feil
   K.-F. deformity
   K.-F. disease
   K.-F. syndrome
Klippel-Feldstein syndrome
Klippel-Trenaunay-Weber
   syndrome
Klüver-Bucy-Terzian
   syndrome
km (kilometer)

kMc (kilomegacycle)
knee
   k. disarticulation (KD)
   k. joint
knee-chest position
knee-elbow position
kneeling-squatting position
Kniest's
   K.'s dysostosis
   K.'s dysplasia
   K.'s syndrome
knock-knees
Knowles pin
Kocher's
   K.'s dilatation ulcer
   K.'s fracture
Kocher-Debré-Sémélaigne
   syndrome
Kock's pouch
Koebner's phenomenon
Köhler's
   K.'s bone disease
   K.'s first disease
   K.'s fracture
   K.'s second disease
   K.'s "teardrop" sign
Köhler-Mouchet disease
Köhler-Stieda-Pellegrini
   syndrome
Kohlrausch's
   K.'s fold
   K.'s valve
Kohm (K or kilohm)
Kohn's pore
König's disease
Kopans
   K. breast lesion
      localization needles
   K. needle
   modified K. breast
   lesion localization
   needles
Kopitz, parallelogram of
Korotkoff's sound

Kosowicz'
  K.' carpal angle
  K.' sign
kotileus
Kovács' method
kPa (kilopascal)
Krabbe's syndrome
Kraske's position
Krause, valve of
Krayenbuhl-Richter line
Krebs cycle
Kretschmann's space
Kreuscher bunionectomy
Kreuzfuchs' method
krinkle mark (or crinkle)
Kristiansen
  K. bone pin
  K. eyelet lag screw
Krukenberg's tumor
krypton
  k. (Kr 81m)
  k. clathrate
  k. hydroquinone complex
KS (Kaposi's sarcoma)
KUB (kidneys, ureters,
  bladder)
Kuchendorf's
  K.'s method
  K.'s position
Kugel's artery
Kugelberg-Welander disease
Kumar, Welti and Ernst method
  (KWE) method
Kümmell's
  K.'s disease
  K.'s kyphosis
  K.'s spondylitis
Kümmell-Verneuil disease

Kundrat's syndrome
Küntscher
  K. cloverleaf nail
  K. intramedullary nail
Kupffer's cell
Kurtzke score
Kurzbauer's
  K.'s method
  K.'s position
kuskokwim
Kussmaul's
  K.'s respirations
  K.'s sign
kV (kilovolt)
kV (kilovoltage)
kVA (kilovolt-ampere)
kVcp (kilovolt constant
  potential)
kVp (kilovolt peak)
kVp (kilovoltage peak)
K-W (Keith-Wagner)
  classification
kw (kilowatt)
kwashiorkor
KWE (Kumar, Welti and Ernst)
  method
K-wires (Kirschner's wire)
kymography
  roentgen k. (RKY)
kymoscope
kyphos
kyphoscoliosis
kyphosis dorsalis juvenilis
kyphotic
  k. curve
  k. deformity
  k. left kidney

Ll

L5 coned view projection
L5-S1 projection
L (Lambert unit)
L (lumbar)
L (lumbar vertebra)
La:A (left atrial to aortic) ratio
Labbé, vein of
labeled
    l. compound
    l. ligand
    l. molecule
labia
    l. majora
    l. minora
labia, pl.
    labium, s.
labium, s.
    labia, pl.
labyrinth
    acoustic l.
    bony l.
    cortical l.
    endolymphatic l.
    ethmoidal l.
    membranous l.
    olfactory l.
    osseous l.
    perilymphatic l.
    statokinetic l.
labyrinthine torticollis
lace-like appearance
laciniate ligament
lacrimal
    l. abscess
    l. canal
    l. canaliculi
    l. caruncle
    l. duct

    l. fold
    l. gland
    l. lake
    l. papilla
    l. process
    l. sac
lacrimo-auriculo-dento-digital
    syndrome
lacrimoconchal suture
lacrimoethmoidal suture
lacrimomaxillary suture
lacrimonasal
lacrimoturbinal suture
lactiferous
    l. ducts
    l. tubule
lactobezoar
lacuna, s.
    lucunae, pl.
lacunar
    l. abscess
    l. infarction
    l. node
    l. skull
lacunula
LAD (left anterior descending
    artery)
Ladd's
    L.'s band
    L.'s syndrome
Ladd-Gross
    L.-G. classification
    L.-G. syndrome
laddering
LAE (left atrial enlargement)
Laennec's cirrhosis
LAG (lymphangiogram)
lag screw

Laimer, fascia of
Laing osteotomy plate
lambda
lambdoidal suture
Lambert (L)
    L., channel of
    L. unit
lamella
lamina
    l. cribrosa
    l. dura
    l. medullaris interna
lamina, s.
    laminae, pl.
laminae, pl.
    lamina, s.
laminagram or laminogram
laminagraphy or laminography
laminated
    l. core
    l. periosteum
    l. silicon steel plates
lamination
laminectomy frame
laminogram or laminagram
laminography or laminagraphy
Landing-Norman disease
landmark
Lane
    L. catheter
    L. plate
Lane's membrane
Langdon Down's syndrome
Langer-Saldino
    achondrogenesis
Langerhans, (islands or islets) of
Lange's position
Lanier, triangle of
Lannelongue-Osgood-Schlatter
    syndrome
Lannois-Gradenigo syndrome
lantern slide
lanthanum oxybromide

LAO (left anterior oblique)
Lapides catheter
lap-type seatbelt fracture
Laquerrière-Pierquin
    L.-P. position
    L.-P. method
lardaceous
    l. kidney
    l. liver
    l. spleen
large-bore biopsy
large
    l. bowel obstruction (LBO)
    l. field of view (LFOV)
    l. particle barium
Larkin's position
Larmor's
    L.'s equation
    L.'s frequency
    L.'s precession frequency
Laron's dwarfism
Larrey's space
Larsen-Johansson syndrome
Larsen's syndrome
laryngeal
    l. carcinoma
    l. cartilage
    l. diverticulum
    l. nodule
    l. polyp
    l. saccule
    l. stenosis
    l. stricture
    l. ventricle
    l. web
larynges, pl.
    larynx s.
laryngismus
    l. paralyticus
    l. stridulus
laryngocele
laryngogram
laryngography
    contrast l.

laryngohypopharynx
laryngomalacia
laryngopharyngeus muscle
laryngoscleroma
laryngoscope
laryngotracheoesophageal cleft
larynx, s.
    larynges, pl.
laser
    l. angioplasty
    l. beam
    l. camera
    l. optical disk
    l. vaporization
laser-generated image
lat. (lateral)
lata fascia
late Hurler's syndrome
latent
    l. image
    l. iron-binding capacity
      (LIBC) test
    l. period
laterad
lateral (lat.)
    l. abscess
    l. alveolar abscess
    l. aneurysm
    l. atlantoaxial joint
    l. atlantoepistrophic joint
    l. autotomogram position
    l. cuneiform
    l. decubitus film
    l. decubitus position
    l. flexion
    l. ligament
    l. malleolus muscle
    l. oblique axial projection
    l. occipitoatlantal ligament
    l. odontoid ligaments
    l. position
    l. projection
    l. prone position

    l. recumbent position
    l. rotation position
    l. transcranial projection
    l. transfacial projection
    l. ventricle
    l. view
lateroconal fascia
lateromedial
    l. oblique projection
    l. position
    l. tangential projection
latex catheter
latissimus
    l. colli muscle
    l. dorsi muscle
latitude
    density l.
    radiographic l.
    x-ray film l.
LATS (long-acting thyroid
   stimulator)
lattice
    l. relaxation time
    l. vibrations
    spin-l. relaxation time
Lattimer's classification
Lauenstein and Hickey
    L. a. H. method
    L. a. H. projection
Lauenstein's position
Lauge-Hanson classification
Laugier's
    L.'s fracture
    L.'s sign
Launois-Cléret syndrome
Laurence-Moon-Biedl
   syndrome
Laurence-Moon-Biedl-Bardet
   syndrome
Lauritson electroscope
law
    Bergonié-Tribondeau l.
    Coulomb's l.

Doerner–Hoskins
distribution l.
Einstein's l.
electrostatic l.
Faraday's l.
Fick's l.
inverse-square l.
Kirchhoff's l.
l. of inertia
l. of reciprocity
l. of refraction
l. of thermodynamics
Newton's l. of action-
reaction
Newton's l. of motion
Ohm's l.
transformer l.
Wolff's l.
Law's
L.'s lateral position
L.'s method
L.'s oblique position
L.'s position
L.'s projection
L.'s view
Lawford's syndrome
Lawrence's
L.'s axial position
L.'s method
L.'s position
L.'s transthoracic position
Lawrence-Seip syndrome
lawrencium (Lw)
Lawson-Thornton plate
"lazy leukocyte" syndrome
LBO (large bowel obstruction)
LCA (left coronary artery)
LCF (left circumflex)
LD (lethal dose)
LD$_{50}$ (median lethal dose)
Le Fort catheter
Le Fort's
Le F.'s I fracture

Le F.'s II fracture
Le F.'s III fracture
lead (Pb)
l. apron
l. equivalent
l. glass
l. gloves
l. gonad shield
l. lines
l. pipe fracture
l. protective chair
l. protectors
l. rubber
l. shutters
lead-containing
lead-impregnated
leading edge
leakage radiation
leakproof adapter
leapfrog position
least-square analysis
leather-bottle stomach
lecithin-sphingomyelin (L:S)
ratio
Lee needle
Lee and Westcott needle
left
l. anterior descending
(LAD) artery
l. anterior oblique (LAO)
position
l. circumflex (LCF)
l. coronary artery (LCA)
l. femoral artery (LFA)
l. lateral (LL)
l. lateral (LLAT) position
l. lower lobe (LLL)
l. lower quadrant (LLQ)
l. occipitoposterior (LOP)
l. occipitotransverse
(LOT)
l. posterior oblique (LPO)
position

left—*Continued*
  l. pulmonary artery (LPA)
  l. renal artery (LRA)
  l. renal vein (LRV)
  l. sacroanterior (LSA)
  l. sacroposterior (LSP)
  l. subclavian artery (LSCA)
  l. subclavian vein (LSV)
  l. to right (L-R)
  l. upper lobe (LUL)
  l. upper quadrant (LUQ)
  l. ventricle (LV)
  l. ventricular cap
  l. ventricular ejection
    fraction (LVEF)
  l. ventricular end-diastolic
    pressure (LVEDP)
  l. ventricular enlargement
    (LVE)
  l. ventricular heave
  l. ventricular hypertrophy
    (LVH)
  l. ventricular systolic
    pressure (LVSP)
left-hand
  l.-h. rule
  l.-h. thumb rule
left-to-right
  l.-to-r. shift
  l.-to-r. shunt
leg-length films
Legendre's node
Legg-Calvé-Perthe's syndrome
Legg-Perthe's disease
leggings
Lehman
  L. catheter
  L. right heart catheter
leiomyoblastoma
leiomyofibroma
leiomyoma
leiomyosarcoma
Lejeune's syndrome
Leksell stereotaxic device

L-electron capture
LEM scintillation camera
Lenard ray tube
lengthwise
lens
  l. axis
  l. speed
  Thorpe plastic l.
lentiform nucleus
lentiginopolypose digestive
  syndrome
lentiginosa profusa syndrome
Lenz' syndrome
Leonard–George
  L.-G. method
  L.-G. position
leontiasis
  l. ossea
  l. ossium
leopard syndrome
leprechaunism
leptomeningeal cyst
lepton
leptospiral jaundice
Lerche's vestibule
Léri's
  L.'s lumbarthria
  L.'s melorheostosis
  L.'s pleonosteosis
Léri-Joanny syndrome
Léri-Weill syndrome
Leriche's syndrome
Leroy's I-cell disease
Lesch-Nyhan syndrome
Lesgraft's space
lesion
  anular l.
  "apple core" l.
  Bankart l.
  bull's eye l.
  "butterfly" l.
  cold l.
  DREZ (dorsal root entry
    zone) l.

"doughnut" l.
"dumbbell" l.
ellipsoid l.
hot l.
napkin ring l.
neoplastic l.
"ring-like" l.
sessile l.
space-occupying l.
wedge-shaped l.
lesser
    l. multangular bone
    l. peritoneal sac
    l. sac of peritoneum
    l. trochanter
    l. tuberosity
LET (linear energy transfer)
lethal dose (LD)
Letterer-Siwe
    L.-S. disease
    L.-S. syndrome
Letterer's reticulosis
leukemia line
levator
    l. anguli oris muscle
    l. ani muscle
    l. labii inferioris muscle
    l. labii superioris alaeque
        nasi muscle
    l. labii superioris muscle
    l. menti muscle
    l. palati muscle
    l. palpebrae superioris
        muscle
    l. veli palatini muscle
    l. muscle
levatores costarum muscle
level
    cancericidal l.
Lévi's syndrome
Levin
    L. tube
    L. visceral catheter
levoangiocardiogram

levoatriocardinal vein
levocardia
    l. with situs inversus
levogram
levorotoscoliosis
Lewis' position
LFA (left femoral artery)
LFOV (large field of view)
Lhermitte's sign
LIBC (latent iron-binding
    capacity)
licorice powder
lid plate
lidofenin
Lieberkühn, crypts of
lienography
Lifecath catheter
Liffert and Arkin osteonecrosis
ligament
    accessory l.
    acromioclavicular l.
    acromiocoracoid l.
    adipose l.
    alar l.
    anterior l.
    anular l.
    apical l.
    arcuate l.
    arterial l.
    auricular l.
    Bertin's l.
    Bigelow's l.
    Brodie's l.
    calcaneofibular l.
    calcaneonavicular l.
    capsular l.
    carpal l.
    carpometacarpal l.
    caudal l.
    check l.
    Cleland's l.
    collateral l.
    conoid l.
    coracoacromial l.

ligament—*Continued*
    coracoclavicular l.
    coracohumeral l.
    costoclavicular l.
    costocolic l.
    costocoracoid l.
    costotransverse l.
    costovertebral l.
    cricopharyngeal l.
    cricothyroid l.
    cricotracheal l.
    cruciate l.
    cruciform l.
    crural l.
    cuboidonavicular l.
    cuneonavicular l.
    deltoid l.
    dentate l.
    falciform l.
    flaval l.
    Gimbernat's l.
    glenohumeral l.
    glenoid l.
    hamatometacarpal l.
    iliofemoral l.
    iliolumbar l.
    iliotrochanteric l.
    inguinal l.
    l. of Botallo
    l. of Ferrein
    laciniate l.
    lateral l.
    lateral occipitoatlantal l.
    lateral odontoid l.
    medial l.
    olecranon l.
    palpebral l.
    patellar l.
    phrenicoesophageal l.
    pisohamate l.
    pisometacarpal l.
    plantar l.
    popliteal l.
    Poupart's l.
    pubocapsular l.

    pubofemoral l.
    radiocarpal l.
    rhomboid l.
    sacroiliac l.
    sacrospinous l.
    sacrotuberous l.
    Santori's l.
    Sappey's l.
    sphenomandibular l.
    sternoclavicular l.
    sternocostal l.
    suspensory l.
    talocalcaneal l.
    talofibular l.
    talonavicular l.
    tendinotrochanteric l.
    transverse crural l.
    transverse l.
    transverse l. of atlas
    trapezoid l.
    Treitz' l.
    ulnar l.
    ulnocarpal l.
    umbilical l.
    uterorectosacral l.
    volar l.
    Walther's oblique l.
    Weitbrecht's l.
    Wrisberg's l.
    Y-l.
    yellow l.
ligamenta, pl.
    ligamentum, s.
ligamentous joint
ligamentum
    l. arteriosum
    l. flavum
    l. nuchae
    l. nuchae ossification
    l. teres
ligamentum, s.
    ligmenta, pl.
ligand
    antibody bound l.
    bound l.

free l.
labeled l.
radiolabeled l.
unlabeled l.
ligation
light
    l. therapy
    l. wave
Lightwood-Albright syndrome
Lightwood's syndrome
Lilienfeld's
    L.'s method
    L.'s position
    L.'s position for the ischium
    L.'s position for the
      shoulder
    L.'s tube
Liliequist, membrane of
"lily-pad" sign
limb venography
limbus vertebra
limulus lysate test
Lin Kuatang-Tz'w
Lindau's
    L.'s disease
    L.'s tumor
Lindau-von Hippel disease
Lindblom's
    L.'s method
    L.'s position
Lindeman needle
Lindemann electrometer
line
    absorption l.
    acanthomeatal l.
    accretion l.
    anterior junctional l.
    anterior mediastinal l.
    auricular l.
    axillary l.
    B septal l.
    bismuth l.
    Blumensaat's l.
    Brailsford l.
    calcaneal l.

Camper's l.
canthomeatal l.
cervico-obturator l.
Chamberlain's l.
clinoparietal l. of Taveras
    Poser
dentate l.
double suture l.
Ellis' l.
epiphyseal plate l.
Etter's l.
field l.
Fischgold's bimastoid l.
Fischgold's biventer l.
Fischgold's digastric l.
Fischgold's l.
Fleischner's l.
flux l.
foramen magnum l.
fracture l.
Fraenkel, white l. of
Frankfort l.
FT l.
gas density l.
glabelloalveolar l.
glabellomeatal l.
gluteal l.
Goodsell l.
Granger's l.
grid l.
Hampton's aortic l.
Hampton's gastric l.
Hilgenreiner l.
iliopectineal l.
infraorbital l.
infraorbitomeatal l.
    (IOML)
infundibuloventricular l.
intercondylar notch l.
intermalleolar l.
interorbital l.
interpupillary l.
intertuberal l.
joint l.
Kaes' l.

line—*Continued*
  Kerley A l.
  Kerley B l.
  Kerley C l.
  Krayenbuhl-Richter l.
  l. focus
  l. imaging
  l. method sensitivity
  l. of demarcation
  l. of force
  l. of Zahn
  l. saturation
  l. scan
  l. space
  l. spectrum
  l. spread function
  l. voltage compensator
  l. width
  lead l.
  leukemia l.
  lorentzian l.
  mammillary l.
  McGregor's l.
  McRae's l.
  mentomeatal l.
  metaphyseal l.
  midtalar l.
  mucoperiosteal l.
  nuchal l.
  oblique orbital l.
  obturator l.
  occlusal l.
  orbitomeatal l. (OML)
  para-aortic l.
  paraesophageal l.
  paraspinal l.
  paratracheal l.
  paravertebral l.
  pericardial l.
  persistent Kerley's l.
  phosphorus l.
  pi l.
  postarrest l.
  posterior junction l.
  psoas l.
  pubococcygeal l.
  retrosternal l.
  reverse S-l. of Golden
  Rugiero's l.
  sacrococcygeal inferior
      pubic l.
  Sahlstedt's l.
  SCIPP l.
  Shenton's l.
  siphon-incisivum l.
  Skinner's l.
  spigelian l.
  subcostal l.
  Swedish l.
  Taylor-Haughton l.
  transpyloric l.
  transtubercular l.
  transverse l.
  transverse ls. of Park
  trough l.
  tuberculo-occipital
      protuberance l.
  Twining's l.
  vertical l. of Ombredanne
  Wimberger's l.
  Y-Y l.
  Z l. of the esophagus
line-to-line movement
linea
  l. aspera
  l. costoarticularis
  l. innominata
  l. sternalis
  l. terminalis
  l. transversae ossi sacri
linea, s.
  lineae, pl.
lineae, pl.
  linea, s.
linear
  l. absorption coefficient
  l. accelerator
  l. accelerator machine

l. amplifier
l. array
l. attenuation
l. attenuation coefficient
l. compartmental system
l. electron accelerator
l. energy transfer (LET)
l. focus
l. fracture
l. grid
l. motion
l. movement
l. partial volume artifact
l. partial volume effect
l. phased arrays
l. photon
l. resolution
l. scan
l. scanning, ultrasound
l. sequenced arrays
l. skull fracture
l. system
l. tomography
lingua, s.
   linguae, pl
linguae, pl.
   lingua, s.
lingual
   l. aponeurosis
   l. gyrus
lingualis muscle
lingula
   l. pulmonis sinistri
lingula, s.
   lingulae, pl.
lingulae, pl.
   lingula, s.
linitis plastica
Lintro-scan mammography
liothyronine
LIP (lymphocytic interstitial pneumonitis)
lipase
lipid

Lipiodol
   ascending L. (iodized oil)
   L. "F"
lipoatrophic
lipocalcinogranulomatosis
lipochondrodystrophy
lipogenesis
lipoglycoproteinosis
lipogranulomatosis
lipoid
   l. cholecystitis
   l. dermatoarthritis
   l. granulomatosis
   l. proteinosis
lipoidosis cutis et mucosae
lipoma
Lipomul (corn oil with d-Alpha tocopheryl acetate, butylated hydroxy-anisole, polysorbate 80, glyceride phosphates, sodium saccharin, sodium benzoate, benzoic acid, sorbic acid)
liposarcoma
Lippes' loop intrauterine device
lipping
   l. and spurring
   l. type of calyceal cavity
   marginal l.
Lippman
   L. corkscrew pin
   L. hip prosthesis
   L. screw
LIQ (lower inner quadrant)
Liquibarine
liquid
   l. crystal thermogram
   l. scintillation system
Liquid Polibar
Liquipake (barium sulfate suspension)
Lisfranc's
   L.'s fracture-dislocation

Lisfranc's—*Continued*
    L.'s joint
lissencephalic
lissencephaly syndrome
listing gait
Listing's plane
lithiasis
lithium
    l. glass
lithotomy
    l. position
    l. Trendelenburg position
lithotripsy
lithotripter or lithotriptor
Littleford-Spector lead
    introducer
liver
    amyloid l.
    biliary cirrhotic l.
    brimstone l.
    bronze l.
    hobnail l.
    l. abscess
    l. edge
    l. extract
    l. glycogen disease
    l. scan
    l. span
    l. studies
    l. transplant
    lardaceous l.
    pigmented l.
    polycystic l.
    sago l.
    stasis l.
    sugar-icing l.
    waxy l.
liver-spleen (LS)
    l. scan
Livingston intramedullary
    bar
LL (left lateral)
LLAT (left lateral)
LLL (left lower lobe)

LL-LL adapters
Lloyd catheter
LLQ (left lower quadrant)
LMR (localized magnetic
    resonance)
lobar
    l. agenesis
    l. bronchus
    l. collapse
    l. consolidation
    l. emphysema
    "l. nephronia"
    l. pneumonia
    l. torsion
lobe
    accessory l.
    appendicular l.
    azygos l.
    caudate l.
    cuneate l.
    flocculonodular l.
    frontal l.
    hepatic l.
    left lower l. (LLL)
    occipital l.
    parietal l.
    piriform l.
    polyalveolar l.
    quadrate l.
    Riedel's l.
    temporal l.
lobi, pl.
    lobus, s.
Lobstein's disease
lobster-claw deformity
lobster-tail catheter
lobular
lobule
lobuli, pl.
    lobulus, s.
lobulus, s.
    lobuli, pl.
lobus, s.
    lobi, pl.

localization
localized
    l. image
    l. image scan
    l. lateral projection
    l. magnetic resonance
       (LMR)
    l. myeloma
    l. tumor
loci, pl.
    locus, s.
Lockwood, superior tendon of
loculated
    l. ascites
    l. cyst
    l. effusion
locum tenens
locus, s.
    loci, pl.
lodestone
Loepp's projection
Löffler's or Loeffler's
    L.'s endocarditis
    L.'s eosinophilia
    L.'s pneumonia
    L.'s syndrome
Löfgren's syndrome
logarithms
Logic 101, 111, and 121 gamma
  counting system
long-acting thyroid stimulator
  (LATS)
long
    l. bone fracture
    l. flexible tip straight
      safety wire guide
    l. TR/TE
    l. transit time
Longdwel catheter
longissimus
    l. capitis muscle
    l. cervicis muscle
    l. dorsi muscle
    l. thoracis muscle

longitudinal
    l. arch
    l. axis
    l. fissure
    l. fracture
    l. magnetization
    l. relaxation time
    l. relaxation time constant
    l. section imaging
    l. section tomography
    l. suture
    l. time constant
    l. tomography
longitudinal or spin-lattice
    l. relaxation time constant
      (T1)
loop
    duodenal l.
    Henle's l.
    Lippes' l.
loopogram (ileostogram)
loose
    l. bodies
    l. fracture
    l. fragments
Looser-Debray-Milkman
  syndrome
Looser's transformation
  zones
LOP (left occipitoposterior)
lopamidol
LoProfile-II balloon catheter
lopsided head
LOQ (lower outer quadrant)
Lorain-Lévi syndrome
lordosis
lordotic
    anteroposterior l.
      projection
    apical l. projection
    l. (A-P) erect projection
    l. curve
    l. position
    l. view

Lorentz's force
lorentzian line
Lorenz and Lilienfeld
  method
Lorenz'
  L.' method
  L.' position
Lorenzo
  L. plate
  L. screw
lorry driver fracture
LOT (left occipitotransverse)
Lottes intramedullary nail
Louis, angle of
lovastatin (Mevacor)
Löw-Beer position
low-density artifact
low-dose scan
low-energy radiation
low-kilovoltage
low-pass filter
Lowe's syndrome
Lowe-Terrey-MacLachlan
  syndrome
lower
  l. bowel series
  l. GI (gastrointestinal)
    series
  l. inner quadrant (LIQ)
  l. lobe bronchus
  l. outer quadrant (LOQ)
  l. ridge slope
Lower's sac
Lower, tubercule of
LPA (left pulmonary artery)
L-plate
LPO (left posterior oblique)
  position
L-R (left to right)
LRA (left renal artery)
LRV (left renal vein)
L/S (lecithin-sphingomyelin)
  ratio
LS (liver-spleen)
LS or L/S (lumbosacral)

LSA (left sacro-anterior)
LSCA (left subclavian artery)
LSCV (left subclavian vein)
LSP (left sacroposterior)
lucency
lucent
Luck finger cap
lückenschädel disease
lucunae, pl.
  lucuna, s.
Ludwig's
  L.'s angina
  L.'s angle
  L.'s plane
Luer plugs
Luer-Lok adapter
luetic
  l. aorta
  l. osteomyelitis
  l. spondylitis
lugged plate
Lugol's solution
LUL (left upper lobe)
lumbar (L)
  l. aortogram
  l. aortography
  l. arch
  l. curve
  l. disk, disc
  l. flexion and extension
    study
  l. fracture
  l. lymph node
  l. myelogram
  l. myelography
  l. puncture
  l. region
  l. spine
  l. vertebra
lumbocostal arch
lumbodorsal fascia
lumboinguinal
lumbosacral (LS or L/S)
  l. angle
  l. angulation

l. articulation
l. cord
l. disk or disc
l. joint
l. plexus
l. projection
l. spine
lumbosacralis muscle
lumbricales
    l. manus muscle
    l. pedis muscle
lumen, s.
    lumina, pl.
lumina, pl.
    lumen, s.
luminance
luminescence
luminous
    l. efficiency
    l. emittance
    l. flux
    l. intensity
Lumoxyd
lumpy jaw
lunate
    l. dislocation
    l. fracture
    l. triquetrum fusion
lunate-scaphoid fusion
Lunderquist
    L. exchange wire guide
    L. exchange guide wire
Lunderquist-Ring torque guide
  wire
lung
    "drowned l."
    esophageal l.
    farmer's l.
    gastric l.
    honeycomb l.
    hyperlucent l.
    l. agenesis
    l. markings
    l. perfusion/ventilation (V/
      Q) study

l. purpura with nephritis
l. root
l. scan
pigeon breeder's l.
"respirator l."
"shock l."
"stiff l."
thresher's l.
lupus pernio
LUQ (left upper quadrant)
Luque instrumentation
Luschka
    foramen of L.
Luschka's
    L.'s crypts
    L.'s joint
    L.'s rib
    L.'s tonsil
luteinizing
Lutembacher's syndrome
luteotrophic
lutetium
Lütkens' sphincter
lux
luxation
luxury perfusion syndrome
LV (left ventricle)
LVE (left ventricular
  enlargement)
LVEDP (left ventricular end-
  diastolic pressure)
LVEF (left ventricular ejection
  fraction)
LVH (left ventricular
  hypertrophy)
LVSP (left ventricular systolic
  pressure)
Lw (lawrencium)
Lyme
    L. arthritis
    L. disease
lymph
    l. sac
    l. space
lymph node

lymph node—*Continued*
  jugulodigastric l.
  l. imaging
  tracheal l.
lymphadenitis
  caseous l.
  enteric l.
  histoplasmic l.
  mesenteric l.
  tuberculoid l.
lymphadenopathy
  axillary l.
  hilar l.
  immunoblastic l.
  mediastinal l.
  mesenteric l.
  tuberculous l.
lymphangiectatic cyst
lymphangiogram (LAG)
lymphangiography (LAG)
  catheter
lymphangioma
  colonic l.
  cystic l.
  intrasplenic l.
  mediastinal l.
lymphangiosarcoma
lymphatic
Lymphazurin (isosulfan blue,
  sodium monohydrogen
  phosphate, potassium
  dihydrogen phosphate)
lymphnodal hamartoma
lymphoblastic
  l. lymphoma
  l. lymphosarcoma
lymphoblastoma
lymphocyte
lymphocytic
  l. interstitial pneumonitis
    (LIP)
  l. leukemia
  l. lymphosarcoma
  l. thyroiditis
lymphoendothelioma

lymphogram
lymphogranuloma
  l. inguinale
  l. malignum
  l. venereum
lymphogranulomatosis
  l. benigna
  l. maligna
lymphography
lymphoma
  alveolar l.
  Burkitt's l.
  clasmocytic l.
  disseminated l.
  giant follicular l.
  granulomatous l.
  histiocytic l.
  Hodgkin's l.
  lymphoblastic l.
  non-Hodgkin's l.
  retroperitoneal l.
  stem cell l.
  undifferentiated l.
lymphomatoid granulomatosis
lymphosarcoma
  fascicular l.
  lymphoblastic l.
  lymphocytic l.
  sclerosing l.
lymphoscintigram
Lysholm grid
Lysholm's
  L.'s position for the cranial
    base
  L.'s position for the optic
    foramen
  L.'s position for the pars
    petrosa
lysis
lysosome
lytic
  l. area
  l. change
  l. degeneration
  l. necrosis

Mm

M (macroscopic magnetization vector)

μ (micron)

mA (milliampere)

MAA (macroaggregated albumin)

MAB (monoclonal antibody)

Macewen's
  M. operation
  M. osteotomy
  M. sign
  M. triangle

Mache unit

Mack-Brunswick medium

Mackenzie-Davidson method

MacLeod's syndrome

MacMillan's position

macroaggregated albumin (MAA)

macroaggregates of radioiodinated albumin (MARIA)

macrocephaly

macrocrania

macrodactyly

macrodystrophia
  m. lipomatosa

macrogenitosomia
  m. praecox
  m. praecox suprarenalis

macroglobulinemia
  Waldenström's m.

macroglossia-omphalocele syndrome

macromolecules

macronodular cirrhosis

macrophage

macroradiogram

macroscopic
  m. magnetization moment
  m. magnetization vector (M)

macroshock

Macrotec (technetium Tc 99m medronate kit)

Madayag needle

Madden's technique

Madelung's
  M.'s deformity
  M.'s subluxation

Madura foot

maduromycosis

Maffucci's syndrome

magenblase

Magendie, foramen of

Magendie's space

magenstrasse

magic numbers

magnesium (Mg)
  m. chloride

magnet
  beam-bending m.
  cryostable m.
  Eindhoven's m.
  permanent m.
  resistive m.
  superconductive m.
  Walker's m.

magnetic
  artificial permanent m.
  m. circuit
  m. dipole
  m. disk, disc
  m. domain

m. field
m. field (H)
m. field gradient
m. field intensity
m. field strength
m. flux
m. flux density
m. focal plane
m. force
m. gradient
m. induction
m. induction field (Bo)
m. induction of flux
   density (B)
m. lines of force
m. material
m. moment
m. permeability
m. permeance
m. pole
m. recording
m. reluctance
m. resonance (MR)
m. resonance imaging
   (MRI)
m. resonance imaging
   system (MR MAX)
m. resonance signal
m. resonance
   spectroscopy (MRS)
m. resonance study
m. retentivity
m. susceptibility
m. tape
magnetization
magnetocardiograph
magnetogyric ratio
magnetoinduction
magnetomotion force
Magnetrode cervical unit
magnetron
Magnevist (gadolinium DTPA)
magnification
   m. angiography

m. factor
m. percentage
m. radiography
radiographic m.
vertebrobasilar m.
magnified
   m. arteriography
   m. carotid arteriography
   m. carotid venography
   m. vertebrobasilar
    arteriography
magnify
magnitude of ripple
Magovern's valve
main stem bronchus
Maisonneuve's fracture
mal
   grand m.
   m. de mer
   petit m.
malabsorption
malacia
   "segmental m."
maladie de Roger
malakoplakia
malalignment
malar (jugal, zygoma, or
  cheek)
   m. fracture
   m. lymph node
Malassez'
   M.' disease
   M.' rest
Malecot catheter
malformation
   Arnold-Chiari m.
   arteriovenous m. (AVM)
   Chiari's m.
   congenital m.
   Ebstein's m.
   Mondini's pulmonary
    arteriovenous m.
   Scheibe's m.
   venous m.

Malgaigne's fracture
malignant
    m. granuloma
    m. hypertension
    m. lymphoma
    m. malnutrition syndrome
    m. melanoma
    m. mixed embryoma
    m. mixed tumor
mallei, pl. (ear bone)
    malleus, s.
malleolar
    m. fossa
    m. screw
malleoli, pl. (ankle bone)
    malleolus, s.
malleolus
    fibular m.
    lateral m.
    m. fracture
    medial m.
    radial m.
    tibial m.
    ulnar m.
malleolus, s. (ankle bone)
    malleoli, pl.
mallet
    m. finger
    m. toe
malleus, s. (ear bone)
    mallei, pl.
Mallinckrodt U.S.P. barium
Mallory-Weiss
    M.-W. syndrome
    M.-W. tear
malocclusion
malomaxillary suture
Maloney
    M. catheter
    M. dilator
malpighian
    m. bodies
    m. capsule
    m. layer
malposed

malrotation
malum
    m. coxae senilis
    m. epiphyseonecroticum
      vertebrale
malunion
malunited fracture
mamillary (or mammillary)
    m. dimpling
    m. duct
    m. line
    m. system
mamillotegmental
    m. tract
mamillothalamic
    m. fasciculus
mammaplasty
mammary
    m. abscess
    m. discharge
    m. dysostosis
    m. dysplasia
    m. gland
    m. implant
    m. node
mammogram
    film screen technique m.
    negative mode m.
    screening m.
    xeroradiographic m.
mammography
    Lintro-scan m.
Mammomat
mammoplasty
    augmentation m.
    reduction m.
Mammorex
Manashil
    M. catheter
    M. sialography catheter
Manchester
    M. Dosage System
    M. ovoids
mandatory
mandible

mandibular
  m. arch
  m. canal
  m. condyle
  m. foramen
  m. fossa
  m. joint
  m. lymph node
  m. notch
  m. ramus
  m. symphysis
mandibulofacial
  m. dysmorphia
  m. dysostosis
mandibulopharyngeal
mandibulosacral dysplasia
Mandl's osteonecrosis
maneuver
  Adson's m.
  Chassard-Lapiné m.
  Engel-Lysholm m.
  Jonnson's m.
  milking m.
  Müller's m.
  Queckenstedt's m.
  toe-touch m.
  Valsalva's m.
  Wolf-Marshak m.
manganese
  m. chloride
  m. chloride Mn-54
Mani
  M. (French) catheter
  M. catheter
  M. cerebral catheter
manipulate
manipulation
  digital m.
  instrument m.
Mankin's method
Mankowsky's syndrome
mannitol
mantle
Manu catheter
manual technique

manubrial artery
manubriosternal joint
manubriosternoclavicular
  abscess
manubrium sterni
Manurkar catheter
manus
maplike skull
Maquet's technique
marble bones
marbleization
march fracture
Marchand's adrenal
Marchesani's syndrome
Marey's sphygomograph
Marfan's syndrome
margin
  costal m.
  infraorbital m.
  midlateral orbital m.
  supraorbital m.
  synovial m.
marginal
  m. lipping
  m. spurs
  m. ulcer
MARIA (macroaggregates of
  radioiodinated albumin)
Marie's
  M.'s ataxia
  M.'s syndrome
Marie-Bamberger syndrome
Marie-Léri syndrome
Marie-Sainton disease
Marie-Strümpell disease
Marjolin's ulcer
Mark IV procedure
markings
  bronchovesicular m.
    (BVM)
Maroteaux-Lamy
  M.-L. pyknodysostosis
  M.-L. syndrome
marrow
  bone m.

Marshall plate
Marshall's syndrome
Martorell–Fabré
  syndrome
Martz' method
mAs (milliAmpere-seconds)
mascara artifact
Maslin's method
Mason classification
mass
    atomic m.
    intraluminal m.
    m. absorption coefficient
    m. acceleration
    m. defect
    m. effect
    m. energy equivalence
    m. impression
    m. lesion
    m. number
    m. sign
    m. spectograph
    m. spectrometer
    m. structure
    relativistic m.
    subcarinal m.
massa
    m. intermedia
massa, s.
    massae, pl.
massae, pl.
    massa, s.
masseter muscle
Massiot's polytome
massive
    m. edema
      hemorrhage
    m. osteolysis
massives
    Bagshaw's m.
MAST suit
mastectomy
    modified m.
    radical m.

    subcutaneous m.
mastocarcinoma
mastochondroma
mastocytoma
mastogram
mastography
mastoid
    m. abscess
    m. air cells
    m. antrum
    m. canaliculus
    m. catheter
    m. lymph node
    m. process
    m. sinus
    m. suture
    m. tip
mastoiditis
    "catarrhal" m.
    sclerotic m.
    suppurative m.
mastopexy
mastoplasty
mastoscirrhus
mastotomy
Matchett-Brown hip prosthesis
matrices or matrixes, pl.
    matrix, s.
matrix, s.
    matrices or matrixes, pl.
matrixes or matrices, pl.
    matrix, s.
maturation
    delayed skeletal m.
    dysharmonic m.
    skeletal m.
Maxicamera II
maxilla
maxillary
    m. antrum
    m. arch
    m. sinus
maxillofacial
Maximar 200 kV machine

maximum
    m. midexpiratory flow rate (MMFR)
    m. permissible concentration (MPC)
    m. permissible dose (MPD)
Maxwell unit
Maxwell's theory of radiation
maxwellian distribution
May's
    M.'s method
    M.'s position
    M.'s view
Mayer's
    M.'s method
    M.'s position
    M.'s projection
    M.'s view
Mayo-Robson position
maze
Mazer stent
mazoplasia
MC (metacarpal)
MCA (middle cerebral artery)
MCA (monoclonal antibody)
McBride acetabulum cup
MCC (metacarpocarpal joints)
McCaskey's catheter
McCort sign
McCune–Albright syndrome
μcg (microgram)
McGoon perfusion catheter
McGregor's
    M.'s baseline
    M.'s line
μc-hr (microcurie-hour)
μCi (microcurie)
MCi (megacurie)
mCi (millicurie)
mCi-hr (millicurie-hour)
McIntosh double-lumen catheter
McIver catheter

McKee
    M. mechanical finger
    M. nail
    M. plate
McKee-Farrar
    M.-F. acetabular cup
    M.-F. prosthesis
McKeever
    M. patella
    M. tibial plateau
McKusick's metaphyseal chondrodysplasia
McLaughlin
    M. four-flanged nail
    M. navicular screw
    M. plate
McLaughlin-Thornton bolt
McMurray's sign
MCP (metacarpophalangeal)
McRae's line
MCTC (metrizamide DT cisternogram)
MDAC (multiplying digital-to-analog converter)
MDP (methylene diphosphonate)
MEA (multiple endocrine adenomatosis) syndrome
meal
    barium m.
    Boyden m.
    opaque m.
mean
    m. circulatory hematocrit
    m. dose
    m. free path
    m. gonad dose
    m. lethal dose
    m. life
    m. marrow dose (MMD)
    m. valve
measured dose
measurement
    Cobb's m.

measurement—*Continued*
    Ferguson's m.
meatal stenosis
meati or meatuses, pl.
    meatus, s.
meatus, s.
    meati or meatuses, pl.
meatuses or meati, pl.
    meatus, s.
mechanical
    m. bull thumb fracture
    m. hand scan
    m. ileus
    m. life support system
    m. obstruction
    m. respirator
    m. traction
    m. ventilation
Meckel's
    M.'s cartilage
    M.'s cave
    M.'s cavity
    M.'s diverticulum
    M.'s ganglion
    M.'s plane
    M.'s scan
    M.'s stone
meconium
    m. aspiration syndrome
    m. ileus
    m. peritonitis
    m. plug syndrome
    m. stain
    m. stained amniotic fluid
MED (minimal erythema dose)
Med-Tech catheter
media, pl.
    medium, s.
mediad
medial
    m. (basilic) vein
    m. aperture
    m. cuneiform
    m. ligament
    m. malleolus

    m. meniscus
    m. oblique axial projection
    m. oblique position
    m. striate artery
    m. stripe
median
    m. atlantoaxial joint
    m. lethal dose (L.D.$_{50}$)
    m. lethal dose (MLD)
    m. lethal time (MLT)
    m. nerve
    m. sagittal plane (MSP)
    m. sternotomy
mediastinal
    m. adenopathy
    m. fibrosis
    m. fluid
    m. flutter
    m. goiter
    m. hemorrhage
    m. lymph node
    m. lymphadenopathy
    m. lymphangioma
    m. pericarditis
    m. pleura
    m. venography
    m. wedge
mediastinography
mediastinoscopy
mediastinum
Medina ileostomy catheter
mediolateral
    m. oblique projection
    m. projection
    m. view
Mediterranean
    M. anemia
    M. fever
medium, s.
    media, pl.
Medopaque
    M. Hond
    M. U
Medotopes
    (radiopharmaceuticals)

Medrat angiography injector
medronate
    m. scan
medulla oblongata
medulla, s.
    medullas or medullae, pl.
medullae or medullas, pl.
    medulla, s.
medullary
    m. canal
    m. carcinoma
    m. cavity
    m. cone
    m. cord
    m. fold
    m. gonadal dysgenesis
    m. groove
    m. plate
    m. rod
    m. space
    m. sponge kidney
medullas or medullae, pl.
    medulla, s.
Medx (manufacturer)
    M. camera
    M. scanner
Meekeren-Ehlers-Danlos
  syndrome
Mees' position
megacalyx
megacardia
megacecum
megacephalic
megacholedochus
megacolon
megacurie (MCi)
megaduodenum
megaelectron volt (MeV)
megaepiphyseal dwarfism
megaesophagus
megahertz (MHz)
megakaryocyte
megalencephalon
megaloblastic
megalobulbus

megalocephaly
megalocheiria
megalocrania
megalodactyly
megaprosopous
megavolt
    m. therapy
megavoltage (MV)
meglumine
    m. and calcium
      metrizoates
    m. diatrizoate
    m. iodipamide
    m. iothalamate
megohm
meibomian gland
Meiboom-Gill sequence
Meige's disease
Meigs' syndrome
Meigs-Cass syndrome
meioses, pl.
    meiosis, s.
meiosis, s.
    meioses, pl.
Meissner's plexus
melanoameloblastoma
melanoma
melanoplakia and small
  intestine polyposis
melanotic
    m. ameloblastoma
    m. sarcoma
melasma suprarenale
Meleda's disease
melenic stool
Melnick-Needles syndrome
melorheostosis leri
melting sign
membrana angularis defect
membranaceous tendon
membrane
    m. of Liliequist
    m. phosphate
    periodontal m.
    placental m.

membrane—*Continued*
  synovial m.
  thyrohyoid m.
  tympanic m. (TM)
membranocartilaginous
membranous
  m. labyrinth
  m. septum
mendelevium (Md)
Mendelson's syndrome
Mendosal suture
Ménétrier's disease
Menghini
  M. needle
  M. thin wall Silverman
    needle
meningeal space
meninges
  arachnoid m.
  dura mater m.
  pia mater m.
meninges, pl.
  meninx, s.
meningioma
  angioblastic m.
  en plaque m.
  falcine m.
  parasagittal m.
  sphenoid wing m.
  suprasellar m.
meningitis
meningo-oculofacial
  angiomatosis
meningo-osteophlebitis
meningoarteritis
meningoblastoma
meningocele
  sacral m.
  spurious m.
meningocephalitis
meningocerebritis
meningocortical
meningocyte
meningoencephalitis
  amebic m.

  eosinophilic m.
  syphilitic m.
meningoencephalocele
meningoencephalomyelitis
meningoencephalomyelopathy
meningoencephalopathy
meningofibroblastoma
meningoma
meningomalacia
meningomyelitis
meningomyelocele
meningomyeloradiculitis
meningopathy
meningorachidian
meningoradicular
meningoradiculitis
meningorrhagia
meningorrhea
meningosis
meningovascular
meninx
  m. fibrosa
  m. tenuis
  m. vasculosa
meninx, s.
  meninges, pl.
meniscal tear
menisci or meniscuses, pl.
  meniscus, s.
meniscosynovial
meniscus sign
meniscus, s.
  meniscuses or menisci, pl.
meniscuses or menisci, pl.
  meniscus, s.
meniscocytosis
Menkes' "kinky-hair"
  syndrome
menopause
menstrual
menstruation
mental
  m. foramen
  m. point
  m. protuberance

m. tubercle
mentalis
mento-occipital position
mentoanterior position
mentomeatal
    m. line
mentoposterior position
mentotransverse position
mEq (milliequivalent)
meralgia paresthetica
"Mercedes-Benz" sign
Mercier
    M. catheter
Mercier's valve
Mercuhydrin
mercuric nitrate
    m. (Hg-197)
    m. (Hg-203)
Mercurio's position
mercury 197
merocrine gland
mesaticephalic
mesencephalon
mesenchymal
mesentera, pl.
    mesenteron, s.
mesenterial intestine
mesenteric
    m. abscess
    m. adenopathy
    m. arteriogram
    m. arteriography
    m. artery
    m. fibrofatty proliferation
    m. gland
    m. infarction
    m. ischemia
    m. lymph node
    m. lymphadenitis
    m. lymphadenopathy
    m. node
    m. thrombosis
    m. vein
mesenteron, s.
    mesentera, pl.

mesial plate
mesiocclusion
mesiodens
mesiodistal
mesoappendicitis
mesoazygos
mesoblastic nephroma
mesocardia
mesocephalic skull
mesocolic lymph node
mesocolon
mesoderm
mesodermal tumor
mesoectodermal dysplasia
mesoesophagus
mesomelic dwarfism of Léri
    and Weill
mesomorphic
meson
mesonephric
    m. duct
    m. ridge
mesonephros
mesosigmoid
mesothelioma
mesothelium
metabolic craniopathy
metabolism
metacarpal (MC)
    m. fracture
    m. head fracture
    m. index
    m. neck fracture
    m. sign
metacarpo-carpal (MCC) joint
metacarpophalangeal (MCP)
  joint
metacarpotalar syndrome
metacarpus
metachromatic leukodystrophy
metachronous
metal catheter
metalix tube
metallic
    m. artifact

metallic—*Continued*
    m. foreign body (MFB)
    m. silver
metanephros
metaphase
metaphyseal
    m. chondrodysplasia
    m. chondroplasia
    m. corner fracture
    m. dysostosis
    m. dysplasia
    m. flaring
    m. irregularity
    m. line
    m. sclerosis
    m. transverse bands
    m. vessel
metaphyses, pl.
    metaphysis, s.
metaphysis, s.
    metaphyses, pl.
metaplasia
    agnogenic myeloid m.
    osseous m.
metaplastic ossification
metasellar
metastable state
metastases, pl.
    metastasis, s.
metastasis, s.
    metastases, pl.
metastasize
metastatic
    m. abscess
    m. carcinoid syndrome
    m. melanoma
    m. pneumonia
    m. tuberculous abscess
    m. tumor
metatarsal (MT) fracture
metatarsalgia
metatarsocuneiform joint
metatarsophalangeal joint (MTPJ)
metatarsus
    m. adductocavus

    m. adductovarus
    m. adductus
    m. atavicus
    m. brevis
    m. inversus
    m. latus
    m. primus brevior
    m. primus varus
    m. varus
metatrophic dwarfism
metatropic dysplasia
metencephalospinal
meteorism
meter-kilogram-second (mks)
methacrylate-bone interface
methiodal sodium
method
    Albers-Schönberg m.
    Alexander's m.
    Anderson's m.
    Andrén's m.
    Arcelin's m.
    Ball-Golden m.
    Ball's m.
    Béclère m.
    Benassi's m.
    Bertel's m.
    Blackett-Healy m.
    body rotation m.
    border detection m.
    Broden's m.
    Budin-Chandler m.
    Bullit's m.
    Cahoon's m.
    Caldwell-Moloy m.
    Cameron's m.
    Camp-Coventry m.
    Camp-Gianturco m.
    Castine-Kinney m.
    Causton's m.
    Chamberlain's m.
    Chassard-Lapiné m.
    Chaussé's III m.
    Chaussé's m.
    Cleaves' m.

Cobb's m.
Colcher-Sussman m.
Cope-m. bronchography
Coutard's m.
Danelius-Miller,
  modification of Lorenz'
  m.
Davis' m.
Dooley-Caldwell-Glass m.
Duncan-Hoen m.
Dunlap, Swanson, and
  Penner m.
Dyke's m.
electrostatic m.
Eraso's m.
Evans' m.
Evart's m.
fast single slice m.
Feist's m.
Feist-Mankin m.
Ferguson's m.
Fick's m.
Fiske's m.
fixed angle m.
Fleischner's m.
Fray's cranial angle m.
Fray's proportional m.
Friedman's m.
Fuchs' m.
Garland-Thomas m.
Garn's m.
Gaynor-Hart m.
Gerota's m.
Gill's m.
Girdany-Golden m.
Girout's m.
Grandy's m.
Granger's m.
Grashey's m.
Gunson's m.
Haas' m.
Hadlock's m. (OB/US)
Harrison-Stubbs m.
Hatt's m.
Henschen's m.

Henschen, Schüller, and
  Lysholm m.
Heublein's m.
Hirtz' m.
Hobbin's m. (OB/US)
Hoffa's m.
Holly's m.
Holmblad's m.
horizontal ray m.
Hough's m.
Hsieh's m.
Hughston's m.
Isherwood's m.
Johnson's m.
Judd's m.
Kandel's m.
Kasabach's m.
Kemp Harper's m.
Kimberlin's m.
Kirdani's m.
Kite's m.
Kovács' m.
Kreuzfuchs' m.
Kuchendorf's m.
Kurzbauer's m.
KWE (Kumar, Welti and
  Ernst) m.
Laquerriere-Pierquin m.
Lauenstein and Hickey m.
Law's m.
Lawrence's m.
Leonard-George m.
Lilienfeld's m.
Lindblom's m.
Lorenz and Lilienfeld m.
Lorenz' m.
Mackenzie-Davidson m.
Mankin's m.
Martz' m.
Maslin's m.
May's m.
Mayer's m.
Meyerding's m.
Miller's m.
modified Fuchs' m.

method—*Continued*
    modified Hickey's m.
    modified Lysholm's m.
    modified Titterington's m.
    modified Waters' m.
    Monte Carlo m.
    Mosley's m.
    multiple line scanning m.
    multiple sensitive point m.
    Nolke's m.
    nuclear magnetic
        resonance spin-warp m.
    orthoroentgenographic m.
    Ottonelo's m.
    Owen-Pendergrass m.
    parallax m.
    parallax motion m.
    Parama's m.
    part-angulation m.
    Pawlow's m.
    Pearson's m.
    Pfeiffer-Comberg m.
    "pinch-cock" m.
    Pirie's m.
    Poppel's m.
    Porcher's m.
    profunda m.
    QRS synchro m.
    Quesada's m.
    reflux m.
    Regaud's m.
    Rhese's m.
    right-angle m.
    Sansregret modification of
        Chaussé III m.
    Schüller's m.
    Seldinger's m.
    sensitive line m.
    sequential line m.
    sequential point m.
    Settegast's m.
    single-tube angulation
        m.
    Sommer-Foegella m.
    Sontag, Snell, and
        Anderson m.
    Staunig's m.
    Stecher's m.
    Stenver's m.
    Strickler's m.
    surface coil m.
    Sweet's m.
    Tanner-Whitehouse-Healy m.
    Tarrant's m.
    Taylor's m.
    Teufel's m.
    Thoms' m.
    Titterington's m.
    transduodenal m.
    Twining's m.
    Ungerleider's m.
    Valdini's m.
    Valvassori's m.
    Vastine-Kinney m.
    vertical ray m.
    Waters' m.
    Wehlin's m.
    Wigby-Taylor m.
    Williams' m.
    Wolf's m.
    Zanelli's m.
    Zimmer's m.
    Zizmor's m.
methyl
    m. cholesterol
    m. methacrylate
methyl-bis-amine
    hydrochloride
methylcellulose gel
methylene
    m. blue
    m. diphosphonate (MDP)
    m. diphosphonate (Tc-
        99m-MDP)
    m. hydroxydiphosphonate
        (MHDP)
methylglucamine
    m. iodipamide

m. iodoxamate
m. ioglycamide
m. iothalamate
m. iotroxamide
m. metrizoate
methysergide
metoclopramide
metopic suture
Metras catheter
metric
    m. system
metrizamide
    m. (Amipaque)
    m. CT cisternogram
        (MCTC)
    m. myelography
metrizamide-assisted
  computed tomography
metrizoate
metrizoic acid
metrography
metrosalpingography
metrotubography
Metufan
MeV (megaelectron volt)
meV (million electron volts)
Mevacor (lovastatin)
Meyenburg-Altherr-Uehlinger
  syndrome
Meyerding's method
Meyer-Schwickerath and
  Weyers syndrome
Meyer's dysplasia of the
  femoral head
Meyer's nomogram
Meynet's node
MF (mycosis fungoides)
MFB (metallic foreign body)
mgh (milligram hours)
MHDP (methylene
  hydroxydiphosphonate)
MHP (1-mercuri-2-
  hydroxypropane)
MHz (megahertz)

MI (mitral insufficiency or
  myocardial infarction)
Michaelis' rhomboid
Michel clips
Michel's deformity
Michotte's syndrome
Mick applicator
micro
    m. curie-hour (μCi-hr)
    m. dip sets
microaneurysm
microangiogram
microcephalic
    m. dwarfism
microcephaly
microcoulomb
microcrania
microcurie (μCi)
microcystic kidney
microdosimetry
Microdot imager
microfarad
microfracture
micrognathia-glossoptosis
  syndrome
microgram (μcg)
microgyrus
Microlite
microlith
micromicrocurie
micron (μ)
micro-organisms
Micropaque
microphotogram
microphthalmia
microphthalmos syndrome
microradiogram
microradiography
microroentgen
microshock
microsphere
Microtrast
microtron
microvivisection

micturition
    m. cystourethrogram
    m. cystourethrography
mid-cristal ventricular septal
   defect
midaxillary
midbrain
midcarpal joint
midclavicular
midcoronal plane
Middeldorpf's tumor
middle
    m. cerebral artery (MCA)
    m. lobe (ML)
    m. lobe bronchus
    m. lobe syndrome
midfoot
midfrontal plane
midgut volvulus
midlateral orbital margin
midline
    m. echo
    m. granuloma
    m. shift
midnight fracture
midoccipital
midplane dose
midsagittal
    m. plane
midtalar line
midtalar-midcalcaneal angle
midtarsal joint
midtegmentum
midthoracic
migrating abscess
Mikaelsson
    M. hook
    M. visceral catheter
Mikulicz'
    M.' angle
    M.' disease
    M.' syndrome
Milch's osteonecrosis

mild-alkali syndrome
miliary
    m. abscess
    m. aneurysm
    m. nodule
    m. tuberculosis
military position
milk
    m. calcium bile
    m. of calcium bile
    m. of calcium renal stone
    m. teeth
milk-alkali syndrome
milk-allergy syndrome
milk-drinker's syndrome
milk-induced colitis
milk-of-calcium
milk-poisoning syndrome
milker's node
milking maneuver
Milkman's syndrome
Milkman-Looser syndrome
Miller
    M. double mushroom
       biliary stent set
    M. double mushroom stent
Miller's
    M.'s method
    M.'s position
    M.'s primary lobule
    M.'s secondary lobule
    M.'s syndrome
Miller-Abbott tube
Milles' syndrome
milliAmpere (mA)
milliAmpere-minute (mAm)
milliAmpere-seconds (mAs)
millicurie (mCi)
millicurie-hour (mCi-hr.)
milliequivalent (mEq)
milligamma
milligram hours (mgh)
milliliter (ml)

millimeter (mm) pattern
millimicrocurie or nanocurie (nc or NCi)
millimicrogram
millimicron
million electron volts (meV)
milliosmoles per kilogram (mOsm/kg)
millirad (mrad)
millirem (mrem)
millirep (mrep)
milliroentgen (mr)
milliroentgen per hour at one meter (mrhm)
millirutherford (mrd)
millisecond (msec) scanner
milliunit (mU)
millivolt (mV)
millosmole (mOsm)
Milroy's disease
mimicking
mimosa pattern
mineral oil aspiration
mini cerebral catheter
miniature radiography
minimal erythema dose (MED)
Minneapolis hip prosthesis
minometer
Mintec generator
minute ventilation
Miokon
miotic
Mirizzi's syndrome
Mirropaque
mirror image lung syndrome
miscibility
miscible
misonidazole (radiosensitizer)
misregistration
mithramycin
mitochondria
mitogenetic radiation
mitosis

mitotane (o,p-DDD)
mitral
   m. atresia
   m. calcification
   m. commissurotomy
   m. configuration
   m. funnel
   m. insufficiency (MI)
   m. leaflet
   m. murmur
   m. prosthesis
   m. regurgitation
   m. stenosis (MS)
   m. valve (MV)
   m. valve prolapse (MVP)
   m. valve replacement (MVR)
mixed
   m. aneurysm
   m. joint
Mixobar
Mixtner catheter
MKS (meter-kilogram-second)
ML (middle lobe)
ml (milliliter)
MLD (median lethal dose)
MLL-MLL adaptors
MLS (multiple line scan)
MLT (median lethal time)
mm (millimeter)
MMD (mean marrow dose)
MMFR (maximum midexpiratory flow rate)
MMM syndrome
M-mode (motion)
   M-m. display
   M-m. echocardiogram (ECHO)
   M-m. scanning
MNG (multinodular goiter)
99Mo (molybdenum)
MoAB (monoclonal antibody)
Moberg arthrodesis

mobile
  m. CT scanner
  m. radiography (portable)
  m. x-ray system
Mobin-Uddin vena caval filter
Möbius' syndrome
modality
mode
  blink m.
  negative m.
modified
  m. barium cookie swallow
  m. F. R. Thompson
    prosthesis
  m. Fuchs' method
  m. Hickey's method
  m. Kopans breast lesion
    localization needle
  m. Lysholm's method
  m. mastectomy
  m. scattering
  m. Titterington's method
  m. Valsalva's maneuver
  m. Waters' method
modulation
  amplitude m.
  brightness m.
  image m.
  m. transfer function (MTF)
  object m.
Moe plate
Moller-Barlow disease
Moller-Boeck disease
Moersch-Woltman syndrome
Mohr's syndrome
Mohr-Wriedt brachydactyly
Mohrenheim's space
Mohs' technique
moiety
molal solution
molality
molar volume
molecular
  m. force

  m. vibrations
molecule
Molnar retention disc
molybdenum-technetium
  generator
Molytech calibrator assay kit
momentum
Mönckeberg's arteriosclerosis
Mondini's pulmonary
  arteriovenous malformation
mongolism
monitor
  beam m.
  m. unit
  radiation m.
monitoring leads
Moniz' carotid siphon
monoarthritic
monochromatic
  m. radiation
monoclonal antibody (MCA or
  MoAB)
monocular stereoscope
monocyte
monoenergetic
  m. radiation
  m. x-ray
mononuclears
Monophen [2-(4-hydroxy-3,5-
  diiodobenzyl)-cyclohexane
  carboxylic acid]
monosodium urate
  monohydrate
Monospot test
monostotic fibrous dysplasia
Monro, foramen of
Monte Carlo method
Monteggia's
  M.'s dislocation
  M.'s fracture
  M.'s fracture-dislocation
  M.'s "reverse" fracture
Montercaux's fracture
moon sign

Moore
  M. adjustable nail
  M. blade plate
  M. hip prosthesis
  M. pin
Moore's fracture
Moore–Blount blade plate
morbus
  m. anglicus
  m. anglorum
  m. ceruleus
  m. coxae senilis
morcellation
Morgagni's
  M.'s crypt
  M.'s cyst
  M.'s hernia
  M.'s sinus
Morgagni, foramen of
Morgagni-Stewart-Morel
  syndrome
Morgagni-Turner-Albright
  syndrome
moribund
Morison's pouch
morphogenesis
morphological
morphology
Morquio's
  M.'s disease
  M.'s syndrome
Morris
  M. biphase screw
  M. catheter
mortice
mortise (ankle)
  m. joint
Morton's
  M.'s foot
  M.'s neuroma
  M.'s plane
  M.'s short first toe
  M.'s syndrome
  M.'s toe

Morujodol
mosaic sign
Moses
  M. curved safe-T-J wire
    guide
  M. guide
Mosley's method
mOsm (milliosmole)
mOsm/kg (milliosmoles per
  kilogram)
Mossbauer's spectrometer
Mosse's syndrome
motility study
motion
  blurring m.
  circular m.
  elliptical m.
  hypocycloidal m.
  linear m.
  m. artifact
  patient m.
  respiratory m.
  spiral m.
mottled
Mouchet's fracture
moulage sign
Moultier's sphincter
Mounier-Kuhn syndrome
movable
  m. core curved safe-T-J
    wire guide
  m. core multiple curved
    safe-T-J wire guide
  m. core straight safety wire
    guide
  m. joint
movement
  arc-to-arc m.
  arc-to-line m.
  circular m.
  hypocycloidal m.
  line-to-line m.
  linear m.
  m. artifacts

movement—*Continued*
  multidirectional m.
  symmetrical-
   unsymmetrical m.
moving grid
moyamoya disease
Moynihan's position
MPC (maximum permissible
  concentration)
MPD (maximum permissible
  dose)
MPI DTPA kit (chelate)
MPJ (metacarpophalangeal
  joint)
MR (magnetic resonance)
mr (milliroentgen)
MR MAX (magnetic resonance
  imaging system)
mrad (millirad)
mrd (millirutherford)
mrem (millirem)
mrep or millirep (milliroentgen
  equivalent physical)
mrhm (milliroentgen/hour at 1
  meter)
MRI (magnetic resonance
  imaging)
MRS (magnetic resonance
  spectroscopy)
MS (mitral stenosis)
MSE (multiple spin echo)
msec (millisecond)
MSP (median sagittal plane)
MT (metatarsal)
MTF (modulation transfer
  function)
MTP (metatarsophalangeal)
MTPJ (metatarsophalangeal joint)
mU (milliunit)
mucinous
  m. carcinoma
  m. tumor
mucocele
mucoepidermoid carcinoma

mucolipidosis
  m. II
  m. III
Mucomyst (acetylcysteine)
mucoperiosteal line
mucoperiosteum
mucopolysaccharidosis
  m. B
  m. I
  m. II
  m. III
  m. IV
  m. V
  m. VI
mucosa, s.
  mucosae or mucosas, pl.
mucosae or mucosas, pl.
  mucosa, s.
mucosal
  m. atrophy
  m. neuroma
mucosas or mucosae, pl.
  mucosa, s.
mucoserous dyssecretosis
mucous
  m. colitis
  m. gland
mucous (adj.)
mucoviscidosis
mucronate
mucus (n.)
Mueller biliary drainage
  catheter
MUGA (multigated acquisition)
  scan
Müller's
  M.'s cyst
  M.'s ducts
  M.'s maneuver
Müller-Damman
  procedure
Müller-Weiss syndrome
müllerian tumor
Mulsopaque

multangula, pl.
  multangulum, s.
multangular (bone)
  greater m. b.
  lesser m. b.
multangulum, s.
  multangula, pl.
multi-med catheter
multi-med triple-lumen
  infusion catheter
multiarticular
multiaxial joint
multichannel analyzer
multicrystal camera
multicystic
  m. kidney
  m. nephroma
  m. structure
multidirectional
  m. movement
  m. polytome
multiecho coronal image
multifaceted
multifidus spinae
multifocal osteomyelitis
multiformat camera
multiforme
  erythema m.
  glioblastoma m.
multigated
  m. acquisition (MUGA)
    analysis scan
  m. angiographic scan
  m. angiography
  m. blood pool (MUGA)
    study
  m. imaging
multigravida
multihole collimator
multilanigraph
multilocular
  m. cystic nephroma
  m. renal cyst
  m. vesicle

multiloculated
  m. abscess
  m. structure
multimodality
  m. display
  m. treatment
multinodular
  m. goiter (MNG)
  m. tuberculosis
multipara
multiparity
multiplanar
  m. imaging
  m. reformation
  m. scanner
multiple
  m. calcified foci
  m. cancellous exostosis
  m. cartilaginous exostosis
  m. congenital
    osteochondromata
  m. curved safe-T-J wire
    guide
  m. enchondromata
    syndrome
  m. endocrine
    adenomatosis (MEA)
    syndrome
  m. fracture
  m. gated acquisition
    (MUGA)
  m. hamartoma syndrome
  m. infarct dementia
  m. lentigines syndrome
  m. line scan (MLS)
  m. line scanning method
  m. line-scan imaging
  m. myeloma
  m. neurofibromatosis
  m. plane imaging
  m. plane integral
    reconstruction
  m. radiography
  m. scleromalacia

multiple—*Continued*
  m. sclerosis
  m. sensitive point method
  m. spin echo (MSE)
  m. spin echo total volume
    imaging
multiplex
multiplying digital-to-analog
  converter (MDAC)
multipurpose tubing adapter
multiscaler
multisection cassette
multislice
  m. full-line scan
  m. modified KWE direct
    Fourier imaging
  m. scanner
multitomography
multiwire proportional
  chamber
mummify
Münchmeyer's syndrome
Munro's abscess
Munro Kerr cesarean section
mural aneurysm
murderer's thumb
Murk-Jansen syndrome
murmur
  amphoric m.
  aneurysmal m.
  aortic m.
  apical diastolic m.
  arterial m.
  asymptomatic m.
  cardiac m.
  congenital m.
  crescendo m.
  diastolic m.
  ejection m.
  innocent m.
  mitral m.
  noninvasive m.
  pansystolic m.

pleuropericardial m.
prediastolic m.
presystolic m.
pulmonic m.
regurgitant m.
subclavicular m.
systolic m.
tricuspid m.
vascular m.
venous m.
Murphy-Pattee test
muscles
  abdomen
    cremaster
    obliquus externus
      abdominis
    obliquus internus
      abdominis
    pyramidalis
    quadratus lumborum
    rectus abdominis
    sphincter pylori
    transversalis
      abdominis
    transversus abdominis
  arm and forearm
    abductor pollicis
      longus
    anconeus
    biceps brachii
    brachialis
    brachioradialis
    coracobrachialis
    extensor carpi radialis
      brevis
    extensor carpi radialis
      longus
    extensor carpi ulnaris
    extensor digiti minimi
    extensor digiti quinti
      proprius
    extensor digitorum
      communis

extensor indicis
extensor ossis
    metacarpi pollicis
extensor pollicis
    brevis
extensor pollicis
    longus
extensor primi
    internodii pollicis
extensor secundi
    internodii pollicis
flexor carpi radialis
flexor carpi ulnaris
flexor digitorum
    profundus
flexor digitorum
    sublimis
flexor digitorum
    superficialis
flexor pollicis longus
palmaris longus
pronator quadratus
pronator teres
radiocarpus
subanconeus
supinator
supinator longus
supinator radii brevis
triceps brachii
back
    accessorius
    biventer cervicis
    cervicalis ascendens
    complexus
    erector spinae
    iliocostalis cervicis
    iliocostalis dorsi
    iliocostalis lumborum
    iliocostalis thoracis
    interspinales
    intertransversarii
    latissimus dorsi
    levator scapulae

longissimus capitis
longissimus cervicis
longissimus dorsi
longissimus thoracis
lumbosacralis
multifidus
multifidus spinae
obliquus capitis
    inferior
obliquus capitis
    superior
rectus capitis
    posterior major
rectus capitis
    posterior minor
rhomboideus major
rhomboideus minor
rotatores
rotatores spinae
sacrolumbalis
sacrospinalis
semispinalis capitis
semispinalis cervicis
semispinalis colli
semispinalis dorsi
semispinalis thoracis
serratus posterior
    inferior
serratus posterior
    superior
spinalis capitis
spinalis cervicis
spinalis thoracis
splenius capitis
splenius cervicis
splenius colli
supraspinatus
suspensorius duodeni
trachelomastoid
transversalis colli
trapezius
ear
    antitragicus

muscles—*Continued*
   helicis major
   helicis minor
   obliquus auriculae
   stapedius
   tensor tympani
   tragicus
   transversus auriculae
  foot
   abductor digiti quinti
   abductor hallucis
   abductor minimi digiti
   adductor hallucis
   adductor obliquus
    hallucis
   adductor transversus
    hallucis
   extensor digitorum
    brevis
   flexor accessorius
   flexor brevis minimi
    digiti
   flexor digiti quinti
    brevis
   flexor digitorum
    brevis
   flexor hallucis brevis
   interosseus dorsalis
    pedis
   interosseus plantaris
   lumbricales pedis
   pronator pedis
   quadratus plantae
   transversus pedis
  general
   arrectores pilorum
  hand
   abductor digiti
    minimi
   abductor digiti quinti
   abductor pollicis
    brevis
   abductor pollicis
    longus

   adductor pollicis
   flexor brevis minimi
    digiti
   flexor digiti quinti
    brevis
   flexor pollicis brevis
   interossei dorsales
    manus
   interossei palmares
   interossei volares
   lumbricales manus
   opponens digiti
    minimi
   opponens digiti quinti
   opponens pollicis
   palmaris brevis
  head and face
   attolins aurem
   attrahens aurem
   auricularis anterior
   auricularis posterior
   auricularis superior
   buccinator
   caninus
   choroideus
   ciliaris
   compressor naris
   corrugator supercilli
   depressor alae nasi
   depressor anguli oris
   depressor labii
    inferioris
   depressor septi
   dilatator naris anterior
   dilatator naris
    posterior
   epicranium
   frontalis
   levator anguli oris
   levator labii inferioris
   levator labii superioris
   levator labii superioris
    alaeque nasi
   levator menti

levator palpebrae
  superioris
masseter
mentalis
nasalis
obliquus oculi inferior
occipitalis
occipitofrontalis
orbicularis oculi
orbicularis oris
orbicularis
  palpebrarum
orbitalis
orbitopalpebralis
procerus
pterygoideus lateralis
pterygoideus medialis
pyramidalis nasi
quadratus labii
  inferioris
quadratus labii
  superioris
quadratus menti
rectus externus or
  lateralis
rectus inferior
rectus internus or
  medialis
rectus superior
retrahens aurem
risorius
temporalis
tensor tarsi
triangularis
zygomaticus major
zygomaticus minor
hip, thigh, lower extremity
  adductor brevis
  adductor longus
  adductor magnus
  articularis genu
  biceps femoris
  crureus
  gemellus inferior

gemellus superior
gluteus maximus
gluteus medius
gluteus minimus
gracilis
iliacus
obturator externus
obturator internus
pectineus
piriformis
psoas major
psoas minor
pyriformis
quadratus femoris
quadriceps extensor
  femoris
quadriceps femoris
rectus femoris
sartorius
semimembranosus
semitendinosus
subcrureus
tensor fasciae femoris
tensor fasciae latae
vastus intermedius
vastus lateralis
vastus medialis
larynx and epiglottis
  aryepiglotticus
  arytenoideus
  cricoarytenoideus
    lateralis
  cricoarytenoideus
    posterior
  cricothyroideus
  thyreoarytenoideus
  thyreoepiglotticus
leg
  extensor digitorum
    longus
  extensor hallucis
    longus
  extensor proprius
    hallucis

muscles—*Continued*
    flexor digitorum
        longus
    flexor hallucis longus
    gastrocnemius
    peroneus brevis
    peroneus longus
    peroneus tertius
    plantaris
    popliteus
    soleus
    tibialis anterior
    tibialis posterior
neck
    amygdaloglossus
    azygos uvulae
    cephalopharyngeus
    circumflexus palati
    constrictor pharyngis
        inferior
    constrictor pharyngis
        medius
    constrictor pharyngis
        superior
    digastricus
    genioglossus
    geniohyoglossus
    geniohyoideus
    glossopalatinus
    hyoglossus
    hyopharyngeus
    laryngopharyngeus
    latissimus colli
    levator palati
    levator veli palatini
    lingualis
    longus capitis
    longus cervicis
    longus colli
    mylohyoideus
    omohyoideus
    palatoglossus
    palatopharyngeus
    pharyngopalatinus

platysma
rectus capitis anterior
rectus capitis anticus
    major
rectus capitis anticus
    minor
rectus capitis lateralis
salpingopharyngeus
scalenus anterior
scalenus medius
scalenus posterior
sphenosalpingostaphylin
sternocleidomatoideus
sternohyoideus
sternothyreoideus
styloglossus
stylohyoideus
stylopharyngeus
tensor palati
tensor veli palatini
tetragonus
thyreohyoideus
uvulae
perineum
    accelerator urinae
    bulbocavernosus
    coccygeus
    compressor urethra
    constrictor urethrae
    corrugator cutis ani
    depressor urethrae
    erector clitoridis
    erector penis
    ischiocavernosus
    ischiococcygeus
    levator ani
    sphincter ani externus
    sphincter ani internus
    sphincter urethrae
        membranaceae
    sphincter vaginae
    sphincter vesicae
    transversus perinei
        profundus

transversus perinei
  superficialis
shoulder
  deltoideus
  infraspinatus
  pectoralis major
  pectoralis minor
  serratus anterior
  serratus magnus
  subclavius
  subscapularis
  supraspinatus
  teres major
  teres minor
thorax
  diaphragma
  infracostales
  intercostales externus
  intercostales internus
  levatores costarum
  subcostales
  transversus thoracis
  triangularis sterni
muscular
  m. cirrhosis
  m. dystrophy
muscularis
musculature
musculoskeletal
musculotendinous
musculus suspensorium
  duodeni
mushroom
  m. catheter
  m. worker's disease
  m. worker's syndrome
mustache sign
Mustard procedure
mutation
mutational dysostosis
MV (megavoltage)
mv (millivolt)
MV (mitral valve)
MVP (mitral valve prolapse)

MVR (mitral valve
  replacement)
MVV (maximal voluntary
  ventilation)
Mx (Medx)
Myà's disease
myalgia
mycetoma pedis
mycosis fungoides (MF)
mycotic aneurysm
myelencephalitis
myelencephalon
myeleterosis
myelin kidney
myelinoclasis
myelitis
myelo-opticoneuropathy
myelo-osteomusculodysplasia
  hereditaria
myeloarchitecture
myeloblast
myelocele
myelocisternoencephalography
myeloclast
myelocoele
myelocone
myelocyst
myelocystocele
myelocystomeningocele
myelodysplasia
myeloencephalic
myelofibrosis
myelofugal
myelogenesis
myelogram
myelography
  cervical m.
  computed m.
  gas m.
  lumbar m.
  m. needle
  metrizamide m.
  opaque m.
  positive contrast m.

myelography—*Continued*
  thoracic m.
myelography needles
myeloid metaplasia
myelolipoma
myelolysis
myeloma
  endothelial m.
  giant cell m.
  indolent m.
  multiple m.
  osteosclerotic m.
  plasma cell m.
  plasma m.
  solitary m.
myelomatosis
myelomeningitis
myelomeningocele
myelomere
myelomyces
myelon
myelopathic
  m. albuminosuria
  m. polycythemia
myelopathy
  apoplectiform m.
  ascending m.
  compression m.
  concussion m.
  descending m.
  focal m.
  funicular m.
  hemorrhagic m.
  interstitial m.
  parenchymatous m.
  sclerosing m.
  spondylotic cervical m.
  systemic m.
  transverse m.
  traumatic m.
myelopetal
myelophage
myelophthisis
myeloplax

myelopoiesis
  ectopic m.
  extramedullary m.
myeloradiculodysplasia
myeloschisisopoiesis
myeloscintogram
myelosuppression
myelotherapy
myenteric plexus of
  Auerbach
Myer-McKeever fracture
Myler catheter
Mylicon (simethicone)
mylohyoid
  m. groove
  m. ridge
mylohyoideus
myo-ossificatio progressiva
  multiplex
myoasthenia
myoblastoma
Myobock artificial hand
myobradia
myocardiac
myocardial
  m. calcification
  m. contusion
  m. infarct imaging
  m. infarction (MI)
  m. ischemia
  m. necrosis
  m. perforation
  m. perfusion
  m. perfusion imaging
myocardiogram
myocardiography
myocardiolysis
myocardiopathy
  alcoholic m.
  chagasic m.
myocardiorrhaphy
myocarditis
  acute bacterial m.
  acute isolated m.

chronic m.
diphtheritic m.
fibrous m.
Fiedler's m.
fragmentation m.
giant cell m.
idiopathic m.
interstitial m.
parenchymatous m.
rheumatic m.
toxic m.
tuberculous m.
myocardium
myocele
myoceptor
myocerosis
myodegeneration
Myodil (ethyl
   iodophenylundecylate)
myodynamics
myodynamometer
myodystrophia congenita
myodystrophy
myoendocarditis
myoepithelial
myoepithelioma
myofascitis
myofibril
myofibrilla, s.
   myofibrillae, pl.
myofibrillae, pl.
   myofibrilla, s.
myogram
myography
myokinesis
myolipoma
myometer
myometrium
myoneural junction

myopathia
   m. osteoplastica
   m. osteoplastica
      progressiva
myopathy
   centronuclear m.
   distal m.
   myotubular m.
   nemaline m.
   ocular m.
   rod m.
myoplastic
myopolar
myosarcoma
myoschwannoma
myositis
   interstitial m.
   m. ossificans
   m. ossificans multiplex
      progressiva
   m. ossificans progressiva
   m. purulenta
   rheumatoid m.
   suppurative m.
myosteoma
myotatic
myotonia atrophica
myotubular myopathy
myxadenoma
myxedema
   circumscribed m.
   papular m.
   pituitary m.
   pretibial m.
myxoblastoma
myxochondrofibrosarcoma
myxochondroma
myxoglobulosis
myxosarcoma

Nn

N electron
N shell
N-(2-6-dimethylphenylcarbamoyl) methyliminodiaetacid; biliary imaging study (HIDA)
NA (Nomina Anatomica)
Na atom
nabothian gland
NACOR (National Advisory Committee on Radiation)
NAD (no active disease)
Naffziger's syndrome
Nägele's pelvis
Nager-de Reynier syndrome
NaI (sodium iodide)
nail
>Austin Moore n.
>Enders n.
>fixation n.
>Hansen-Street diamond-shaped n.
>interlocking IM (intramedullary) n.
>Jewett n.
>n. blade appliance
>Neufeld n.
>Plummer n.
>Smillie n.
>Smith-Peterson n.
>triflanged n.
nail-patella syndrome
nanocephalic dwarfism
nanocurie or millimicrocurie (nc or nCi)
nanogram (ng)
nanomelia

napkin ring
>n. defect
>n. deformity
>n. lesion
nares, pl.
>naris, s.
naris, s.
>nares, pl.
narrow
>n. beam half-thickness
>n. lumbar spinal canal syndrome
>n. polyposis
narrow-angle tomography
nasal
>n. bone
>n. catheter
>n. fossa
>n. septum
>n. suture
nasalis
nasion postcondylare plane
naso-oral
nasoantral
nasofrontal duct
nasogastric (NG)
>n. catheter
>n. tube
nasolabial lymph node
nasolacrimal
>n. canal
>n. duct
nasomaxillary suture
nasopalatine canal
nasopharyngeal
>n. carcinoma (NPC)
>n. torticollis

nasopharyngography
nasopharynx
nasopineal angle
nasoseptal
nasoseptitis
nasosinusitis
nasospinale
nasotracheal catheter
nasoturbinal
NAT (nonaccidental trauma)
National Advisory Committee
  on Radiation (NACOR)
National Council for Radiation
  Protection and
  Measurements (NCRP)
National Electrical
  Manufacturers Association
  (NEMA)
Natritope
natural radioactivity
navicular
    n. fracture
    n. joint
    n. projection
nc or nCi (nanocurie or
  millimicrocurie)
NCAS (neocarzinostatin)
NCRP (National Council for
  Radiation Protection and
  Measurements)
Neal catheter
near
    n. field
    n. syncope
    n. ultraviolet
nearthrosis
nebula frontalis
NEC (necrotizing enterocolitis)
neck extension position
necrosis
    aseptic n.
    avascular n.
    Friedrich's n.

necrotizing enterocolitis (NEC)
NED (no evidence of disease)
needle
    Ackermann biopsy n.
    arterial venous
      catheterization n.
    B-D thin-wall n.
    Baltaxe-Mitty-Pollack
      coaxial n.
    Barth biliary drainage n.
    bird's eye n.
    Blakemore n.
    butterfly n.
    Chiba biopsy n.
    Chiba transhepatic
      cholangiography n.
    Cloward n.
    Cone n.
    Cook modified
      percutaneous entry n.
    Cook percutaneous entry
      teflon catheter n.
    Cook winged percutaneous
      entry n.
    Cournand n.
    Craig n.
    Curry n.
    Dos Santos n.
    Franseen lung biopsy n.
    Franseen n.
    gas-tight n.
    Goetz n.
    Greene biopsy n.
    Haaga biopsy n.
    Hinck myelography n.
    Hinck spinal n. with depth
      guide
    Hunt n.
    Indian Club n.
    Jamshidi n.
    Kahn n.
    Kopans n.
    Lee and Westcott n.

Lee n.
Lindeman n.
Madayag n.
Menghini n.
Menghini thin-wall
  Silverman n.
modified Kopans breast
  lesion localization n.
myelography n.
n. wire guide obturator
original Turner biopsy n.
pencil point percutaneous
  entry n.
PercuGuide n.
percutaneous n.
Pfister nephrostomy n.
portal vein n.
Potts modified
  percutaneous entry n.
Quincke-Babcock spinal n.
radium n.
Riley n.
Ring drainage catheter n.
Ring n.
Robb n.
Rotex n.
Seldinger n.
shark jaw biopsy n.
sheathed Chiba n.
splenic n.
standard catheter n.
Teflon sheath n. sets
translumbar aortic
  catheter n.
trocar n.
TruCut n.
Tuohy n.
Turkel n.
Turner biopsy n.
vanSonnenberg biopsy n.
  set
Vim-Silverman n.
Westcott n.

Zavala lung biopsy n.
Neer
  N. humeral head
    prosthesis
  N. shoulder prosthesis
Neer's
  N.'s I fracture
  N.'s II fracture
negative
  n. charge
  n. direction
  n. electron
  n. emission
  n. ion
  n. mode
  n. mode mammogram
  n. pi meson
  n. terminal
  n. torsion
negatoscope
negatron
  n. emission
negligence
negligible individual
Neil-Gilmour classification
Nélaton catheter
Nélaton's
  N.'s dislocation
  N.'s fold
  N.'s sphincter
Nelson's
  N.'s segment
  N.'s syndrome
NEMA (National Electrical
  Manufacturers Association)
nemaline myopathy
neocarzinostatin (NCAS)
Neo-Cholex (fat emulsion
  containing pure vegetable
  oil)
neodymium (Nd)
Neohydrin Hg-203
Neo-Hydriol fluid (viscous)

Neo-Iodipin
Neo-Iopax
Neo-Methiodal
neon
neonatal osteomyelitis
neoplasia
neoplastic
   n. appearance
   n. fibrosis
   n. fracture
   n. lesion
Neoscan (gallium citrate Ga67)
Neo-Skiodan
neostigmine
Neo-Tenebryl
nephradenoma
nephrelcosis
nephridia, pl.
   nephridium, s.
nephridium, s.
   nephridia, pl.
nephritic
nephritides or nephritises, pl.
   nephritis, s.
nephritis, s.
   nephritises or nephritides,
   pl.
nephritises or nephritides, pl.
   nephritis, s.
nephroabdominal
nephroangiography
nephroblastoma
   cystic differentiated n.
   polycystic n.
nephrocalcinosis infantum
nephrogram phase
nephrography
nephrohypertrophy
nephrolithiasis
nephroma
   mesoblastic n.
   multicystic n.
   multilocular cystic n.
nephromegaly

nephronophthisis
nephropathy
nephroses, pl.
   nephrosis, s.
nephrosis
   Finnish-type n.
nephrosis, s.
   nephroses, pl.
nephrosonography
nephrostolithotomy
nephrostomy catheter
nephrotomogram
nephrotomography
   bolus injection n.
   infusion n.
nephrotoxicity
nephrourogram
nephrourography
neprhoma
   embryonal n.
neptunium (Np)
nerve
   n. root sleeves
   vidian n.
Neufeld nail
Neuhauser-Berenberg
   syndrome
neural
   n. arch
   n. canal
   n. foramen
neurilemmitis
neurilemoma
neurinoma
neurinomatosis centralis
neuroanatomy
neuroangiographic
neuroangiomatosis
   encephalofacialis
neuroarthromyodysplasia
neuroarthropathy
neuroastrocytoma
neuroblastoma
neurocentral joint

neurocytoma
neurodiagnostic scanner
neuroectodermal
neuroembryology
neurofibromatosis
neurofibrosarcoma
neurogenic
    n. arthropathy
    n. bladder
    n. fracture
    n. sarcoma
    n. tumor
neuroglia, pl.
    neuroglion, s.
neurogliocytoma
neuroglion, s.
    neuroglia, pl.
neurohypophyseal
neurological
neuroma
    acoustic n.
    mucosal n.
    trigeminal n.
neuromeningeal
neuromuscular scoliosis
neuron
neuro-oculocutaneous
  angiomatosis
neuropathic
    n. arthropathy
    n. joint
neuropraxia
neuroradiologic
neuroradiology
neuroroentgenography
neurosarcoma
neurosciences
NeuroSector real-time
  ultrasound (U/S or US)
neuroses, pl.
    neurosis, s.
neurosis, s.
    neuroses, pl.
neurotica arthropathia

neurotomography
neurotrophic osteopathy
neurovasculotropic
  osteoporosis
neutral
    n. atom
    n. position
neutralization plate
neutrino
neutron
    epithermal n.
    fast n.
    intermediate n.
    n. absorption process
    n. activation analysis
    n. bombardment
    n. number
    slow n.
    thermal n.
neutrophil
nevi, pl.
    nevus, s.
nevoid basal cell carcinoma
  syndrome
nevus, s.
    nevi, pl.
New England Baptist
  acetabular cup
Newton
    N. cerebral catheter
    N. cerebral curved safe-T-J
      wire guide
    N. cerebral straight safety
      wire guide
Newton's
    N. law of action-reaction
    N. law of motion
Newvicon camera
NFS (no fracture shown)
ng (nanogram)
NHL (non-Hodgkin's
  lymphoma)
niche
    Barclay's n.

niche—*Continued*
  Haudeck's n.
Nicholas' disease
nickel chloride (Ni-63)
Nicoll
  N. blade plate
  N. bone graft
nidus
Nielsen's disease
Niemann-Pick syndrome
Nierhoff-Hübner syndrome
Nievergelt-Erb syndrome
Nievergelt-Pcarlman syndrome
Nievergelt's syndrome
nightstick fracture
NIH angiographic catheter
niobium (Nb)
Niopam
nipple
  n. inversion
  n. markers
  n. shadow
NIRL (negligible individual
  radiation level)
Nishimoto-Takeuchi-Kudo
  disease
Nissen plate
Nissen's
  N.'s fundoplication
  N.'s gastrectomy
  N.'s procedure
nitrofurantoin
nitrogen
NMR (nuclear magnetic
  resonance)
NMT (Nuclear Medicine
  Technology)
NMTCB (Nuclear Medicine
  Technology Certification
  Board)
no
  n. active disease (NAD)
  n. evidence of disease
    (NED)

n. fracture shown (NFS)
n. line of demarcation
No (nobelium)
Noack's syndrome
nobelium (No)
Noble's position
nocardiosis
nodal arrhymthia
node
  Aschoff-Tawara n.
  periaortic n.
nodes
  abdominal lymph n.
  anorectal lymph n.
  aortic lymph n.
  aortic n.
  aortic-pulmonic lymph n.
  aortocaval n.
  apical lymph n.
  appendicular lymph n.
  Aschoff-Tawara n.
  atrioventricular (AV) n.
  axillary lymph n.
  azygos lymph n.
  Bouchard's n.
  brachial lymph n.
  bronchopulmonary lymph
    n.
  buccal lymph n.
  buccinator lymph n.
  carinal n.
  caval lymph n.
  celiac lymph n.
  central lymph n.
  cervical lymph n.
  circumcardiac lymph n.
  Cloquet's n.
  colic lymph n.
  cubital lymph n.
  Delphian n.
  deltoideopectoral n.
  diaphragmatic lymph n.
  Dürck's n.
  Edward's n.

epicolic lymph n.
facial lymph n.
Flack's n.
foraminal n.
gastric lymph n.
gastroepiploic lymph n.
gastro-omental lymph n.
gluteal lymph n.
gouty n.
Haygarth's n.
Heberden's n.
hemal n.
Hensen's n.
hepatic lymph n.
hilar lymph n.
ileocolic lymph n.
iliac circumflex lymph n.
inguinal lymph n.
intercostal lymph n.
interiliac lymph n.
interpectoral lymph n.
jugular lymph n.
jugulodigastric lymph n.
jugulo-omohyoid lymph n.
juxtaintestinal n.
Keith's n.
lacunar n.
Legendre's n.
lumbar lymph n.
lymph n.
malar lymph n.
mammary n.
mandibular lymph n.
mastoid lymph n.
mediastinal lymph n.
mesenteric lymph n.
mesocolic lymph n.
Meynet's n.
milker's n.
n. of anterior border of
    epiploic foramen
n. of Aschoff and Tawara
n. of neck of gallbladder
n. of Ranvier

nasolabial lymph n.
obturator lymph n.
occipital lymph n.
Osler's n.
pancreatic lymph n.
pancreaticoduodenal
    lymph n.
pancreaticosplenic lymph
    n.
para-aortic n.
paracardial lymph n.
paracolic lymph n.
paramammary lymph n.
pararectal lymph n.
parasternal lymph n.
paratracheal lymph n.
parauterine lymph n.
paravesicular lymph n.
parotid lymph n.
Parrot's n.
pectoral lymph n.
pelvic lymph n.
pericardial lymph n.
peroneal n.
phrenic lymph n.
popliteal lymph n.
postaortic lymph n.
postcaval lymph n.
prececal lymph n.
prelaryngeal n.
pretracheal n.
prevascular lymph n.
prevesicular lymph n.
primitive n.
pulmonary
    juxtaesophageal lymph
    n.
pulmonary lymph n.
pyloric lymph n.
rectal lymph n.
retroaortic lymph n.
retroauricular lymph n.
retrocecal lymph n.
retrocrural n.

nodes—*Continued*
  retroperitoneal lymph n.
  retropharyngeal lymph n.
  retropyloric n.
  Rosenmüller's n.
  Rotter's n.
  sacral lymph n.
  Schmidt's n.
  Schmorl's n.
  sentinel n.
  sigmoid lymph n.
  signal n.
  singer's n.
  sinoatrial n.
  sinus n.
  splenic lymph n.
  subcarinal n.
  submandibular lymph n.
  submental lymph n.
  syphilitic n.
  teacher's n.
  tracheal lymph n.
  tracheobronchial lymph n.
  triticeous n.
  Troisier's n.
  Virchow's n.
  vital n.
nodular subepidermal fibrosis
nodule
  acinar n.
  air-containing n.
  alveolar n.
  autonomous n.
  cold n.
  hot n.
  interstitial n.
  miliary n.
  pulmonary n.
  solitary n.
  thyroid n.
noduli, pl.
  nodulus, s.
nodulus, s.
  noduli, pl.

noise
noisy
Nolke's
  N.'s method
  N.'s position
Nomina Anatomica (NA)
nominal single dose (NSD)
nomogram
nomography
nonaccidental trauma (NAT)
nonarticular fracture
noncalcified
noncommunicating
  hydrocephalus
nonconductive
nondiagnostic
nondynamic slices
nonenhanced CAT scan
nonfiberoptic bronchoscopy
nonflocculating
nongated CT scan
nongoiterous
nongranulocyte
nongummatous
non-Hodgkin's lymphoma
  (NHL)
nonhomogeneous
noninvasive murmur
noninverted transposition
nonionic
  n. contrast media
  n. dimers
  n. monomers
nonionizing
nonlinear
  n. artifact
  n. partial volume artifact
nonlinearity
nonlipid reticuloendotheliosis
nonmagnetic
Nonne's syndrome
Nonne-Milroy-Meige
  syndrome
nonobstructive

non-ohmic resistor
nonopaque
nonossifying fibroma
nonosteogenic fibroma
nonoverlapping
nonparous
nonperfusion
nonrachitic bowleg in children
nonradiopaque
nonrotation of the colon
nonscreen
    n. film
    n. holder
nonseminomatous tumor
nonsequestrating osteomyelitis
nonspecific
    n. pneumonitis
    n. retroperitoneal
        inflammation
nonstriated muscle
nonsuppurative osteomyelitis
nontoxic
    n. goiter
    n. multinodular goiter
        (NTMNG)
nonuniformity
nonunion
nonvisualization
nonvisualized
Noonan's syndrome
noradrenaline
norepinephrine
Norland-Cameron photon
  densitometry
norma
    n. anterior
    n. basilaris
    n. facialis
    n. frontalis
    n. inferior
    n. lateralis
    n. occipitalis
    n. posterior
    n. sagittalis

    n. superior
    n. temporalis
    n. ventralis
    n. verticalis
normal
    n. AP view
    n. pressure hydrocephalus
        (NPH)
    n. standard dose (NSD)
    n. ventriculotruncal
        alignment
normalized plateau slope
Nosophen
nostril
Nosydrast
Nosylan
notch
    angular n.
    articular n.
    capitate n.
    cardiac n.
    cerebellar n.
    clavicular n.
    coracoid n.
    costal n.
    ethmoidal n.
    fibular n.
    infratragal n.
    interclavicular n.
    intercondylar n.
    intervertebral n.
    jugular n.
    mandibular n.
    n. sign
    radial n.
    scapular n.
    sciatic n.
    semilunar n.
    spinoglenoid n.
    sternal n.
    suprascapular n.
    suprasternal n.
    supratragal n.
    tentorial n.

notch—*Continued*
  trochlear n.
  vertebral n.
notochord
notomelus
Novopaque
NPC (nasopharyngeal
  carcinoma)
NPH (normal pressure
  hydrocephalus)
NRC (Nuclear Regulatory
  Commission)
NSD (nominal single dose)
NSD (normal standard dose)
NTMNG (nontoxic
  multinodular goiter)
"nubbin" sign
nuchal
  n. line
  n. rigidity
nuchofrontal projection
Nuck's canal
nuclear
  n. angiography
  n. cardiology
  n. decay
  n. disintegration
  n. emulsion
  n. energy
  n. fission
  n. force
  n. fusion
  n. imaging
  n. medicine
  n. notation
  n. particle
  n. probe
  n. pulse amplifier
  n. radiation
  n. reaction
  n. reactor
  n. relaxation
  n. scan
  n. scanner

n. scintigraphy
n. signal
n. spin
n. spin quantum number
n. structure
nuclear magnetic resonance
  (NMR)
    n. m. r. Fourier
      transformation
    n. m. r. image
    n. m. r. phantoms
    n. m. r. relaxation rate
      enhancement
    n. m. r. scanning sequence
    n. m. r. signal intensity
    n. m. r. spectral parameter
    n. m. r. spectrometer
    n. m. r. spin-warp method
    n. m. r. tomography
    pulsed n. m. r.
Nuclear Medicine
    N. M. Technology (NMT)
    N. M. Technology
      Certification Board
      (NMTCB)
    Society of Clinical N. M.
Nuclear Regulatory
  Commission (NRC)
nuclease
nuclei or nucleuses, pl.
    nucleus, s.
nucleide
nucleiform
nucleography
nucleoid
nucleoliform
nucleon number
nucleoprotein
nucleoreticulum
nucleoside
nucleotherapy
nucleotide
nucleus
    amygdaloid n.

atomic n.
caudate n.
daughter n.
lentiform n.
n. pulposus
parent n.
red n.
nucleus, s.
    nucleuses or nuclei, pl.
nucleuses or nuclei, pl.
    nucleus, s.
nuclide
nullipara
nulliparous
Nulsen-Spitz valve
number
    Avogadro's n.

effective atomic n.
Euler's n.
Hounsfield's n.
n. profile
nursemaid's elbow
nutation
Nutricath (catheter)
nutrient
    n. artery
    n. foramen
nutritional deficiency
    osteoporosis
Nyegaard
Nyquist theorem
nystagmus

Oo

OA (osteoarthritis)
oat cell carcinoma
O'Beirne's sphincter
obelion
Obersteiner-Redlich space
object
    o. modulation
object-film distance (OFD)
object-to-image receptor
  distance (OIRD)
oblique
    o. anteroposterior
      projection
    o. axial position
    o. (coned view) projection
    o. erect projection
    o. fracture
    o. head
    o. heart
    o. interlobar fissure
    o. orbital line
    o. position
    o. projection
    o. transfacial projection
    o. view
obliquity
obliquus
    o. auriculae
    o. capitis inferior
    o. capitis superior
    o. externus abdominis
    o. internus abdominis
    o. oculti inferior
obliterate
obliteration
    cortical o.
    fibrous o.
    o. of supra-aortic branches

obliterative
    o. brachiocephalic arteritis
    o. endocarditis
    o. pleuritis
oblongata, s.
    oblongatae or oblongatas,
      pl.
oblongatae or oblongatas, pl.
    oblongata, s.
oblongatas or oblongatae, pl.
    oblongata, s.
Obrinsky's syndrome
obscure
obstetrical position
obstipation
obstruction
    atrial o.
    biliary o.
    bronchial o.
    cystic duct o.
    esophageal o.
    intestinal o.
    intraductal o.
    mechanical o.
    renal o.
    small bowel o. (SBO)
    transhepatic o.
    ureteral o.
    ureteropelvic junction
      (UPJ) o.
    ureterovesical junction o.
    urinary tract o.
obstructive
    o. carcinoma
    o. cardiomyopathy
    o. cirrhosis
    o. collapse
    o. diverticulitis

obstructive—*Continued*
   o. emphysema
   o. hydrocephalus
   o. jaundice
   o. pulmonitis
   o. thrombus
obstruent
obtund
obturator
   o. artery
   o. externus muscle
   o. foramen
   o. groove
   o. internus muscle
   o. line
   o. lymph node
   o. muscle
   o. nerve
   o. sign
   o. vein
obviate
"obui-himo" syndrome
occipital
   o. anteroposterior
     projection
   o. artery
   o. bone
   o. groove
   o. gyrus
   o. horn
   o. lobe
   o. lymph node
   o. nerve
   o. pole
   o. projection
   o. sinus
   o. sulcus
   o. vein
   o. vertebra
occipitalis muscle
occipitalization
occipitoanterior position
occipitoatloid
occipitoaxoid

occipitobasilar
occipitobregmatic
occipitocervical
occipitofrontal projection
occipitofrontalis muscle
occipitomastoid suture
occipitomental (OM) position
occipitoparietal suture
occipitoposterior position
occipitosacral position
occipitotemporal gyrus
occipitothalamic radiation
occipitotransverse position
occiput
   o. anterior position
   o. posterior position
   o. sacral position
   o. transverse position
occlude
occluder
   Tuohy-Bost o.
occluding
   o. fracture frame
   o. thrombus
occlusal
   o. film technique
   o. line
   o. position
   o. projection
occlusion
occular
   o. muscle palsy
   o. myopathy
occult
   o. blood
   o. fracture
occulta
occupational lung disease
OCG (operative
   cholangiogram)
OCG (oral cholecystogram)
ochronosis
Ochsner's
   O.'s muscle

O.'s position
octet rule
ocular myopathy
oculoauricular dysplasia
oculoauriculovertebral
  dysplasia
oculocerebrorenal syndrome
oculodento-osseous dysplasia
oculodentodigital syndrome
oculoplethysmography
  (OPG)
oculo-urethro-articular
  syndrome
oculovertebral dysplasia
OD (outside diameter)
Odelberg's disease
Odelca camera unit
Odman-Ledin catheter
O'Donoghue's triad
odontic
odontoameloblastoma
odontoblastoma
odontogenic fibromyxoma
odontogram
odontography
odontoid
    o. apophysis
    o. process
    o. projection
    o. vertebra
odontoma
odontopathy
odontoradiography
odynophagia
Oe (oersted)
oersted (Oe)
OFD (object-film distance)
off-center
    o. field
    o. position
off-line processing
offset corrections
OGD (old granulomatous
  disease)

Ohio Nuclear Delta
  (manufacturer)
    O. N. D. 2000 scanner
    O. N. D. 50 FS scanner
ohm
Ohm's law
ohmic resistor
ohmmeter
OIH (orthoiodohippurate)
oil-based
oil-cooled tube
OIRD (object-to-image receptor
  distance)
old granulomatous disease
  (OGD)
olecranon
    o. fossa
    o. fracture
    o. ligament
    o. process
    o. screw
olegranuloma
oleic acid
    o. a. I-125 capsules
    o. a. iodine-131
oleoperitoneography
oleothorax
Oleotope
olfactory
    o. bulb
    o. foramen
    o. gland
    o. gyrus
    o. labyrinth
    o. nerve
    o. sulcus
    o. tract
oligoarthritis
oligoarticular
oligocystic
oligodactylia syndrome
oligodactyly
oligodendrocyte
oligodendroglioma

oligohydramnios
oliva
    o. cerebellaris
oliva, s.
    olivae, pl.
olivae, pl.
    oliva, s.
olive
    cerebellar o.
    inferior o.
    superior o.
olive-tip catheter
olivocerebellar tract
olivopontocerebellar
olivospinal
Ollier's
    O.'s disease
    O.'s syndrome
Ollier-Trenaunay-Klippel
  syndrome
OM (occipitomental)
omagra
omarthritis
Ombanja
OMBL (orbitomeatal baseline)
Omega
    O. C balloon transluminal
      angioplasty catheter
    O. NV balloon transluminal
      angioplasty catheter
omega-shaped sella
omenta, pl.
    omentum, s.
omental
    o. apron
    o. bursa
    o. cyst
    o. hernia
    o. sac
omentoportography
omentum
    gastrocolic o.
    gastrosplenic o.
    pancreaticosplenic o.

    splenogastric o.
omentum, s.
    omenta, pl.
OML (orbitomeatal line)
Ommaya
Omnipaque (iohexol)
omoblastoma
omocephalus
omodynia
omohyoideus muscle
omoplata
omosternum
omovertebral process
omphalocele
omphalomesenteric
    o. artery
    o. duct
    o. vein
    o. vessels
oncocytoma
oncology
    radiation o.
oncotherapy
Oncotrac
ondometer
one million electron volts
  (meV)
one thousand electron volts
  (keV)
one-part percutaneous entry
  needle
one-way stopcock
onychodystrophy
onycholysis
onycho-osteoarthral dysplasia
oocyesis
oogeneses, pl.
    oogenesis, s.
oogenesis, s.
    oogeneses, pl.
OOP (out of plaster)
oophorectomy
oophoron
opacification

opacified
Opacin
opacity
    Caspar's ring o.
Opacol
opaque
    o. arthrography
    o. enema
    o. injection
    o. meal
    o. media
    o. myelography
    o. suture
Oparenol
o,p-DDD (mitotane)
OPD syndrome
    (otopalatodigital) syndrome
open
    o. bronchus sign
    o. fracture
    o. spina bifida
    o. type of sella
open-core transformer
open-mouth
    o. odontoid view
    o. projection
    o. view
opening of Moniz' siphon
operating voltage
operative
    o. cholangiogram (OCG)
    o. cholangiography (OCG)
operculum
OPG (oculoplethysmography)
OPG (orthopantomography)
ophryon
ophthalmic
    o. artery
    o. nerve
    o. vein
ophthalmography
ophthalmology
ophthalmopathy
opisthion

opisthocranion
opisthognathism
opisthotonos position
OPLL (ossification of the
    posterior longitudinal
    ligament)
Oppenheim's gait
opponens
    o. digiti minimi muscle
    o. digiti quinti muscle
    o. minimi digiti muscle
    o. pollicis muscle
opposed fields
Opraflex incise drape
oprocemic acid
optic
    o. canal
    o. chiasm glioma
    o. chiasma
    o. cup
    o. density
    o. disk
    o. foramen
    o. granuloma
    o. groove
    o. nerve
    o. papilla
    o. radiation
    o. recess
    o. scanner
    o. tract
    o. vesicle
optimal
optimum
Optiplanimat automated unit
ora, pl. (mouth)
    os, s. (mouth)
Orabilex
orad
Oragrafin
    O. calcium (ipodate
      calcium)
    O. sodium (ipodate
      sodium)

O'Rahilly, classification of
oral
    o. cholecystogram (OCG)
    o. choleystography (OCG)
    o. fractionated dose
    o. urography
oral-facial-digital (OFD)
    syndrome
Oratrast (barium sulfate,
    sucrose, sodium saccharin,
    and suspending agents)
Oravue
orbicularis
    o. oculi muscle
    o. oris muscle
    o. palpebrarum muscle
orbit
    blow-out fracture of the o.
orbita
orbital
    o. abscess
    o. aneurysm
    o. arch
    o. artery
    o. base
    o. electron
    o. fat
    o. fissure
    o. fracture
    o. gyrus
    o. hemangioma
    o. plane
    o. plate
    o. pneumotomography
    o. region
    o. ridge
    o. sulcus
  orbitalis muscle
orbitography
Orbitome tomographic system
orbitomeatal
    o. baseline (OMBL)
    o. line (OML)

    o. plane
orbitopalpebralis muscle
orbitoparietal oblique
    projection
Orbix x-ray unit
organ tolerance dose (OTD)
organic brain syndrome
organized thrombus
organoaxial rotation
organography
organomegaly
orientation
    corneal o.
    sagittal o.
    transverse o.
orifice
orificium
original Turner biopsy needle
Oriodide-131
Ormond's syndrome
orofaciodigital (OFD)
    o. syndrome I
    o. syndrome II
orogenital syndrome
oromaxillary
oronasal
oropharyngeal
    o. isthmus
    o. membrane
orothopantomograph
Orr-Loygue technique
Orthicon
    O. television camera
    O. tube
orthodiagram
orthodiagraphy
orthodiascopy
orthoiodohippurate (OIH)
orthopantomography (OPG)
orthopnea position
orthoroentgenographic method
orthoroentgenography
orthoskiagraph

orthostereoscope
orthotomography
orthotonos
orthovoltage
Ortner's syndrome
os
    cervical o.
    o. calcis (calcaneus)
    o. centrale
    o. coxae
    o. cuneiforme intermedium
    o. cuneiforme laterale
    o. cuneiforme mediale
    o. externum
    o. hamatum
    o. innominatum
    o. intercuneiform
    o. intermedium
    o. intermetatarseum
    o. ischii
    o. lunatum
    o. magnum
    o. multangulum majus
    o. multangulum minus
    o. naviculare pedis
      retardatum
    o. odontoideum
    o. peronacum
    o. peroneum
    o. pisiforme
    o. pretrapezium
    o. pubis
    o. scaphoideum
    o. styloideum
    o. subfibulare
    o. subtibiale
    o. suprapetrosum of
      Meckel
    o. tibiale externum
    o. trapezium secundarium
    o. triangulare
    o. trigonum
    o. trochlearis
    o. uteri
    o. vesalianum
os, s. (mouth)
    ora, pl. (mouth)
Osbil
Osborne precision stopcocks
    and manifolds
oscillating
    o. Bucky
    o. electron
    o. grid
oscillography
oscilloscope
osculum
Osgood-Schlatter
    O.-S. disease
    O.-S. syndrome
Osler's
    O.'s disease
    O.'s node
    O.'s syndrome
OSMED
    (otospondylomegaepiphyseal
    dysplasia)
osmium (os)
osmolality
osmolarity
osmoses, pl.
    osmosis, s.
osmosis, s.
    osmoses, pl.
osmotic pressure
ossature
osseocartilaginous
osseosonometry
osseous
    o. defect
    o. demineralization
    o. labyrinth
    o. metaplasia
    o. necrosis
    o. ray formation
    o. spicule

osseous—*Continued*
  o. sunburst
  o. synostosis
  o. thinning
  o. tophi
ossicle
  auditory o.
  Kerckring's o.
ossicula intercalaria
ossicular
  o. ligament
  o. muscle
ossificans
ossification
  cartilaginous o.
  dichotomous o.
  ectopic o.
  endochondral o.
  heterotopic o. (HO)
  intracartilaginous o.
  intramembranous o.
  metaplastic o.
  o. of the posterior
    longitudinal ligament
    (OPLL)
  pathologic o.
  perichondral o.
  periosteal o.
  pulmonary o.
  vertebral o.
ossified diathesis
ossifluence
ossifying
  o. fibroid
  o. fibroma
  o. inflammation
  o. interstitial myositis
  o. leiomyoma
  o. ligamentous spondylitis
  o. nodule
  o. periostitis
  o. pneumonitis
osteal resonance
ostealgia

osteanagenesis
osteectopia
osteitis
  o. condensans
  o. condensans ilii
  o. cystica multiplex
  o. cystica multiplex
    tuberculosa
  o. deformans
  o. fibrosa cystica
  o. fibrosa cystica
    disseminata
  o. pubis
  radiation o.
  rubella o.
  sclerosing o.
ostembryon
ostempyesis
osteoaneurysm
osteoarthritis (OA)
  o. coxae
  o. juvenilis
osteoarthrosis
  intervertebral o.
  o. interspinalis
osteoblastoma
osteocampsia
osteocartilaginous exostosis
osteocele
osteocephaloma
osteochondral fracture
osteochondritis
  o. deformans juvenilis
  o. deformans tibiae
  o. dissecans
  o. ischiopubica
  o. necroticans
  o. subepiphysaria
  o. vertebralis infantilis
osteochondroarthrosis
  deformans endemica
osteochondrodesmodysplasia
osteochondrodysplasia
  deformans

osteochondrodystrophia fetalis
osteochondrodystrophy
osteochondrolysis
osteochondroma
osteochondromatosis
osteochondromuscular
 dystrophy
osteochondromyxoma
osteochondropathia
 o. cretinoidea
 o. ischiopubica
osteochondrosarcoma
osteochondrosis
osteoclastoma
osteoclysis
osteocomma
osteocope
osteocystoma
osteodermopathic hyperostosis
 syndrome
osteodynia
osteodysmetamorphosis
 foetalis
osteodysplasia
osteodystrophia
 o. cystica
 o. fibrosa
 o. fibrosa unilateralis
 o. generalisata
osteodystrophy
 Albright's o.
 renal o.
osteoencephaloma
osteoepiphysis
osteofibroma
osteofibrosis deformans
 juvenilis
osteogenesis
 o. imperfecta
 o. imperfecta B
 o. imperfecta congenita
 o. imperfecta lethalis
 o. imperfecta psathyrotica
 o. imperfecta tarda

osteogenic sarcoma
osteoglophonic dwarfism
osteogram
osteography
osteohalisteresis
osteohypertrophic varicose
 nevus syndrome
osteoid osteoma
osteolipochondroma
osteoliposarcoma
osteolytic sarcoma
osteoma
 fibrous o.
 o. cutis
 o. eburneum
 o. medullare
 o. multiplex
  intermusculare
 o. sarcomatosum
 o. spongiosum
 osteoid o.
 parosteal o.
 "tropical ulcer" o.
osteomalacia
osteomalacic pelvis
osteomiosis
osteomyelitis
 calvarial o.
 Candida o.
 fungal o.
 Garré's sclerosing o.
 hematologic o.
 iliac o.
 luetic o.
 multifocal o.
 neonatal o.
 nonsequestrating o.
 nonsuppurative o.
 o. sicca
 o. variolosa
 pyogenic o.
 tuberculous o.
osteomyelodysplasia
osteomyelography

osteomyxochondroma
osteon
osteoncus
osteo-onycho dysostosis
osteo-onychodysplasia
osteopathia
    o. acidotica
      pseudorachitica
    o. fibrosa generalisata
    o. hypertrophicans toxica
    o. striata
osteopathy
osteopecilia
osteopedion
osteopenia
osteoperiostitis familiaris
osteopetrosis
osteophyma
osteophyte
osteophytic
osteophytosis
osteoplastic
osteopoikilosis
osteoporosis
    congenital o.
    endocrine o.
    hyperparathyroid o.
    iatrogenic o.
    idiopathic juvenile o.
    neurovasculotropic o.
    nutritional deficiency o.
    o. circumscripta
    o. of disuse
    postmenopausal o.
    senile o.
    spinal o.
    subchondral o.
osteoporosis-osteomalacia
  syndrome
osteoprogenitor cell
osteopsathyrosis
    o. congenita
    o. foetalis
    o. idiopathica tarda
osteopulmonary arthropathy

osteoradionecrosis
osteosarcoma
    parosteal o.
    telangiectatic o.
Osteoscan
osteosclerosis congenita
osteosclerotic myeloma
osteoscope
osteosis eburnisans
  monomelica
osteospongioma
osteosteatoma
osteosynovitis
osteotabes
Österreicher-Turner syndrome
osthexia
ostia, pl.
    ostium, s.
ostium
    o. abdominale
    o. primum
    o. secundum
    o. uteri
ostium, s.
    ostia, pl.
OTD (organ tolerance dose)
otic
    o. grandion
    o. vesicle
otitic hydrocephalus
otitis media
    chronic adhesive o. m.
    fibro-osseous o. m.
otocranium
otocyst
otography
otomandibular dysostosis
otomastoiditis
otopalatodigital (OPD)
  syndrome
otosclerosis
    cochlear o.
    fenestral o.
otospondylomegaepiphyseal
  dysplasia (OSMED)

Otto's
    O.'s pelvis
    O.'s syndrome
Otto-Krobak pelvis
Ottonelo's method
out of plaster (OOP)
out-of-field artifact
out-of-phase
outer tunnel
Outerbridge scale
outflow tract
outside diameter (OD)
ova, pl.
    ovum, s.
oval
    o. window
    o. pigtail catheter
ovale
    foramen o.
    foramen o. septi atriorum
ovarian
    o. artery
    o. ascites-pleural effusion
      syndrome
    o. cyst
    o. dwarfism
    o. follicle
    o. ligament
    o. mumps
    o. short-stature syndrome
    o. teratoma
    o. tumor
    o. vein
    tubo-o. obstruction
    tubo-o. opacification
ovary
    absent o.
    dermoid cyst of o.
    polycystic o.
overbite
overbridged sella
overcirculation
overcouch
    o. exposure

    o. tube
    o. view
overdevelopment
overexpansion
overexposure
overflow incontinence
overhanging margin of bone,
    sign of
Overhauser effect
overhead
    o. film
    o. fracture frame
overinflation
overlapping of slices
overloading
overpenetrated film
overrange
overreading
overriding
    o. aorta
    o. fracture
overscan
overshoot artifact
overtoe
overvoltage
oviduct
ovoid-shaped
ovulation
ovum, s.
    ova, pl.
Owen-Pendergrass method
Owen's
    O.'s position
    O.'s view
Owens catheter
ox gall enema
oxidation
oxycephaly
oxygenated
oxygenation
oxyphil adenoma
oxytocin
    o. challenge

Pp

P 32 collodial chromic phosphate
P 231 (radiophosphorus)
P electron
P shell
PA and lateral
    PA and l. position
    PA and l. projection
Pa (pascal)
PA (posteroanterior) position
Pa (protactinium)
PA (pulmonary artery)
PAC automatic calculator
pacchionian
    p. bodies
    p. depression
    p. granulation
pacemaker catheter
Paceport catheter
pachyderm vorticella
pachydermia
pachydermoperiostitis
pachydermoperiostosis
pachygnathous
pachymeningitis
Pacific Northwest Radiological Society (PNRS)
pacing
    p. catheter
    p. electrodes
packing fraction
PACS (picture archiving and communication systems)
pad sign of Case
Padgett's tentorial sinus
Page's kidney
Paget's
    P. disease
    P. disease of the breast

    P. quiet necrosis of bone
Paget-Schroetter syndrome
pagetoid
PAH (para-aminohippurate)
painful
    p. apicocostrovertebral syndrome
    p. ophthalmoplegia
pair
    Helmholtz p.
    p. annihilation
    p. production
palatal
    p. abscess
    p. arch
palate
palatine
    p. foramen
    p. process
    p. suture
    p. tonsil
palatoethmoidal
palatoglossus
palatography
palatomyography
palatopharyngeal sphincter
palatopharyngeus muscle
palatum
    p. dura
    p. ogivale
paleoradiology
Paley manifold
palindromic rheumatism
palladium
palliative
    p. irradiation
    p. treatment
palmar
    p. aponeurosis

palmar—*Continued*
    p. projection
palmaris
    p. brevis muscle
    p. longus muscle
    p. longus tendon
palmitate
palmitic acid
palmoplantar keratosis
palpebral ligament
panacinar emphysema
panagram
panagraphy
Pancoast's
    P.'s sign
    P.'s syndrome
    P.'s tumor
pancreas-blood-bone
    syndrome
pancreatic
    p. abscess
    p. calcification
    p. carcinoma
    p. cholera
    p. cyst
    p. duct
    p. head
    p. lymph node
    p. malignancy syndrome
pancreaticoduodenal lymph
    node
pancreaticosplenic
    p. lymph node
    p. omentum
pancreatogram
pancreatography
pancreozymin
pancytopenia
    Fanconi's p.
pancytopenia-dysmelia
panendoscope
pangynecogram
pangynecography
panhypopituitarism
panlobular emphysema

panmural
    p. cystitis
    p. fibrosis
panmyelopathy, Fanconi's
panmyelosis
Panner's disease
pannus
panography
panoral
    p. radiogram
    p. radiography
panoramic
    p. radiography
    p. tomography
    p. view
panoramix
Panorex
    P. view
pansystolic murmur
pantographic view
pantomographic view
pantomography
    concentric p.
    eccentric p.
Pantopaque (ethyl
    iodophenylundecylate)
    P. iophendylate
    P. radiopaque oil
pantothenic acid
PAP (primary atypical
    pneumonia)
Paparella catheter
papaverine hydrochloride
paper
    p. dot scan
    p. drape
papilla
    lacrimal p.
    optic p.
    p. of Vater
papillary ducts
papilledema
papilloma
    choroid plexus p.
    squamous cell p.

papillomata
papillomatosis
Papillon-Léage and Psaume
  syndrome
Papillon-Lèfevre syndrome
papular myxedema
papulosquamous
PAPVR (partial anomalous
  pulmonary venous return)
para-aminohippurate (PAH)
para-aminohippuric acid
para-aminosalicylic acid
  (PAS)
para-aortic
  p. line
  p. node
para-aortic/splenic
parabutyl IDA (BIDA)
paracardial
  p. lymph nodes
paracathode ray
paracentesis
parachute
  p. jumper's dislocation
  p. mitral valve
paracolic lymph nodes
paracolonic gutter
paracondyloid process
paradox
paradoxical incontinence
paraduodenal fossa
paraesophageal
  p. hernia
  p. line
paraffinoma
parafrenal abscess
parahilar
parahippocampal gyrus
parallax
  p. method
  p. motion method
  p. view
parallel
  p. circuit
  p. grid

p. opposing portals
p. ray
parallel-hole collimator
parallelogram of Kopitz
paralysis
paralytic ileus
Parama's method
paramagnetic
  p. bodies
  p. ion
  p. relaxation
  p. shift
paramammary lymph node
paramediastinal
parameter
parametrial abscess
parametric abscess
paranasal
  p. sinus
paraneoplastic
paranephric abscess
pararectal lymph node
pararenal
  p. abscess
  p. compartment
  p. fat
  p. space
parasagittal
  p. meningioma
  p. plane
parasella
parasellar
paraseptal emphysema
parasinoidal space
paraspinal
  p. hematoma
  p. line
  p. muscle
parasternal
  p. hernia
  p. lymph node
parastremmatic
  p. dwarfism
  p. dysplasia
parasutural sclerosis

parasympathetic
parathyroid gland
paratracheal
    p. line
    p. lymph node
    p. stripe
paratrooper's fracture
paratyphoid spondylitis
paraureteral
parauterine lymph node
paravaterian
paravertebral line
paravesical fossa
paravesicular lymph node
parenchyma or parenchyme
parenchymal or
   parenchymatous
    p. cyst
    p. hemorrhage
    p. kidney
    p. myelopathy
    p. myocarditis
parenchymatous or
   parenchymal
parent
    p. element
    p. nuclide
parent-infant traumatic stress
   (PITS) syndrome
paresis
    pharyngeal p.
    Todd's p.
parietal
    p. abscess
    p. fenestra
    p. foramen
    p. foramina
    p. fossa
    p. lobe
    p. peritoneum
    p. plate
    p. pleura
    "p. star"
    p. stellate

    p. suture
parietoacanthal projection
parietography
parietomastoid suture
parieto-occipital fissure
parieto-orbital oblique
   projection
parietotemporal projection
Park Blade septostomy
   catheter
Park's aneurysm
Park, transverse lines of
Parkes Weber syndrome
Parkinson's position
Parma's position
parosteal
    p. osteoma
    p. osteosarcoma
    p. sarcoma
parotid
    p. calculus
    p. gland
    p. lymph node
    p. mass
parotiditis, s.
    parotiditises, pl.
parotiditises, pl.
    parotiditis, s.
parovarian
paroxysmal
    p. nocturnal
      hemoglobulinuria (PNH)
    p. polyserositis
Parrot's
    P.'s achondroplasia
    P.'s disease
    P.'s node
    P.'s paralysis
    P.'s pseudoparalysis
    P.'s sign
Parrot-Kaufmann syndrome
parry fracture
Parry-Romberg syndrome
pars

p. distalis
p. interarticularis
p. intermedia
p. nervosa
p. petrosa
p. plana
p. tuberalis
pars, s.
   partes, pl.
part-angulation method
part-film distance
part-thickness
partes, pl.
   pars, s.
partial
   p. anomalous pulmonary
     venous return (PAPVR)
   p. flexion
   p. persistent truncus
     arteriosus
   p. saturation (PS)
   p. scan
   p. thread wood screw
   p. volume artifact
particle
   alpha p.
   beta p.
   high-velocity p.
   ionizing p.
   p. waves
   viral p.
partition coefficient
PAS (para-aminosalicylic acid)
pascal (Pa)
passbox
paste-like
pastille radiometer
Patau's syndrome
patella (knee cap)
   floating p.
   high-lying p.
   p. alta
   p. baja
Patella's disease

patella, s.
   patellas or patellae, pl.
patellae or patellas, pl.
   patella, s.
patellar
   p. fossa
   p. fracture
   p. ligament
   p. tendon
patellas or patellae, pl.
   patella, s.
patelliform
patellofemoral groove
patency
patent
   p. airway
   P. Blue V
   p. bronchus sign
   p. ductus arteriosus (PDA)
   p. ductus arteriosus
     urachus
Paterson-Kelly
   P.-K. syndrome
   P.-K. webs
Paterson-Parker Dosage
  System
pathogenic
pathognomonic
pathologic
   p. atrophy
   p. fracture
   p. ossification
   p. tissue
pathway
   Embden-Meyerhof
     glycolytic p.
   visual p.
patient motion
pattern
   alveolar p.
   "broken bough" p.
   convolutional p.
   corkscrew p.
   cystic p.

pattern—*Continued*
    "fingerprint" p.
    frequency p.
    gas p.
    "hair brush" p.
    haustral p.
    "herring-bone" p.
    intestinal gas p.
    "mimosa" p.
    rugal p.
    solid p.
    start test p.
    tertiary p.
    three-dimensional
        physiologic flow p.
patulous
pauciarthritis
pauciarticular
paucity of air
Pauli's exclusion principle
Pautrier's abscess
Pauwels' fracture
Pavlov's stomach
Pawlik's triangle
Pawlow's
    P.'s method
    P.'s position
Payr-Strauss sphincter
Pb (lead)
PBF (pulmonary blood flow)
PBI (protein bound iodine)
P-B-I-Rezikit
PC (pentose cycle)
pc or pCi (picocurie)
PCA (posterior cerebral artery)
pCi or pc (picocurie)
P-comm (posterior
    communicating)
PCP (pneumocystis carinii
    pneumonia)
PCR (Philips computed
    radiography)
PCTA (percutaneous coronary
    transluminal angioplasty)
PCXR (portable chest X-ray)

PDA (patient ductus
    arteriosus)
PDA (posterior descending
    artery)
PDD (cisplatin)
PDR (pediatric radiology)
PDU (pulsed Doppler
    ultrasonography)
PE (photographic effect)
PE (pulmonary embolism)
PE Plus-II catheter
peak
    Bragg p.
    characteristic p.
    p. kilovoltage (kVp)
    p. value
peak-to-peak
Péan's position
pearly tumor of the skull
Pearson's
    P.'s method
    P.'s position
PECHO (prostatic echogram)
pectineal fascia
pectineus muscle
pectoral
    p. aplasia-dysdactyly
        syndrome
    p. girdle
    p. lymph node
pectoralis
    p. major muscle
    p. minor muscle
pectus
    p. carinatum
    p. excavatum
    p. gallinatum
    p. recurvatum
pediatric
    p. Harwood-Nash cerebral
        catheter
    p. Hinck Headhunter
        cerebral catheter
    p. pigtail catheter
    p. radiology (PDR)

p. straight catheter
pedicle (peduncle)
pedis
peduncle (pedicle)
pedunculi, pl.
    pedunculus, s.
pedunculus, s.
    pedunculi, pl.
peel-away introducer
PEEP (positive end-expiratory
    pressure)
PEG (pneumoencephalogram)
PEG
    (pneumoencephalography)
peg-and-socket joint
Pel-Ebstein disease
Pelizaeus-Merzbacher disease
Pelken's
    P.'s sign
    P.'s spur or sign
Pellegrini-Stieda disease
Pellegrini's disease
pellucid
pellucidum
pelves, pl.
    pelvis, s.
pelvic
    p. abscess
    p. aneurysm
    p. cavity
    p. fascia
    p. girdle
    p. gutter
    p. inlet
    p. kidney
    p. lymph node
    p. ring fracture
    p. scan
    p. sonogram
    p. spot
    p. ultrasound
pelvicephalography
pelvicephalometry
pelvimetry
pelviography

pelvioradiography
pelvioscopy
pelvirectal abscess
pelviroentgenography
pelvis
    Kilan's p.
    Otto-Krobak p.
    p. spinosa
    renal p.
pelvis, s.
    pelves, pl.
pencil
    p. dosimeter
    p. point percutaneous
        entry needle
"pencil-in-cup" deformity
"pencil-like" deformity
"penciling" bone
Pendred's syndrome
pendulous breast sign
pendulum heart
penetrating
    p. foreign body
    p. ulcer
penetration fraction
penetrology
penetrometer
    Benoist p.
penile
    p. catheter
pentagastrin
pentetate
    p. indium disodium in 111
    p. calcium trisodium Yb-
        169
pentose cycle (PC)
pentrometer
penumbra
PEP (polyestradiol phosphate)
pepsin
peptic
    p. aspiration pneumonitis
    p. ulcer disease (PUD)
Per-Abrodil
Per-Radiographol

percent depth dose
perceptibility
Perchloracap
percholorate
    p. discharge test
    potassium p.
PercuGuide needle
percussion
percutaneous
    p. antegrade pyelogram
    p. antegrade pyelography
    p. antegrade urogram
    p. antegrade urography
    p. carotid arteriography
    p. catheter
    p. coronary transluminal
      angioplasty (PCTA)
    p. hepatobiliary
      cholangiography
    p. interventional
      radiobiology
    p. liver biopsy
    p. needle
    p. needle biopsy (PNB)
    p. nephrostomy
    p. puncture
    p. transhepatic biliary
      drain (PTHBD)
    p. transhepatic
      cholangiogram (PTC)
    p. transhepatic
      cholangiography (PTC)
    p. transhepatic puncture
    p. transluminal angioplasty
      (PTA)
    p. transluminal coronary
      angiography (PTCA)
    p. transtracheal
      bronchography
    p. ultrasonic
      nephrolithotripsy
      (PUNL)
perforate
perforating
    p. fibers of Sharpey

    p. fracture
    p. ulcer
performed
perfusion
    luxury p. syndrome
    myocardial p.
    p. lung scan
    p. scan
    p. study
    peripheral p.
periacetabular
perianal hematoma
perianeurysmal fibrosis
periaortic node
periapical
    p. abscess
    p. granuloma
periappendiceal abscess
periarthritis humeroscapularis
periarticular fracture
periaxial space
peribiliary fat
peribronchial
pericallosal artery
pericardiac
    p. pleura
pericardial
    p. calcification
    p. effusion
    p. fat pad
    p. hernia
    p. line
    p. lymph node
    p. sac
pericardial-pseudocirrhosis of
  the liver
pericardiocentesis
pericarditis
    bacterial p.
    carcinomatous p.
    mediastinal p.
    suppurative p.
    tuberculous p.
    uremic p.
pericardium

pericholecystic abscess
perichondral ossification
perichondrium
pericolonic
    p. abscess
    p. gutter
perigraft abscess
perihepatic
    p. abscess
    p. space
perihilar
perilunate dislocation
perilymphatic labyrinth
perimetrium
perinaeum or perineum, s.
    perinea or perineae, pl.
perinea or perineae, pl.
    perinaeum or perineum, s.
perineal
    p. aponeurosis
    p. space
perineosacral
perinephric
    p. abscess
    p. air injection
    p. cyst
    p. hematoma
perinephritic
perineum also perinaeum, s.
    perinea or perineae, pl.
perineuronal space
perinodal
perinuclear
    p. cisterna
    p. space
periodic
    p. abdominalgia
    p. fever
    p. polyserositis
    p. table
periodontal
    p. abscess
    p. membrane
periostea, pl.
    periosteum, s.

periosteal
    p. chondroma
    p. desmoid
    p. dysplasia
    p. ossification
    p. reaction
periosteum, s.
    periostea, pl.
periostitis
    florid reactive p.
    "lace-like" p.
    p. deformans
    p. tuberositas tibiae
    sesamoid p.
peripheral
    p. angiogram
    p. angiography
    p. arteriogram
    p. arteriography
    p. circulation
    p. edema
    p. perfusion
    p. vascular (PV)
    p. venogram
    p. venography
periphery
peripleuritic abscess
perirenal
    p. abscess
    p. air study
    p. compartment
    p. fascia
    p. fascitis
    p. fat
    p. hemorrhage
    p. insufflation
    p. "P" sign
perisellar
perisigmoidal abscess
peristalses, pl.
    peristalsis, s.
peristalsis, s.
    peristalses, pl.
peristaltic
    p. jump

peristaltic—*Continued*
p. rushes
p. waves
peritendinitis calcarea
peritendinous
peritoneal
p. abscess
p. cavity
p. fluid
p. lymphadenopathy
p. sac
peritoneography
peritoneum
peritonitis
peritonsillar abscess
peritubal syndrome
perityphilitis
periureteral
p. abscess
p. fibrosis
perivascular
Perjodal
Perlmann's tumor
perlunate dislocation
permanent magnet
permeability
magnetic p.
p. constant
permissible dose
pernicious anemia
perodactylia
perodactyly
peromelia
peromelus
peronarthrosis
peroneal node
peroneotibial
peroneus
p. brevis muscle
p. longus muscle
p. tertius muscle
peroral retrograde
pancreaticobiliary
ductography
perpendicular plate

perpetual arrhythmia
persistent
p. fetal circulation
syndrome
p. Kerley's line
pertechnetate
Perthes-Jüngling disease
pertrochanteric fracture
Perurdil
pes
p. abductus
p. adductus
p. anserinus
p. cavus (foot)
p. convex (rocker-bottom
foot)
p. hippocampi
p. plano-valgus
p. planus (flatfoot)
p. pronatus
p. valgus (flatfoot)
p. varus (pigeon toe)
pessary
PET (positron emission
tomography) scan
petit mal
petrobasilar suture
petroclinoid
petromastoid canal
petro-occipital joint
petropharyngeus
petrosa, s.
petrosae, pl.
petrosae, pl.
petrosa, s.
petrosal
p. process
p. sinus
petrosphenobasilar suture
petrospheno-occipital suture
petrosquamous fissure
petrotympanic fissure
petrous
p. apex
p. pyramid

p. ridge
p. temporal
p. tip
PETT (positron emission transverse tomography)
PETT (positron emission transaxial tomography)
Peutz-Jeghers syndrome
Peyer's patch(es); also, Peyer's gland
Peyronie's disease
Peyrot's thorax
Pezzer catheter
PFA (profunda femoris artery)
Pfaundler-Hurler
    P.-H. gargoylism
    P.-H. syndrome
PFEAAC (posterior fossa extra-axial arachnoid cyst)
Pfeiffer's
    P.'s acrocephalosyndactyly
    P.'s board
    P.'s syndrome
Pfeiffer-Comberg method
PFFD (proximal femoral focal deficiency) syndrome
Pfister nephrostomy needle
Pfizer (manufacturer)
    P. 0450 scanner
    P. 200 FS scanner
    P. whole-body CT system
PFT (phenylalanine mustard [melphalan] fluorouracil, tamaxifen)
pH (hydrogen in concentration)
phagocytosis
phakoma
phakomatosis
phalangeal
    p. arthrosis
    p. fracture
    p. joint
    p. microgeodic syndrome
    p. sign

p. tuft
phalanges or phalanxes, pl.
    phalanx, s.
phalanx, s.
    phalanxes or phalanges, pl.
phalanxes or phalanges, pl.
    phalanx, s.
phallic shield
phantom
    p. bone
    p. clavicle
    p. image
    p. pain
    p. resolving power
pharmacoradiology
Pharmaseal catheter
pharyngeal
    p. aponeurosis
    p. diverticulum
    p. paresis
    p. tumor
pharyngoepiglottic fold
pharyngoesophageal
    p. diverticulum
    p. sphincter
pharyngoesophagraphy
pharyngography
pharyngolaryngeal
pharyngomaxillary space
pharyngopalatine
pharynx
phase
    p. difference
    p. encoding
    p. imaging
    p. sensitive detector
phasic arrhymthia
phenidone
Pheniodol [3-(4-hydroxy-3,5-diiodophenyl)-2-phenylpropionic acid]
phenobutiodyl
phenolphthalein
phenolsulfophthalein (PSP)

phenoltetrachlorophthalein
phenomenon
    flip-flop p.
    interference p.
    Koebner's p.
    pulmonary vascular
      autoregulatory p.
    Raynaud's p.
    "vacuum" p.
phenotype
    Turner's p.
phentetiothalein
phenylalanine mustard
    (melphalan) fluorouracil,
    tamaxifen (PFT)
phenyldiphenyloxadiazole
    (PPD)
phenylketonuria
phenyloxazolyl
phenylpyruvic oligophrenia
pheochromocytoma
Philipps'
    P.' contact therapy unit
    P.' position
Philips
    P. computed radiography
      (PCR)
    P. intensifier
    P. system
Phillips catheter
phlebogram
phlebography
phlebolith
phlegmon
phlegmonous
    p. abscess
    p. gastritis
PHO/CON tomographic multi-
    plane scanner
Pho/Dot
PHO/Gamma LEM low energy
    mobile scintillation camera
PHO/Gamma V scintillation
    camera

phocomelia
phoenix abscess
phonate
phonation study
phonocardiogram
phonocardiography
phosphate
phosphatemia
Phospho-Soda (sodium
    biphosphate, sodium
    phosphate)
Phosphocaps
Phosphocol P-32
phosphor
phosphorated
phosphorescence
phosphorescent
phosphorus
phosphorus-32 (P 32)
phosphorus lines
phosphorus-32
    diisofluorophosphate
Phosphotec (technetium
    Tc99m pyrophosphate kit)
Phosphotope
photo scan
photocathode
photochemical radiation
photoconductive material
photodisintegration
photodisplay unit
photodot scanner
photoelectric
    p. absorption
    p. attenuation
    p. circuit
    p. effect
    p. emission
    p. interaction
    p. threshold
photoelectron
photoflow
photofluorogram
photofluorography

photographic
    p. dosimetry
    p. effect (PE)
    p. radiometer
photomeson
photomicrography
photomultiplier tube
photon
    Compton p.
    Compton's scattering p.
    degraded p.
    linear p.
    p. bombardment
    p. energy
    p. fluence
    p. flux
    p. mottle
    "p. poor"
    p. starvation
photoneutron
photonuclear
    p. effect
    p. reaction
photopeak
photorecording
photoroentgenography
photoscanner
photosensitivity
photosensitization
phototimer
phototube output circuit
phrenic lymph node
phrenicocolic
phrenicoesophageal
    p. ligament
phrenicovertebral angle
phrenocostal
    p. sinus
    p. space
phrenopyloric syndrome
PHRT (procarbazine, hydroxyurea radiotherapy) protocol
phrygian cap

physeal growth
physical half-life
physicist
physics
physiochemical
physiologic
    p. dead space
    p. rest position
physiological saline
physiology
pi
    p. lines
    p. mesons
pia mater
pial funnel
PICA (posterior inferior cerebellar artery)
Pick's
    P.'s atrophy
    P.'s cirrhosis
    P.'s disease
    P.'s hallucinations
    P.'s triad
    P.'s vision
pick-up tube
Picker (manufacturer)
    P. Magna scanner
    P. Pace-1 gamma-counting system
    P. Synerview 600 scanner
    P. system
"picket fence" sign
pickwickian syndrome
picocurie (pc or pCi)
Picture Archiving and Communications System (PACS)
picture frame-like
PIE (pulmonary infiltrates with eosinophils)
PIE (pulmonary infiltration [with] eosinophilia)
PIE (pulmonary interstitial edema)

PIE (pulmonary interstitial
  emphysema)
Piedmont fracture
Pierquin's position
Pierre-Marie disease
Pierre-Marie-Bamberger
  syndrome
Pierre Robin's syndrome
pietoficatio cutis
piezoelectric
  p. crystals
  p. effect
pig bronchus
pig-tailed
  p. catheter
  p. guide wire
pigeon
  p. breast
  p. breast deformity
  p. breeder's disease
  p. breeder's lung
  p. toe
Pigg-O-Stat immobilization
  device
pigmented liver
pigtail catheter
Pilcher catheter
pile
pillar
  p. projection
  p. view
pillion fracture
pilonidal cyst
pilot scan
Pilotip catheter
pin
  Bohlman p.
  Compere p.
  Deyerle p.
  four-flanged p.
  Hagie p.
  Hansen-Street p.
  Hatcher p.

Knowles p.
Moore p.
p. vise
Rush p.
Steinmann p.
Street p.
Turner p.
Turner-McElvenny p.
von Saal p.
Zimmer p.
pin-cushion distortion
pin-hole
  p.-h. collimator
  p.-h. photography
  p.-h. picture
pin-point imaging
Pindborg's tumor
pine-tree bladder
pineal
  p. body
  p. germinoma
  p. gland
pinealoblastoma
pinealoma
ping-pong fracture
pink
  p. tetralogy of Fallot
  p. tooth
pinocytosis
pion
  p. beam
  p. dosimetry
PIP (postinflammatory
  polyposis)
PIP (proximal interphalangeal)
  joint
pipestem ureter
PIPIDA (pisopropylacetanilido-
  iminodiacetic acid) scan
PIPIDA scan (now called
  DISIDA)
PIPJ (proximal interphalangeal
  joint)

Pipkin classification
Pirie's
  P.'s bone
  P.'s method
  P.'s transoral projection
  P.'s view
piriform (pyriform)
  p. cortex
  p. lobe
  p. sinus
piriformis muscle
pisiform
pisiform-hamate fusion
pisohamate ligament
pisometacarpal ligament
pisopropylacetanilido-
  iminodiacetic acid (PIPIDA)
  scan
pisotriquetral joint
PIT (plasma iron turnover)
pitchblende
Pitocin (oxytocin with
  chlorobutanol and acetic
  acid)
Pitressin (vasopressin with
  chlorobutanol and acetic
  acid)
PITS (parent-infant traumatic
  stress) syndrome
pitting
  "pepper-pot" p.
pituitary
  anterior p.
  p. adenoma
  p. ameloblastoma
  p. basophilism
  p. cachexia
  p. dwarfism
  p. fossa
  p. gland
  p. hypogonadism
  p. myxedema
  p. nanism

  p. stalk
Pituitrin
pivot
  p. joint
  p. view
pixel (picture element)
  p. highlighting
  p. histogram
placenta praevia or previa
placental membrane
placentogram
placentography
plafond fracture
plagiocephalic
plagiocephaly
plagioprosopia
plain
  p. film
  p. film technique
plana (flat surface)
planar
  p. imaging
  p. spin imaging
Planck's
  P.'s constant
  P.'s quantum theory
plane
  Addison's p.
  Aeby's p.
  auriculoinfraorbital p.
  axiopetrosal
  Baer's p.
  Blumenbach's p.
  Bolton-nasion p.
  Broadbent-Bolton p.
  Broca's p.
  coronal p.
  cross-sectional p.
  Daubenton's p.
  dextrosinistral p.
  Frankfort's p.
  frontal p.
  German horizontal p.

plane—*Continued*
   Hensen's p.
   Hodge's p.
   horizontal p.
   interparietal p.
   intertubercular p.
   Listing's p.
   Ludwig's p.
   Meckel's p.
   median sagittal p. (MSP)
   midcoronal p.
   midfrontal p.
   midsagittal p.
   Morton's p.
   nasion-postcondylare p.
   p. integral projection
     reconstruction
   p. joint
   p. sensitivity
   parasagittal p.
   Pöschl's p.
   sagittal p.
   sternoxiphoid p.
   transtubercular p.
   transverse p.
   Virchow's p.
plane-pair resolution
planigram
planigraphic principle
planigraphy
planimetry
plantar
   p. aponeurosis
   p. arch
   p. flexion
   p. ligament
   p. muscle
   p. perforating disease
   p. surface
   p. view
   p. wart
plantaris
plantodorsal
   p. position

   p. projection
   p. view
planum
   Calvé's vertebra p.
   p. sphenoidale
plasma
   p. cell granuloma
   p. cell myeloma
   p. iron turnover (PIT)
   p. volume (PV)
plasmacytoma
plasmapheresis
plasmocytoma
plaster
   p. cast
   p. of Paris cast
plastic
   p. catheter
   p. exudate
   p. induration of the penis
plastic-sheathed needle-
   catheter
plate
   axial p.
   Badgley p.
   blade p.
   Blount p.
   buttress p.
   clinoid p.
   condylar p.
   Conley mandibular p.
   cribriform p.
   deck p.
   Deyerle p.
   dorsal p.
   dynamic compression p.
   Eggers p.
   Elliott p.
   epiphyseal p.
   film p.
   flat p.
   floor p.
   foot p.
   Fresnel zone p.

growth p.
Haglund p.
Hoen p.
Jewett p.
Kessel p.
Laing osteotomy p.
Lane p.
Lawson-Thornton p.
McLaughlin p.
medullary p.
mesial p.
Moe p.
neutralization p.
p. spacing
parietal p.
perpendicular p.
roof p.
Sherman p.
tarsal p.
Thornton p.
ventral p.
Vitallium (cobalt-
    chromium alloy) p.
volar p.
Wilson p.
Wilson spinal p.
Wright p.
zone p.
plate-like atelectasis
plateau
platelets
platinocyanide
platinum
platybasia
platypelloid pelvis
platysma
platyspondylia
    p. generalisata
playback amplifier
pleating of bowel wall of
    colon
pledget
pleiotropism
pleomorphic adenoma

pleonosteosis
    Léri's p.
    p. familiaris
plesiosectional tomography
plesiosette
plesiotherapy
plesiotomography
plethysmography
    impedance p. (IPG)
pleura
    apical p.
    cervical p.
    costal p.
    diaphragmatic p.
    mediastinal p.
    parietal p.
    pericardiac p.
    pulmonary p.
    visceral p.
pleura, s.
    pleuras or pleurae, pl.
pleuracentesis
pleurae or pleuras, pl.
    pleura, s.
pleural
    p. cap
    p. cavity
    p. drainage tube
    p. effusion
    p. exudate
    p. fluid
    p. meniscus sign
    p. sac
pleuras or pleurae, pl.
    pleura, s.
pleurisy
pleuritis
pleurodynia
pleurography
pleuropericardial murmur
pleuroperitoneal
plexus
    Batson's p.
    brachial p.

plexus—*Continued*
　choroid p.
　diaphragmatic p.
　lumbosacral p.
　p. of Santorini
　solar p.
　venous p.
plica
　p. circulares
　p. colliculi
　p. sublingualis
plicate
plication
PLIF (posterior lumbar
　interbody fusion)
Plumbicon tube
Plummer nail
Plummer's disease
Plummer-Vinson syndrome
plunger
pluridirectional tomography
　(PT)
plurigraph
plutonium
Pm (promethium)
PML (progressive multifocal
　leukoencephalopathy)
PNB (percutaneous needle
　biopsy)
pneumarthrogram or
　pneumoarthrogram
pneumarthrography or
　pneumoarthrography
pneumatic space
pneumatization
pneumatocele
pneumatogram
pneumatography
pneumatosis
　p. cystoides coli
　p. intestinalis
　p. pulmonum
pneumoalveolography
pneumoangiogram

pneumoangiography
pneumocardiogram
pneumocardiography
pneumocephalus secondary to
　cranial osteoma
pneumococcal empyema
pneumoconiosis
pneumocystis
pneumocystis carinii
　pneumonia (PCP)
pneumocystography
pneumocystotomography
pneumoencephalogram (PEG)
pneumoencephalography
　(PEG)
　cerebral p.
pneumoencephalomyelogram
pneumoencephalomyelography
pneumoencephalopathy
pneumofasciogram
pneumogastrography
pneumogram
pneumographic
pneumography
　cerebral p.
　retroperitoneal p.
pneumogynogram
pneumolith
pneumomediastinogram
pneumomediastinography
pneumomediastinum
pneumomycosis
pneumomyelography
pneumonia
　acute interstitial p.
　apical p.
　aspiration p.
　bronchial p.
　contusion p.
　double p.
　Eaton's p.
　embolic p.
　fibrous p.
　Friedländer p.

influenzal p.
interstitial p.
lobar p.
metastatic p.
traumatic p.
viral p.
pneumonitis
    desquamative interstitial p.
    granulomatous p.
    lymphocytic interstitial p.
    (LIP)
    ossifying p.
pneumonogram
pneumonography
pneumopericardium
pneumoperitoneography
pneumoperitoneum
pneumopyelogram
pneumopyelography
pneumoradiography
    retroperitoneal p.
pneumoretroperitoneum
pneumoroentgenogram
pneumoroentgenography
pneumothorax (PTX)
    diagnostic p.
pneumotomography
pneumoventriculogram
pneumoventriculography
PNH (paroxysmal nocturnal
    hemoglobulinuria)
PNRS (Pacific Northwest
    Radiological Society)
pocket
    p. chamber
    p. dosimeter
    p. ionization chamber
podagra
poikiloderma atrophicans
point
    auricular p.
    mental p.
    p. imaging
    p. scanning

    p. sensitivity
    p. spread function
Poisson's
    P.'s distribution
    P.'s noise fluctuations
poker
    p. deformity
    "p." spine
Poland's syndactyly
polarity
Polaroid unit
Polibar
poliomyelitis
polonium
Polya's procedure
polyadenome "en nappe"
polyalveolar lobe
polyarthritic
polyatresia congenita
polyaxial joint
polychondritis
polychondropathy
polychromatic
polycycloidal tomography
polycystic
    p. kidney
    p. kidney of the newborn
    p. liver
    p. nephroblastoma
    p. ovary
polycystoma
polycythemia
    p. rubra
    p. vera
polydystrophic
    p. dwarfism
    p. oligophrenia
polyenergetic x-ray
polyester
polyestradiol phosphate (PEP)
polyethylene catheter
polyethylene glycol
polygonal cell
polyhedral

polymelia
polymer
polymorphonuclear
polymyalgia rheumatica
polymyositis
polyossificatio congenita
  progressiva
polyostotic
    adenomatous p.
    p. fibrous dysplasia
    p. infantilia
    p. osteitis fibrosa
polyp
    fibroangiomatous p.
    intussuscepting p.
    sessile p.
polyperiostitis hyperesthetica
polyphalangia
polyphase generator
polypoid
polyposis
polypous gastritis
polyradiculitis
polyradiculoneuritis
polystan catheter
polystan venous return
  catheter
polysyndactyly
polysynostosis
polysynovitis
polytendinitis
polytendinobursitis
polytenosynovitis
polytome
    Massiot's p.
    multidirectional p.
polytomogram
polytomography
polytopic enchondral
  dysostosis
polyvinylpyrrolidone (PVP)
POMP (prednisone, vincristine
  [Oncovin]), methotrexate, 6-
  mercaptopurine)
Pompe's disease

pond fracture
pons
    p. cerebelli
    p. hepatis
pons, s.
    pontes, pl.
pons-oblongata
pontes, pl.
    pons, s.
pontine glioma
pontocaine
POP (popliteal)
popliteal (POP)
    p. cyst
    p. fossa
    p. ligament
    p. lymph node
    p. muscle
    p. pterygium syndrome
    p. space
popliteus
POPOP-1,4-bis-2-(5-
  phenyloxazolyl)-benzene
Poppel's
    P.'s method
    P.'s sign
Porak-Durante syndrome
porcelain gallbladder
Porcher's method
porencephalic cyst
pores of Kohn
pori acoustici, pl.
    porus acousticus, s.
pori, pl.
    porus, s.
porphyry spleen
port-film distance
porta
    p. hepatis
    p. lienis
    p. omenti
    p. pulmonis
portable (port.)
    p. chest x-ray (PCXR)
portacamera

portal
    p. canal
    p. vein (PV) needle
    p. venography
Portner-Koolpe biliary biopsy
  set
portocaval shunt
portogram
portography
portophlebography
portosplenogram
portosplenography
portovenography
portwine
    p. marks
    p. stain
porus
    p. acusticus
    p. acusticus internus
    p. sudoriferus
porus, s.
    pori, pl.
Posada's fracture
Pöschl's plane
position
    abduction p.
    Adams' p.
    adduction p.
    Albers-Schönberg p.
    Albert's p.
    Alexander's
      anteroposterior p.
    Alexander's lateral p.
    anatomical p.
    anterior lordotic p.
    AP (anteroposterior) p.
    apical p.
    Arcelin's p.
    arm extension p.
    axial p.
    axiolateral p.
    basilar p.
    batrachian p.
    Bèclére's p.
    Benassi's p.

bending-forward p.
Bertel's p.
Blackett-Healy p.
Blackett-Healy prone p.
Blackett-Healy supine p.
Bonner's p.
Boyce's p.
Bozeman's p.
Brickner's p.
Broden's p.
brow-down p.
brow-up p.
Buie's p.
butterfly p.
Cahoon's p.
Caldwell's p.
Camp-Coventry p.
Casselberry's p.
Causton's p.
centric p.
Chamberlain-Towne p.
Chassard-Lapiné p.
chest p.
Cleaves' p.
Clements-Nakayama p.
coiled p.
Coyle's trauma p.
cross-table lateral p.
Danielius-Miller p.
decortical p.
decubitus p.
Depage's p.
dorsal decubitus p.
dorsal elevated p.
dorsal inertia p.
dorsal lithotomy p.
dorsal oblique p.
dorsal p.
dorsal recumbent p.
dorsal rigid p.
dorsodecubitus p.
dorsoplantar oblique p.
dorsoplantar p.
dorsorecumbent p.
dorsosacral p.

position—*Continued*
    dorsosupine p.
    Duncan's p.
    Edebohls' p.
    Elliot's p.
    emprosthotonos p.
    English p.
    erect p.
    eversion p.
    exaggerated Waters' p.
    extension p.
    face-down p.
    Feist-Mankin p.
    fencing p.
    fetal p.
    Fick's p.
    Fleischner's p.
    flexion p.
    four-cavities p.
    Fowler's p.
    Friedman's p.
    frog-leg p.
    frog-like p.
    frontal anterior p.
    frontal posterior p.
    frontal transverse p.
    frontoanterior p.
    fronto-occipital p.
    frontoposterior p.
    frontotransverse p.
    Fuchs' anteroposterior p.
    Fuchs' oblique p.
    Fuchs' p.
    Gaynor-Hart p.
    genucubital p.
    genufacial p.
    genupectoral p.
    Granger's 17 degrees p.
    Granger's 23 degrees p.
    Granger's 107 degrees p.
    Granger's p.
    Grashey's p.
    Gunson's p.
    Haas' p.

    Haas' prone p.
    half-axial p.
    hallux-valgus p.
    hanging-head p.
    head-dependent p.
    head-low p.
    Henschen's p.
    Hickey's p. for the femur
    Hickey's p. for the mastoid
      process
    hinge p.
    Hirtz' p.
    Holmblad's p.
    horizontal p.
    hornpipe p.
    Hsieh's p.
    hyperextension p.
    inferosuperior p.
    inlet p.
    inversion p.
    inverted jackknife p.
    Isherwood's p.
    jackknife p.
    Johnson's p.
    Jones' p.
    Judd's p.
    kidney p.
    knee-chest p.
    knee-elbow p.
    kneeling-squatting p.
    Kraske's p.
    Kuchendorf's p.
    Kurzbauer's p.
    Lange's p.
    Laquerrière-Pierquin p.
    Larkin's p.
    lateral autotomogram p.
    lateral decubitus p.
    lateral p.
    lateral prone p.
    lateral recumbent p.
    lateral rotation p.
    lateromedial p.
    Lauenstein's p.

Law's lateral p.
Law's oblique p.
Law's p.
Lawrence's axial p.
Lawrence's p.
Lawrence's transthoracic
  p.
leapfrog p.
left anterior oblique (LAO)
  p.
left lateral (LLAT) p.
left posterior oblique
  (LPO) p.
Leonard-George p.
Lewis' p.
Lilienfeld's p.
Lilienfeld's p. for the
  ischium
Lilienfeld's p. for the
  shoulder
Lindblom's p.
lithotomy p.
lithotomy Trendelenburg
  p.
LLAT (left lateral) p.
lordotic p.
Lorenz' p.
Löw-Beer p.
LPO (left posterior
  oblique) p.
Lysholm's p. for the
  cranial base
Lysholm's p. for the optic
  foramen
Lysholm's p. for the pars
  petrosa
MacMillan's p.
May's p.
Mayer's p.
Mayo-Robson p.
medial oblique p.
Mees' p.
mentoanterior p.
mento-occipital p.

mentotransverse p.
Mercurio's p.
military p.
Miller's p.
Moynihan's p.
neck extension p.
neutral p.
Noble's p.
Nolke's p.
"nose-chin" p.
"nose-forehead" p.
oblique axial p.
oblique p.
obstetrical p.
occipitoanterior p.
occipitofrontal p.
occipitomental p.
occipitoposterior p.
occipitosacral p.
occipitotransverse p.
occipitovertical p.
occiput anterior p.
occiput posterior p.
occiput sacral p.
occiput transverse p.
occlusal p.
Ochsner's p.
off-center p.
opisthotonos p.
orthopnea p.
Owen's p.
PA and lateral p.
PA (posteroanterior) p.
Parkinson's p.
Parma's p.
Pawlow's p.
Péan's p.
Pearson's p.
Philipps' p.
physiologic rest p.
Pierquin's p.
plantodorsal p.
posterior border p.
posterior lordotic p.

position—*Continued*
    posteroanterior (PA) p.
    postvoid p.
    Proetz' p.
    profile p.
    prone jackknife p.
    prone p.
    pulmonary wedge p.
    radiographic p.
    Rapp's p.
    reclining p.
    recumbent lateral p.
    recumbent p.
    rest p.
    retrosternal p.
    reverse Caldwell p.
    reverse Trendelenburg p.
    reverse Waters' p.
    Rhese's p.
    Rhese's p. for the optic
      foramen
    Rhese's p. for the
      paranasal sinuses
    right anterior oblique
      (RAO) p.
    right lateral p.
    right posterior oblique
      (RPO) p.
    Robson's p.
    Rose's p.
    sacroanterior p.
    sacroposterior p.
    sacrotransverse p.
    sacrum anterior p.
    sacrum posterior p.
    Samuel's p.
    scapula anterior p.
    scapula posterior p.
    scapuloanterior p.
    scapuloposterior p.
    Schüller's p.
    scorbutic p.
    Scultetus' p.
    seated-erect p.

semi-Fowler p.
semiaxial p.
semiaxial transoral p.
semierect p.
semiprone p.
semireclining p.
semirecumbent p.
Settegast's p.
shock p.
Simon's p.
Sims' p.
sitting p.
spine right and left ps.
Staunig's p.
Stecher's p.
steep Trendelenburg p.
Stenver's p.
Stern's position
submentovertex p.
submentovertical p.
superoinferior p.
supine p.
supraorbital p.
swimmer's p.
Tarrant's p.
Taylor's p.
ten-degree off-lateral p.
Teufel's p.
Titterington's p.
tonsil p.
Towne-Chamberlain p.
Towne's p.
transabdominal p.
transaxillary p.
transorbital p.
transthoracic p.
Trendelenburg's p.
tripod p.
Twining's p.
ulnar flexion p.
upright p.
upside-down p.
Valdini's p.
Valentine's p.

ventral p.
vertical p.
verticomental p.
verticosubmental p.
Walcher's p.
Waters' p.
Waters-Waldron p.
weight-bearing p.
Wigby-Taylor p.
Williams' p.
Wolfenden's p.
Zanelli's p.
positive
    p. beam limitation
    p. charge
    p. contrast myelography
    p. direction
    p. elbow fat pad sign
    p. electron
    p. ion
    p. navicular fat stripe sign
    p. rim sign
    p. rolandic sharp wave
    p. stretch sign
    p. terminal
    p. torsion
    p. wash-out test
positrocephalogram
positron
    p. decay
    p. emission tomography
      (PET)
    p. emission transaxial
      tomography (PETT)
    p. emission transverse
      tomography (PETT)
    p. scan
    p. scintillation camera
positron-coincidence
positronium
post
    p. release radiography
    p. voiding (PV)
post-thoracentesis

post-thoracotomy
post-traumatic
    p.-t. spondylitis
postadrenalectomy pituitary
  adenoma
postaortic lymph node
postarrest line
postassium chloride (k42)
postaxial
postbulbar
postcalcarine
postcaval
    p. lymph node
    p. ureter
postcentral channel
postcesarean
    p. menouria
    p. vesicouterine fistula
postcholecystectomy
  syndrome
postcommissurotomy
  syndrome
postcondylare
postcricoid
postdysenteric rheumatoid
posterior
    p. border position
    p. bowing syndrome
    p. cerebral artery (PCA)
    p. clinoid process
    p. communicating (P-
      comm)
    p. descending artery
      (PDA)
    p. fossa
    p. fossa extra-axial
      arachnoid cyst
      (PFEAAC)
    p. gutters
    p. inferior cerebellar
      artery (PICA)
    p. intraoccipital joint
    p. junction line
    p. lordotic position

posterior—*Continued*
    p. lumbar interbody fusion (PLIF)
    p. profile projection
    p. sagittal index (PSI)
    p. sagittal view
    p. superior iliac spine (PSIS)
    p. thoracic puncture procedure
    p. tibial (artery) (PT)
    p. trabeculated septum
    p. view
posterior-anterior (PA)
posteroanterior (PA)
    p. (coned view) projection
    p. (scout film) projection
    p. axial projection
    p. erect projection
    p. lordotic projection
    p. projection
    p. view
posterolateral
    p. view
posteromedial projection
postevac. (postevacuation)
postevacuation (postevac.)
postexercise
postfatty meal
postfibrinous fibrosis
postganglionic
postgastrectomy syndrome
posticus
postinflammatory polyposis (PIP)
postirradiation
postischemia
postmastectomy
postmyocardial infarction syndrome
postoperative
    p. cholangiography
postpartum
    p. hypophyseogenic myxedema

    p. hypopituitarism
    p. pituitary necrosis
postpericardiotomy syndrome
postpneumonectomy tuberculous empyema
postprandial syndrome
postprocessing corrections
postradiation dysplasia (PRD)
postreduction (PR)
    p. film
postrelease radiography
poststenotic aneurysm
poststress
postureter
postvesicular lymph node
postvoid
    p. radiography
    p. residual (PVR)
potassium (K)
    p. bromide
    p. chloride (K 42)
    p. iodide
    p. perchlorate
    p. permanganate powder
potential
    p. difference
    p. electric
    p. energy
    p. gradient
potentiometer
Pott's
    P.'s aneurysm
    P.'s caries
    P.'s curvature
    P.'s disease
    P.'s fracture
    P.'s procedure
    P.'s puffy tumor
Potter's
    P.'s syndrome
    P.'s thumb
Potter-Bucky
    P.-B. diaphragm
    P.-B. grid

Potts modified percutaneous
    entry needle
Potts-Smith-Gibson
    anastomosis
pouch of Douglas
pound weight
Poupart's ligament
Pouteau's fracture
power
    p. factor
    p. formula
    p. loss
    p. rule
    p. supply
Pozzi's senile pseudorickets
PP (proximal phalanx)
PPD
    (phenyldiphenyloxadiazole)
PPO (2,5-diphenyloxazole)
PR (postreduction)
Pr (praseodymium)
Prader-Labhart-Willi-Fanconi
    syndrome
Praestholm
praseodymium (Pr)
PRD (postradiation
    dysplasia)
preamplifier
preaortic lymph node
preauricular
precaval lymph node
prececal lymph node
precervical
precession
precessional frequency
precordium
predetector
prediastolic murmur
prednisone, vincristine
    [Oncovin], methotrexate, 6-
    mercaptopurine (POMP)
predominance
pre-epiglottic space
prefrontal artery
preganglionic

Preiser's disease
prelaryngeal node
preliminary film
premammary abscess
premolar
prepatellar
preperitoneal fat line
preponderance
preprocessing correction
prepubertal
    panhypopituitarism
preputial gland
prepyloric
    p. sphincter
    p. ulcer
presacral space
presbyesophagus
pressure
    p. atrophy
    p. fracture
    p. mark
    p. point
    stump p.
pressurized
presystolic murmur
pretibial myxedema
pretracheal
    p. node
    p. space
prevalence
prevascular space
prevertebral space
prevesical space
prevesicular lymph node
primary
    p. atypical pneumonia
      (PAP)
    p. beam
    p. circuit
    p. embryonic
      hypertelorism
    p. familial xanthomatosis
    p. filter
    p. hypertrophic
      osteoarthropathy

primary—*Continued*
  p. indurative cavernositis
    of the penis
  p. micro-orchidism
  p. ovarian insufficiency
  p. radiation
  p. ray
  p. splenic neutropenia
    with arthritis
  p. tuberculous complex
  p. tumor
  p. x-ray circuit
primigravida
primipara
primitive node
primordial
  p. cyst
  p. dwarfism
princeps pollicis
principle
  air-gap p.
  Dodge's p.
  Fick's p.
  Grossman's p.
  Pauli's exclusion p.
  planigraphic p.
  tomographic p.
Prinzmetal's
  P.'s angina
  P.'s angor
Priodax
priority
  p. processing
  p. reconstruction
prism
Pro-Banthine (propantheline
  bromide)
PRO-MACE (prednisone,
  methotrexate, Adriamycin,
  cyclophosphamide,
  etoposide [VP-16-23])
probe
  fiberoptic p.
  scintillation p.
Probitron (geiger counter)

procarbazine, hydroxyurea
  radiotherapy (PHRT)
  protocol
procedure
  Anderson's p.
  Bristow's p.
  CABG p. (pronounced
    "cabbage")
  coronary artery bypass
    graft (CABG) p.
  Glenn's p.
  Gotmori-Takamatsu p.
  Hartmann's p.
  Hill's p.
  Jannetta's p.
  Mark IV p.
  Müller-Damman p.
  Mustard's p.
  Nissen's p.
  Polya's p.
  push-back p.
  V-Y p.
  variceal sclerosing p.
  Vineberg's p.
  Whipple's p.
  Zancolli's p.
procerus
process
  acromion p.
  alveolar p.
  anterior clinoid p.
  articular p.
  bremsstrahlung p.
  capitular p.
  clinoid p.
  condyloid p.
  conoid p.
  consolidative p.
  coracoid p.
  coronoid p.
  ensiform p.
  epitransverse p.
  frontal p.
  glenoid p.
  hamulus p.

inferior articular p.
inflammatory p.
intercondylar p.
lacrimal p.
mastoid p.
neutron absorption p.
odontoid p.
olecranon p.
palatine p.
paracondyloid p.
petrosal p.
posterior clinoid p.
pterygoid p.
spinous p.
styloid p.
superior articular p.
supraclinoid p.
supracondyloid p.
temporal p.
transverse p.
uncinate p.
ungual p.
vermiform p.
xiphoid p.
zygomatic p.
processus lunatus
Proetz' position
profile
    p. position
    p. ray view
    p. scan
Profile Plus catheter
profunda
    p. femoris artery (PFA)
    p. method
profundus
progenitor
progeria
    p. adultorum
    p. syndrome
    p.-like syndrome
Progestasert intrauterine
  device (IUD)
progesterone
prognathism

prognoses, pl.
    prognosis, s.
prognosis, s.
    prognoses, pl.
programmable
progressive
    p. diaphyseal dysplasia
    p. dyspnea
    p. fibromyositis
    p. hemifacial paralysis
    p. multifocal
      leukoencephalopathy
      (PML)
    p. muscular tautness
    p. portal fibrosis
    p. pulmonary dystrophy
projection
    abduction p.
    acanthiomeatal p.
    acanthioparietal p.
    acute flexion axial p.
    adduction p.
    anterior circulation p.
    anterior p.
    anterior profile p.
    anteroposterior above
      diaphragm p.
    anteroposterior axial p.
    anteroposterior basal p.
    anteroposterior below
      diaphragm p.
    anteroposterior external p.
    anteroposterior lordotic p.
    anteroposterior oblique p.
    anteroposterior odontoid
      p.
    anteroposterior p.
    apical lordotic p.
    apical p.
    axial p.
    axial supine p.
    axial transcranial p.
    axillary p.
    axiolateral p.
    ball-catcher's p.

projection—*Continued*
    basilar p.
    basovertical p.
    Bertel's p.
    biplane p.
    Blineau's p.
    blow-out p.
    Bridgman's p.
    Caldwell's p.
    caudal p.
    cephalad angled p.
    cephalic p.
    cervicothoracic p.
        (Fletcher's)
    Chassard-Lapiné p.
    Chaussé's p.
    chewing p.
    "Cleopatra" p.
    composite dorsoplantar p.
    coned-down p.
    craniocaudal p.
    cross-sectional transverse
        p.
    decubitus p.
    distal p.
    dorsoplantar p.
    eccentric p.
    eccentric-angle parieto-
        orbital p.
    en face p.
    erect anteroposterior p.
    erect fluoro spot p.
    erect oblique p.
    erroneous p.
    extraoral p.
    filtered-back p.
    Fletcher's p.
        (cervicothoracic)
    flexion/extension p.
    Fourier two-dimensional p.
    frontal p.
    geometrical p.
    half-axial p.
    inferior p.

    inferior-superior p.
    inferior-superior tangential
        p.
    inferosuperior axial p.
    inferosuperior p.
    intraoral p.
    L5 coned view p.
    L5-S1 p.
    lateral (Bridgman's) p.
    lateral (Friedman's) p.
    lateral oblique axial p.
    lateral p.
    lateral transcranial p.
    lateral transfacial p.
    lateromedial oblique p.
    lateromedial tangential p.
    Lauenstein and Hickey p.
    localized lateral p.
    Loepp's p.
    lordotic (A-P) erect p.
    lumbosacral p.
    Mayer's p.
    medial oblique axial p.
    mediolateral oblique p.
    mediolateral p.
    navicular p.
    nuchofrontal p.
    oblique (cone view) p.
    oblique anteroposterior p.
    oblique erect p.
    oblique transfacial p.
    occipital anteroposterior
        p.
    occipital p.
    occipitofrontal p.
    occlusal p.
    odontoid p.
    open-mouth p.
    orbitoparietal oblique p.
    orbitoparietal p.
    p. formula
    p. reconstruction imaging
    PA and lateral p.
    palmar p.

parieto-orbital oblique p.
parieto-orbital p.
parietoacanthal p.
parietotemporal p.
perineosacral p.
pillar p.
Pirie's transoral p.
plantodorsal p.
posterior profile p.
posteroanterior (coned view) p.
posteroanterior (scout film) p.
posteroanterior axial p.
posteroanterior erect p.
posteroanterior lordotic p.
posteroanterior p.
posterolateral p.
posteromedial p.
proximal p.
RADFILE p.
radiographic p.
recumbent lateral p.
Rhese's prone p.
right anterior oblique (RAD) p.
right lateral (RLAT) p.
Runström's p.
scanned p.
scaphoid p.
scout film (posteroanterior) p.
semiaxial anteroposterior p.
semiaxial p.
semiaxial transcranial p.
semierect p.
skyline p.
Stenver's for tips (prone) p.
stereo right lateral p.
stereoscopic p.
submentovertex p.
submentovertical axial p.

submentovertical p.
superimposition p.
superoinferior p.
supine p.
supraorbital p.
"sunrise" p.
swimmer's p.
tangential p.
Templeton and Zim carpal tunnel p.
thalamocortical p.
Towne-Chamberlain p.
transabdominal (A-P) p.
transcranial p.
transfacial p.
translateral p.
transoral p.
transtabular AP/PA p.
transthoracic p.
tunnel p.
ulnar deviation p.
vertebral arch p.
vertex p.
verticomental p.
verticosubmental p.
Vogt's bone-free p.
volar p.
Waters' p.
weight-bearing p.
prolapse
    holosystolic p.
    mitral valve p. (MVP)
    systolic p.
prolapsed bladder
proliferative
    p. arthritis
    p. fibrosis
prolongation
promethium (Pm)
prominence
prominent
promontory
pronate
pronation

pronator
    p. pedis
    p. quandratus muscle
    p. teres muscle
prone
    p. jackknife position
    p. position
pronephros
propagation
propantheline bromide
properitoneal
    p. fat line
    p. fat stripe
prophase
proportional
    p. counter
    p. region
proptosis
propyliodone
propylthiouracil (PTU) tablets
prostate
    p. calculus
    p. capsule
    p. enlargement
    p. gland
    p. urethra
prostatic
    p. calcification
    p. catheter
    p. echogram (PECHO)
    p. vesicle
prostatography
prostheses, pl.
    prosthesis, s.
prosthesis
    Austin Moore hip p.
    Beall p.
    F. R. Thompson p.
    Freeman-Swanson p.
    Matchett-Brown hip p.
    modified F. R. Thompson
    Swanson p.
prosthesis, s.
    prostheses, pl.

prosthetic valve
Prostigmin (neostigmine)
protactinium (Pa)
protein
    p. absorption
    p. bound iodine (PBI)
proteinemia
proteolysis
protirelin
proton
    p. density
    p. relaxation time
    p. spin-lattice relaxation
proton-synchrotron
protoplasm
protrusio acetabuli
protuberance
    external occipital p.
proximal
    p. convoluted tubule
    p. femoral focal deficiency
      (PFFD) syndrome
    p. interphalangeal (PIP)
      joint
    p. phalanx (PP)
    p. projection
    p. tibial
prune-belly syndrome
PRZF (pyrazofurin)
PS (partial saturation)
PS (pulse sequence)
psammoma bodies
psammosarcoma
psammotherapy
pseudarthrosis
pseudo-Crouzon familial
    craniostenosis
pseudo-elephantiasis
    neuroarthritica
pseudo-Hurler polydystrophy
pseudo-Hurler's syndrome
pseudo-obstruction
pseudo-optic foramen
pseudo-Turner's syndrome

pseudoachondroplastic
  dysplasia
pseudoacromegalic syndrome
pseudoactinomycosis
pseudoarthrosis
pseudobrachydactyly
pseudocamptodactyly
pseudocoarctation of the
  aorta
pseudocoxalgia
pseudodiverticulum
pseudoepiphysis
pseudoforamen
pseudofracture
pseudogout
  (chondrocalcinosis)
pseudohydrocephalus
pseudolymphoma
pseudomembranous
    p. colitis
    p. enterocolitis
    p. gastritis
pseudomucinous
  cystadenocarcinoma
pseudomyxoma peritonei
pseudonuchal infantilism
pseudopodal
pseudopolyp
pseudopolyposis
pseudopost-Billroth I sign
pseudo-
  pseudohypoparathyroidism
pseudosarcoma
pseudospondylolisthesis of
  Junghans
pseudotruncus arteriosus
pseudotumor
pseudoxanthoma elasticum
  (PXE)
PSI (posterior sagittal index)
PSIS (posterior superior iliac
  spine)
psoas
    p. abscess

p. fascia
p. line
p. major
p. minor
p. muscle
p. shadow
psoriatic
    p. arthritis
    p. spondylitis
PSP (phenolsulfonphthalein)
psychogenic
    p. constipation
    p. megacolon
    p. rheumatism
psychosocial dwarfism
PT (pluridirectional
  tomography)
PT (posterior tibial) artery
PTA (percutaneous
  transluminal angioplasty)
PTBD (percutaneous
  transhepatic biliary
  drainage)
PTC (percutaneous
  transhepatic
  cholangiography)
PTCA (percutaneous
  transluminal coronary
  angiography)
pterion
pterygium
    p. syndrome
    p. universalis
pterygoarthromyodysplasia
pterygoid
    p. apophysis
    p. fossa
    p. hamulus
    p. plate
    p. process
pterygoideus
    p. lateralis
    p. medialis
pterygomaxillary fissure

pterygopalatine
  p. canal
  p. fossa
pterygospinous
PTHBD (percutaneous
  transhepatic biliary drain)
ptosis-epicanthus syndrome
PTU (propylthiouracil)
PTX (pneumothorax)
ptyalography
ptyalolithiasis
puberal seminiferous tubule
  failure
puberty
pubes, pl.
    pubis, s.
pubic
  p. arch
  p. bone
  p. rami fracture
  p. ramus
  "p." sign
  p. symphysis
  p. varus
pubis, s.
    pubes, pl.
pubocapsular ligament
pubococcygeal line
pubofemoral ligament
Puck cutfilm changer
PUD (peptic ulcer disease)
pudendal
  p. artery
  p. canal
  p. ulcer
Puder-Hayer valve system
Pulmolite Technetium Tc 99M
  aggregated albumin
pulmonary
  p. abscess
  p. airway
  p. alveolar microlithiasis
  p. alveolar proteinosis
  p. amyloidosis

p. anectasis
p. angiography
p. anthrax
p. aplasia
p. arteriography
p. arteriovenous
  malformation
p. arteritis
p. artery (PA)
p. artery bending
p. artery catheter
p. aspergillosis
p. aspiration
p. atelectasis
p. atresia
p. barotrauma
p. blood flow (PBF) study
p. blood volume
p. capillary wedge
  pressure
p. coccidoidomycosis
p. collapse
p. congestion
p. contusion
p. cyst
p. density
p. dysmaturity
p. edema
p. embolism (PE)
p. embolus (PE)
p. emphysema
p. extravascular lung water
p. fibrosis
p. fissure
p. flow
p. gangrene
p. granuloma
p. hamartoma
p. hematoma
p. hemorrhage
p. hemosiderosis
p. hives
p. hyperaeration
p. hypertension

p. hypertrophic osteoarthropathy
p. hypoplasia
p. infarction
p. infiltrate
p. infiltration with eosinophilia (PIE)
p. insufficiency
p. interstitial edema (PIE)
p. interstitial emphysema (PIE)
p. interstitial fibrosis
p. juxtaesophageal lymph node
p. laceration
p. lymph node
p. meniscus sign
p. mitral valve
p. nodule
p. notch sign
p. oligemia
p. ossification
p. osteoarthropathy
p. osteopathia
p. parenchymal trauma
p. pedicle
p. perforation
p. pleura
p. renal syndrome
p. ridge
p. scar
p. semilunar valve
p. sequestration
p. sling
p. stenosis
p. support
p. target sign
p. thrombosis
p. trunk
p. tuberculosis
p. valve
p. valve stenosis
p. vascular autoregulatory phenomenon
p. vasculature
p. venolumbar syndrome
p. venous hypertension (PVH)
p. venous pressure (PVP)
p. venous redistribution (PVR)
p. ventilation study
p. wedge position
pulmonic
    p. murmur
    p. regurgitation
    p. stenosis
pulpal abscess
pulsating current
pulse
    p. amplifier
    p. Doppler
    p. generator
    p. length (width)
    p. sequence (PS)
    p. width code
    selective radiofrequency p.
pulse-height analyzer
pulse-height spectrometry
pulse-height spectrum
pulsed
    p. Doppler ultrasonography (PDU)
    p. gradient
    p. NMR
    p. radiofrequency field
    p. response resonance
pulsed-wave Doppler (PWD)
pulseless disease
pulsion
pulvinar thalami
punched-out lytic lesion
punctate calcification
punctum dilator
puncture
    arterial p.
    cisternal p.
    direct cardiac p.

puncture—*Continued*
  lumbar p.
  percutaneous p.
  percutaneous transhepatic
    p.
PUNL (percutaneous ultrasonic
  nephrolithotripsy)
Purkinje's imaging
purpura
  Henoch's p.
  Henoch-Schönlein p.
push-back procedure
putamen
Putti's
  P.'s syndrome
  P.'s triad
putty kidney
PV (peripheral vascular)
PV (plasma volume)
PV (portal vein)
PV (postvoiding)
P&V (pyloroplasty and
  vagotomy)
PVH (pulmonary venous
  hypertension)
PVP (polyvinylpyrrolidone)
PVP (pulmonary venous
  pressure)
PVR (postvoid residual)
PVR (pulmonary venous
  redistribution)
PXE (pseudoxanthoma
  elasticum)
pyarthrosis
Pychokon-R
Pyelectan
pyelectasis
pyelocaliectasis
pyelocalyceal
pyelofluoroscopy
pyelogram
  hydrated p.
  retrograde p. (RP)
pyelography
  antegrade p.

ascending p.
drip infusion p.
hydrated p.
intravenous p. (IVP)
percutaneous antegrade p.
retrograde p. (RP)
washout p.
pyelointerstitial
Pyelombrine
pyelonephritic kidney
pyelonephritis
  atrophic p.
  emphysematous p.
  focal p.
  xanthogranulomatous p.
Pyelosil
pyemic abscess
pyknodysostosis
pyknosis
Pyle's disease
Pyle-Cohn disease
pylephlebostenosis splenica
pylori or pyloruses, pl.
  pylorus, s.
pyloric
  p. antrum
  p. atresia
  p. canal
  p. channel
  p. lymph node
  p. orifice
  p. portion
  p. sphincter
  p. stenosis
  p. string sign
  p. tit, sign of
  p. torus defect
  p. ulcer
  p. valve
  p. vestibule
pyloroplasty and vagotomy
  (P&V)
pylorospasm
pylorus, s.
  pylori or pyloruses, pl.

pyloruses or pylori, pl.
 pylorus, s.
Pylumbrin
pyogenic
 p. abscess
 p. arthritis
 p. granuloma
 p. osteomyelitis
pyogram
pyohemopneumothorax
PYP (pyrophosphate)
pyramid
pyramidal
 p. blush
 p. fracture

 p. tract
pyramidalis nasi
pyrazofurin (PRZF)
pyridoxilene glutamate (PGA)
pyridoxine
pyridoxylideneglutamate
pyriform (piriform)
 p. thorax
pyriformis
pyrogen
Pyrolite sodium
pyrophosphate (PYP)
 p. imaging
 p. scan

Qq

Q angle
QC (quality control)
QCT (quantitative computed tomography)
QCT (quantitative CT)
QF (quality factor)
q.n. (every night)
QPC (quadrigeminal plate cistern)
QRS synchro method
quadrant
quadrantectomy, axillary dissection, and radiotherapy (QUART)
quadrate lobe
quadrature detector
quadratus
    q. femoris
    q. labii inferioris muscle
    q. labii superioris
    q. lumborum
    q. lumborum fascia
    q. menti
    q. plantae
quadriceps
    q. extensor femoris
    q. femoris muscle
quadrigeminal
    q. lamina
    q. plate cistern (QPC)
quadrigeminate
quadriplegic standing fracture frame
quadruple syndrome
quality
    q. control (QC)

q. factor (QF)
quanta, pl.
    quantum, s.
quantification
Quantisorb 125-I
quantitative
    q. bone mineral analysis
    q. brain imaging
    q. cardiology
    q. computed tomography (QCT)
    q. CT (QCT)
    q. CT densitometry
    q. regional lung function study
    q. tracer study
quantum
    q. energy
    q. mottle
    q. number
    q. theory
    q. unit
    q. yield
quantum, s.
    quanta, pl.
QUART (quadrantectomy, axillary dissection, and radiotherapy)
quarter
    q. offset
quarter-quarter offset
quartz glass
Quatrefages' angle
Queckenstedt's
    Q.'s maneuver
    Q.'s sign

quenching gas
Quervain's fracture
Quesada's method
Quick CT scanner
quiescent

Quincke's meningitis
Quincke-Babcock spinal needle
Quinton catheter
    Q. Mahurkar dual-lumen c.

Rr

R (roentgen)
RA (radioactive)
Ra (radium)
RA (rheumatoid arthritis)
RA (right atrium)
RaafCath catheter
RAB (remote afterloading
  brachytherapy)
rabbetting
rabbit
rabbit-ear sign
Rabinov sialography catheter
racemose aneurysm
rachicentesis
rachigraph
rachischisis
rachitis
Racobalamin
rad (radiation absorbed dose)
RAD (right anterior
  descending) coronary artery
RAD (roentgen administered
  dose)
RADFILE projection
radial
    r. epiphysis
    r. fossa
    r. groove
    r. head
    r. malleolus
    r. notch
    r. tuberosity
radialis indicis volaris
radian
radiant energy
radiation
    acoustic r.
    actinic r.

alpha r.
annihilation r.
auditory r.
background r.
beta r.
"braking" r.
bremsstrahlung r.
Cerenkov r.
characteristic r.
corpuscular r.
cosmic r.
direct r.
dose equivalent r.
effective direct r. (EDR)
electromagnetic r.
external r.
gamma r.
genetic effect of r.
heterogeneous r.
homogeneous r.
infrared r.
intercavitary r.
interstitial r.
ionizing r.
irritative r.
K r.
leakage r.
low-energy r.
Maxwell's theory of r.
mitogenetic r.
monochromatic r.
monoenergetic r.
nuclear r.
occipitothalamic r.
oncology r.
optic r.
photochemical r.
primary r.

r. absorbed dose (rad)
r. burn
r. coil
r. colitis
r. counter
r. dosimetry
r. effect
r. energy
r. enteropathy
r. equivalent man (REM)
r. exposure
r. exposure limit
r. gastritis
r. hazard
r. hepatitis
R. Laboratory (RL)
r. leakage
r. level (NIRL)
r. monitor
r. of corpus callosum
r. oncology
r. osteitis
r. pneumonia
r. production
r. protection
r. reaction (RR)
r. response (RR)
r. sickness
r. symbol
r. syndrome
r. therapy (RTx or RT)
r. therapy oncology group (RTOG)
r. window
recoil r.
remnant r.
scatter r.
solar r.
specific r.
spontaneous r.
stem r.
stray r.
striomesencephalic r.
striothalamic r.

supervoltage therapy r.
terrestrial r.
thalamic r.
thermal r.
ultraviolet r.
visible r.
white r.
radiation-sensitive
radical
r. mastectomy
r. neck dissection (RND)
radicle
radiculogram
radiculopathy
radii or radiuses, pl.
radius, s.
Radio-Cholografin
radio-opacity
radio-osteonecrosis
Radio-Teridax
radioactinium
radioactive (RA)
r. albumin
r. applicator
r. capture
r. colloidal gold (Au198)
r. decay
r. disintegration
r. effluents
r. element
r. equilibrium (Eq.)
r. fallout
r. gallium (Ga)
r. gold (Au)
r. half-life
r. iodine (I)
r. iodine uptake (RAIU)
r. iron
r. isotope
r. nuclides
r. patient
r. phosphorus
r. series
r. source

radioactive (RA)—*Continued*
  r. strontium (Sr)
  r. tagging
  r. technetium (99m Tc)
  r. thorium (Th)
  r. tracer
  r. uptake
radioactivity
  artificial r.
  induced r.
  natural r.
radioallergosorbent test
  (RAST)
radioanaphylaxis
radioassay
radioautogram
radioautography
radiobe
radiobioassay
radiobiological
radiobiologist
radiobiology
  interventional r.
  percutaneous
    interventional r.
radiocalcium
radiocarbon
radiocarcinogenesis
radiocardiogram (RKG or RCG)
radiocardiography (RKG or
  RCG)
radiocarpal
  r. angle
  r. articulation
  r. joint
  r. ligament
radiocarpus
radiochemical
  r. analysis
  r. purity
radiochemistry
radiochemotherapy
radiochemy
radiocholecystogram

radiocholecystography
radiochroism
radiochromatographic
radiochromatography
radiochrometer
radiocinematograph
radiocobalt
radiocolloid
radiocurable
radiocyanocobalamin solution
radiocystitis
radiode
radiodense
radiodensity
radiodermatitis
radiodiagnosis
radiodiagnostic
radiodiaphane
radiodontia
radiodontist
radioecology
radioelectrocardiogram (REKG
  or RECG)
radioelectrocardiography
  (REKG or RECG)
radioelectroencephalograph
  (REEG)
radioelement
radioencephalogram
radioencephalography
radioepidermitis
radioepithelitis
radiofluorine
radiofrequency (RF)
  r. coil
  r. electrophrenic
    respiration
  r. pulse
radiogallium (Ga 72)
radiogenic
radiogold
radiogram
radiographic
  r. baseline

r. contrast
r. density
r. distortion
r. effect
r. grid
r. image
r. latitude
r. magnification
r. mode
r. mottle
r. penetration
r. position
r. projection
r. quality
r. resolution
r. technique
r. view
Radiographol
radiography
    air contrast r.
    biomedical r.
    body section r.
    bone age r.
    "chalky" r.
    diagrammatic r.
    electron r.
    gamma r.
    industrial r.
    kinescope r.
    magnification r.
    miniature r.
    multiple r.
    panoral r.
    panoramic r.
    postrelease r.
    postvoid r.
    r. filter
    scanned projection r.
    scout r.
    spill r.
    "split film" r.
    stereoscopic r.
radiohepatographic
radiohumeral

radioimmunity
radioimmunoassay (RIA)
radioimmunodiffusion
radioimmunoelectrophoresis
radioimmunoprecipitation test
radioinduction
radioiodinated
    r. human serum albumin
      (RIHSA)
    r. orthoiodohippurate
    r. serum
    r. serum albumin (RISA)
radioiodine
    r. test
radioiron
    r. half-life
    r. incorporation rate
radioisotope
    r. bone scan
    r. calibrator
    r. caliper
    r. camera
    r. cisternography
    r. liver scan
    r. liver/spleen scan
    r. medicine (RIM)
    r. osteogram
    r. placentogram
    r. renogram
    r. scan
    r. scanner
    r. scanning
    r. technologist
    r. thyroid scan
radioisotopes
    aggregated radioiodinated
      albumin (human) I-131
    ammonium molybdate
      (Mo-99)
    arsenate 74 (As-74)
    barium carbonate (C-14)
    cadmium chloride (Cd-
      109)
    calcium chloride (Ca-45)

radioisotopes—*Continued*
   calcium chloride (Ca-47)
   californium 252
   carbon 14
   ceric nitrate (Ce-141)
   cesium 137 (Cs-137)
   chlorine 36 (Cl-36)
   chlormerodrin (Hg-197)
   chlormerodrin (Hg-203)
   chromic chloride (Cr-51)
   Chromitope chloride
   Chromitope sodium
     (chromate Cr-51
     sodium)
   chromium 51
   cobalt 57 (Co-57)
   cobalt 58 (Co-58)
   cobalt 60 (Co-60)
   cobaltous chloride (Co-57)
   cobaltous chloride (Co-60)
   cupric acetate (Cu-64)
   cyanocobalamin (Co-57)
   cyanocobalamin (Co-60)
   diotyrosine (I-125)
   Dipath
   ferric chloride (Fe-55)
   ferric chloride (Fe-59)
   ferrous ascorbate
   ferrutope (Fe-59)
   fluorine 18
   fluoride
   gold 198 (Au-198)
   Hipputope I-131 (radio-
     iodinated sodium
     iodohippurate [^{131}I])
   hydrochloric acid (Cl-36)
   hydrogen 3 (tritium)
   indium 111
   indium 111 chloride
   indium 113m
   iodine 123 (I-123)
   iodine 125 (I-125)
   iodine 131 (I-131)
   iodine 132 (I-132)
   Iodocaps I-125 or I-131

   iridium (Ir-192)
   iron 55 (Fe-55)
   iron 59 (Fe-59)
   ISO/Meridrin Hg-197, Hg-
     203
   krypton (Kr-81)
   manganese chloride Mn-54
   mercuric nitrate Hg-197
   mercuric nitrate Hg-203
   mercury 197
   molybdenum (Mo-99)
   Natritope
   Neohydrin (Hg-203)
   nickel chloride Ni-63
   Oleotope
   Oriodide-131
   Phosphocaps
   phosphorus 32 (P-32)
   phosphotec
   radiogold (198-Au)
   radioiodinated serum
     albumin (human) I-125
   radioiodinated serum
     albuminia (human) I-131
   Radio-Teridax
   radiosodium
   radiotriolein
   radium 226 (Ra-226)
   raoleic acid
   Robengatope
   rubidium chloride (Rb-86)
   selenium 75
   selenomethionine (Se-75)
   sodium 23 (Na-23)
   sodium 24 (Na-24)
   sodium chromate (Cr-51)
   sodium iodide (I-125)
   sodium iodide (I-131)
   sodium phosphate (P-32)
   sodium molybdate (Mo-
     99)
   stannous chloride (Sn-113)
   stannous chloride (Sn-
     119m)
   strontium 85

strontium 87
strontium 90
strontium nitrate (Sr-85)
sulfuric acid (S-35)
technetium-99m
tellurium (Te)
tetrafluoroborate
thallium chloride (Tl-201)
thallium nitrate (Tl-204)
thorium 232 (Th-232)
thulium chloride (Tm-170)
tin 113 (Sn-113)
tin 119m (Sn-119m)
titanium dioxide 47 (Ti-47)
tolpovidone (I-131)
triolein (I-131)
Triomet
tritium
xenon (Xe-133)
ytterbium 90 (Yb-90)
ytterbium chloride (Yb-169)
zinc chloride (Zn-65)
radioisotopic
radiokymography
radiolabeled ligand
radiolead
radiolesion
radioligand
radiologic
    r. technician
    r. technologist (RT)
radiological emergency assistance
Radiological Health Data (RHD)
radiologist
radiology information system (RIS)
radiology operations system (ROS)
Radiology Society of North America (RSNA)
radiolucency
radiolucent

radiolus
radiometallography
radiometer
    pastille r.
    photographic r.
radiometric
radiomicrometer
radiomimetic
radion
radionecrosis
radioneuritis
radionitrogen
radionuclide
    first-pass r.
    r. angiocardiography
    r. angiography
    r. cholescintigram
    r. cholescintigraphy
    r. cisternography
    r. cystography
    r. cystourethrogram
    r. emission tomography
    r. imaging
    r. injection
    r. kinetics
    r. purity
    r. scan
    r. venography (RNV)
    r. ventriculography (RVG)
    r. voiding cystourethrography
radionuclides
    18F (fluorine)
    32P (phosphorus)
    42K (potassium)
    51Cr (chromium)
    52Fe (iron)
    57Co (cobalt)
    58Co (cobalt)
    59Fe (iron)
    60Co (cobalt)
    67Ga (gallium)
    68Ga (gallium)
    75Se (selenium)
    81Kr (krypton)

radionuclides—*Continued*
    85Kr (krypton)
    85Sr (strontium)
    87mSr (strontium)
    90Y (yttrium)
    99m-Tc (technetium)
    99Mo (molybdenum)
    111In (indium)
    113mIn (indium)
    123I (iodine)
    125I (iodine)
    127Xe (xenon)
    131I (iodine)
    133Ba (barium)
    133Xe (xenon)
    137Cs (cesium)
    169Yb (ytterbium)
    192Ir (iridium)
    195Au (gold)
    197Hg (mercury)
    198Au (gold)
    199Au (gold)
    201Tl (thallium)
    203Hg (mercury)
radiopacity
radiopaque
    r. bougie
    r. catheter
    r. foreign body
    r. intestinal tube
    r. substance
    r. suture
radioparency
radioparent
radiopathology
radiopelvimetry
radiopharmaceuticals
    125I-sodium iothalamate
    131I-iodohippurate
    aggregated
        a. albumin
        a. radioiodinated (I
            131) albumin
    albumin microspheres

Albumotope (I-131)
    (albumin, iodinated I-
    131 serum)
aldosterone (3H)
    radioimmunoassay
Androstenedione
Angiotensin I (125I)
Aureoloid 198
Aureotope
Aus-tect Test System,
    rheophoresis
Ausab
Auscell
Ausria
calcium chloride
chlormerodrin
Chromalbin (chromium CR
    51 and human albumin)
Chromitope sodium
    (chromate Cr 51,
    sodium)
Circulating T3 test set
citrate
Cobatope-57 (cobaltous
    chloride Co 57)
colloidal gold
colloidal phosphorus
cortisol (125I)
    radioimmunoassay kit
cromalbin
cyanocobalamin (Co-57)
cyanocobalamin (Co-60)
dehydroepiandrosterone
Dicopac kit
digitoxin test set
digoxin I-125
    immunoassay diagnostic
    kit
diphenylhydantoin
diphosphonate
DPH (diphenylhydantoin,
    phenytoin)
DTPA (diethylenetriamine
    penta-acetic acid)

Epi-testosterone
estradiol
estriol (125I)
estrogen (E1/E2)
estrone
ethan-1-hydroxyl-1, 1
  diphosphonate (EHD)
ethiodized oil
ferric chloride
ferrous
  f. citrate Fe 59
  f. sulfate
fluorine 18
folate
gallium citrate (Ga 67)
gamma reference source
  sets
gastrin immutope kit
gold colloid
Haverhill (^{198}Au)
HIDA (N-[2,6-dimethyl]
  iminodiacetic acid)
hippuran I-131 injection
Hipputope (radio-
  iodinated sodium
  iodohippurate [^{131}I])
iocetamic acid
iodated I-125
iodated I-131
iodipamide meglumine
  injection
iodohippurate sodium
Iodotope (sodium iodide I-
  131)
iopanoic tablets
Irosorb-59 diagnostic
  kit
latent iron-binding
  capacity (LIBC) test
liothyronine
Macrotec (technetium Tc-
  99m medronate kit)
Medotopes
  (radiopharmaceuticals)

meglumine and calcium
  metrizoates
methylene diphosphonate
  (MDP)
methylene
  hydroxydiphosphonate
  (MHDP)
Molytech calibrator assay
  kit
Neohydrin Hg-203
oleic acid
  o. I-125 capsules
  o. iodine-131
pentetate calcium
  trisodium Yb-169
Perchloracap
Phosphocol P-32
Phosphotec
Phosphotope
potassium perchlorate
progesterone
protirelin
pulmolite technetium
Quantisorb 125-I
Racobalamin
Renotec
Reptilase-R
Res-O-Mat
RIA-Mat Angiotensin
Robengatope
rose bengal sodium
RUBA-tect rubella
  diagnostic test
Rubacell
Rubratope 57
  (cyanocobalamin Co 57)
Rubratope 60
selenomethionine Se-75
Sensor
Seralute
Sethotope
  (selenomethionine Se
  75)
sincalide

radiopharmaceuticals—*Continued*
  sodium
    s. chromate
    s. iodide
    s. iodohippurate I-131
    s. iothalamate I-125
    s. pertechnetate Tc-99m
    s. phosphate
    s. rose bengal I-131
    s. tyropanoate
  stannous
    s. sulfur colloid
    s. diphosphonate
    s. pyrophosphate
  Stillmeadow 198 Au
  strontium
    s. nitrate Sr-85
    s. Sr-87m
  sulfur colloid (SC)
  Tc-99m
    T. ceretec (Hg-197)
    T. ceretec (Hg-203)
    T. dimercaptosuccinic (DISIDA) scan
    T. dimethylacetanilide-iminodiacetic acid (HIDA)
    T. disofenin (DISIDA) scan
    T. fibriscint
    T. glucoheptonate
    T. HSA
    T. hydroxydiphosphonate (HDP)
    T. lung aggregate
    T. macroaggregated albumin (MAA)
    T. methylene diphosphonate (MDP)
    T. microlite
    T. microspheres
    T. osteolite
    T. osteoscan (HDP)
  TechneColl kit
  TechneScan MAA kit (aggregated human albumin)
  technetated (Tc 99m) aggregate albumin
  testosterone RIA antiserum
  Tesuloid (technetium Tc-99m sulfur colloid)
  Tetrasorb
  thallium-201 chloride
  thiethylperazine maleate
  Thypinone (protirelin)
  Thyrolute
  Thyrostat-3
  tolpovidone
  tracer microspheres
  Trilute 125I uptake test
  triolein
  vitamin B_{12}
  Xeneisol
  xenon (Xe-133)
  xenon gas
  ytterbium (Yb-69) DTPA
radiopharmacy
radiophosphate (32 p)
radiophosphorus (P 231)
radiophotography
radiophylaxis
radiopotassium
radiopotentiation
radiopraxis
radioprotective drugs
radiopulmogram
radiopulmonography
radioreceptor assay (RRA)
radioresistance
radioresistant
radioresponsive
radiosclerosis

radioscope
radioscopy
radiosensitive
radiosodium
radiospirometry
radiostereoscopy
radiosterilization
radiostrontium
radiosulfur
radiosurgery
radiotechnetium
    r. polyphosphate
radiotelemetry
radiotellurium
radiothanatology
radiotherapeutics
radiotherapist
radiotherapy (RT)
    computerized r.
    interstitial r.
    intracavitary r.
radiothermy
radiothorium
radiotoxemia
radiotracer
radiotransparent
radiotriolein
radiotropic
radioulnar
    r. articulation
    r. joint
    r. synostosis
RADISH (rheumatoid arthritis
    diffuse idiopathic skeletal
    hyperostosis)
radium (Ra)
    r. 226 (Ra 226)
    r. application
    r. beam therapy
    r. dosimetry
    r. equivalent
    r. implant
    r. insertion
    r. needle

    r. therapy (RT)
radius
    Bohr r.
    r. grid
radius, s.
    radii or radiuses, pl.
radiuses or radii, pl.
    radius, s.
Radner's vein
radon (Rn)
    r. seed implant
RAE (right atrial enlargement)
Raeder-Harbitz syndrome
railway catheter
Raimondi
    R. catheter
    R. ventricular catheter
rainbow fracture frame
RAIU (radioactive iodine
    uptake) test
rales
ram's horn sign
rami, pl.
    ramus, s.
ramus
    inferior r.
    ipsilateral r.
    ischial r.
    mandibular r.
    pubic r.
    superior r.
ramus, s.
    rami, pl.
random
Ranke complex
RAO (right anterior oblique)
    projection
raoleic acid
raphe
rapid
    r. processing film
    r. processing mode (RPM)
rapid-drip study
rapid-sequence scanning

Rapido-mat
Rapp's position
rare earth
rarefaction
Rashkind catheter
Rashkind's
    R.'s procedure
    R.'s technique
Rasmussen's aneurysm
RAST (radioallergosorbent
    test)
rate meter
Rathbun's disease
Rathke's
    R.'s pouch
    R.'s pouch tumor
ratio
    cardiothoracic r. (CTR)
    gyromagnetic r.
    lecithin/sphingomyelin (L/
        S) r.
    magnetogyric r.
    perimeter r.
    r. grid
    r. transformer
    rectosigmoid r.
    signal-to-noise r. (SNR)
    target-to-nontarget r.
    ventilation-perfusion r.
        (VQR)
"rat-tail" deformity
ratty
Rauber's sign
raw data
ray
    alpha r.
    B r.
    Becquerel r.
    beta r.
    cathode r.
    central r.
    corresponding r.
    cosmic r.
    delta r.
    fluorescent r.

gamma r.
glass r.
Goldstein's r.
grenz r.
infraroentgen r.
Lenard r. tube
paracathode r.
parallel r.
primary r.
roentgen r.
secondary r.
vertical r.
Wehnelt (W) r.
Raybar 75
Rayleigh scattering
Raynaud's
    R.'s gangrene
    R.'s phenomenon
    R.'s syndrome of the upper
        limb
Rayopak
Rayvist
RBC (red blood cell) scan
RBE (relative biologic
    effectiveness)
RBL (Reid's baseline)
RBZ (rubidazone [zorubicin])
RC (retrograde cystogram)
RCA (right coronary artery)
RCCA (right common carotid
    artery)
RCM (red cell mass)
RCV (red cell volume)
rd (rutherford)
RDMS (Registered Diagnostic
    Medical Sonographer)
RDS (respiratory distress
    syndrome)
re-entrance angle
reabsorption
reactance
reaction
    biomolecular r.
    Eisenmenger's r.
    endergic r.

exergic r.
nuclear r.
periosteal r.
thermonuclear r.
reactor
    nuclear r.
read-out
    r. delay
reading
    r. fracture frame
real-time
    r. scan
    r. ultrasonography
    r. ultrasound
REB (roentgen-equivalent
  biological)
recanalization
receiver
    r. coil
receptacle
recess
    azygoesophageal r.
    epitympanic r. (EPR)
RECG or REKG
  (radioelectrocardiogram)
reciprocating grid
reciprocity
    r. failure
    r. law
recoil
    electron r.
    radiation r.
Recombivax
reconstructed
    r. field of view
reconstruction
    Fourier transformation r.
    plane integral projection r.
    r. algorithm
    r. filter
    r. speed
    single slice line integral
      projection r.
    single slice projection r.
    "target" r.

two-dimensional line
  integral projection r.
two-dimensional
  projection r.
"zoom" r.
reconstructive imaging
reconstructor
    dynamic planar r.
    dynamic spatial r.
record/playback head
recorded detail
recovery
    inversion r.
    inversion r. sequence
    r. phase
    r. time
    saturation r.
    silver r.
recrudescence
rectal
    r. abscess
    r. catheter
    r. lymph node
    r. polyp
    r. sphincter
    r. transducer
rectangular
rectification
    r. half-wave
    self-r.
    solid-state r.
rectifier
    full-wave r.
    self-r.
    silicon r.
    solid-state diode r.
    thermionic r.
    valve tube r.
rectifying
    r. circuit
    r. insufficiency
    r. system
    r. tube
rectilinear
    r. coordinates

rectilinear—*Continued*
  r. scan
  r. scanner
rectosigmoid
  r. index
  r. junction
  r. ratio
rectum
rectus
  r. abdominis
  r. capitis anterior
  r. capitis anticus major
  r. capitis anticus minor
  r. capitis lateralis
  r. capitis posterior major
  r. capitis posterior minor
  r. externus or lateralis
  r. femoris
  r. inferior
  r. internus or medialis
  r. muscle
  r. superior
recumbency
recumbent
  r. lateral projection
  r. position
  r. view
recurrent
  r. lenticulostriate artery
  r. polyserositis
recurvatum deformity
red
  r. blood cells (RBCs)
  r. cell mass (RCM)
  r. cell survival time
  r. cell volume (RCV)
  r. nucleus
  r. prussiate of potash
  r. Robinson catheter
  r. rubber catheter
Redi-Flow contrast media
redistribution study
reducing fracture frame
reduction mammoplasty

redundancy
redundant
REEG
  (radioelectroencephalography)
reeling gait
reference image
reflections
reflex
  r. atelectasis
  r. bone atrophy
  r. sympathetic dystrophy
    syndrome
  r. tandems
reflux
  duodenogastric bile r.
  esophageal r.
  gastroesophageal r.
  hepatojugular r. (HJR)
  intrarenal r.
  jugular r.
  r. esophagitis
  r. method
  r. nephropathy
  ureteric r.
  ureterovesical r.
  urethrovesical differential
    r.
  vaginal r.
  vesicoureteral r.
  vesicoureteric r.
reformation
reformatting
refraction
  law of r.
refractory
Regaud's method
region
  abdominal r.
  axillary r.
  frontal r.
  hypochondriac r.
  iliac r.
  inguinal r.
  lumbar r.

orbital r.
proportional r.
r. of interest (ROI)
regional
    r. enteritis
    r. extravascular lung water
    r. lung function test
    r. ventilation-perfusion
      (VQ or V/Q) study
Registered Diagnostic Medical
    Sonographer (RDMS)
Registered Technologist in
    Nuclear Technology (RT
    N[ARRT])
Registered Technologist in
    Radiation Technology (RT
    R[AART])
regression analysis
regurgitant murmur
regurgitation
    aortic r. (AR)
    gastric r.
    mitral r.
    pulmonic r.
    tricuspid r.
    valvular r.
    vesicoureteral r.
Reichel-Jones-Henderson
    syndrome
Reid's
    R.'s baseline (RBL)
    R.'s lobule
Reil
    circular sulcus of R.
    island of R.
Reimann's periodic disease
reinforced balloon dilation
    catheter
reintussusception
Reiter's
    R.'s arthritis
    R.'s disease
    R.'s triad
relapsing polychondritis

relationship
    Karplus r.
relative
    r. aperture
    r. biologic effectiveness
      (RBE)
relativistic mass
relaxation
    r. process
    r. rate
    r. time
relay
relief skull
REM (radiation equivalent
    man)
rem (roentgen equivalent man)
Remak's sign
remnant radiation
remote
    r. afterloading
      brachytherapy (RAB)
    r. control diagnostic
      system
REMP (roentgen-equivalent-
    man period)
renal
    r. abscess
    r. aneurysm
    r. angiography
    r. aortography
    r. arteriography
    r. artery stenosis
    r. biopsy
    r. calculi
    r. capsule
    r. carbuncle
    r. cell carcinoma
    r. cholesteatoma
    r. cortex
    r. cyst
    r. double curve visceral
      catheter
    r. duplication
    r. dysplasia

renal—*Continued*
   r. echogram
   r. failure
   r. fascia
   r. fossa
   r. function
   r. halo sign
   r. hematuria
   r. infarction
   r. ischemia
   r. localization
   r. margins
   r. medullary contamination
   r. obstruction
   r. osteodystrophy
   r. outline
   r. pelvis
   r. plasma flow
   r. pyramid
   r. radionuclide study
   r. scan
   r. scintigraphy
   r. "string bead"
      appearance
   r. transit time
   r. transplant
   r. tubular acidosis
   r. venography
   r. venous wash-out time
Rendu-Osler syndrome
Rendu-Osler-Weber syndrome
  syndrome
reniform
renipelvic
reniportal
Reno-M
Reno-M-30 (meglumine
  diatrizoate 30%)
Reno-M-60 (meglumine
  diatrizoate 60%)
Reno-M-Dip (meglumine
  diatrizoate injection 30%)
renocystogram
renofacial syndrome

Renografin
   R.-60 (meglumine
      diatrizoate 52%, sodium
      diatrizoate 8%)
   R.-76 (meglumine
      diatrizoate 66%, sodium
      diatrizoate 10%)
renogram
renography
Renotec
renovascular
Renovist (diatrizoate
  methylglucamine 34.3%,
  sodium diatrizoate 35%)
Renovist II (sodium diatrizoate
  29.1%, meglumine diatrizoate
  28.5%)
Renovue (iodamide
  meglumide)
REP (roentgen equivalent
  physical)
repetition time (TR)
rephasing
   r. gradient
replacement
   r. fibrosis
   r. "O" rings
repolarization
Reptilase-R
RES (reticuloendothelial
  system)
Res-O-Mat
rescanned
resecting fracture
resection
reservoir
reset switch
residual volume/total lung
  capacity (RV/TLC)
residuum
resin
   r. triiodothyronine uptake
      (RT3U)
   r. uptake (RU)

resistance
  r. drop
  r. loss
resistive magnet
resistivity
resistor
  non-ohmic r.
  ohmic r.
  variable r.
resolution
  axial r.
  contrast r.
  density r.
  energy r.
  hole-pair limiting r.
  image r.
  linear r.
  plane-pair r.
  radiographic r.
  scanogram r.
  spatial r.
  spatiotemporal r.
  target r.
  temporal r.
  ultrasound r.
resolving time (counter)
resonance
  amphoric r.
  bandbox r.
  bell-metal r.
  cough r.
  cracked-pot r.
  electron paramagnetic r.
    (EPR)
  electron spin r. (ESR)
  field focusing nuclear
    magnetic r.
  focused nuclear magnetic
    r. (FONAR)
  hydatid r.
  magnetic r. (MR)
  osteal r.
  pulsed-response r.
  r. capture

  r. condition
  r. frequency
  r. generator
  r. theory
  shoulder-strap r.
  skodaic r.
  topical magnetic r.
    (TMR)
  tympanic r.
  tympanitic r.
  vesicular r.
  vesiculotympanic r.
  vocal r.
  whispering r.
  wooden r.
resonant frequency
resorption
respiratory
  r. abronchiole
  r. arrhythmia
  r. distress syndrome
    (RDS)
  r. excursion
  r. motion
  r. support
  r. synctyial virus (RSV)
  r. tract
rest position
restraining
  r. board
retained
  r. foreign body
  r. gastric antrum
    syndrome (RGAS)
rete
  r. mirabile conjugatum
  r. mirable geminum
  r. mirable simplex
retention
  r. catheter
  r. cyst
retentivity
reticular
reticulation

reticuloendothelia, pl.
  reticuloendothelium, s.
reticuloendothelial
  r. cell
  r. imaging
  r. system (RES)
reticuloendotheliosis
reticuloendothelium, s.
  reticuloendothelia, pl.
reticulosarcoma
reticulum cell sarcoma
retinal
  r. angiomatosis
  r. commotio
  r. detachment
  r. tear
retinoblastoma
retinopathy of premature birth
retrahens aurem muscle
retreatment tumor, nodes, and
  metastasis (rTNM)
Retro-Conray
retro-ocular space
retroaortic lymph node
retroareolar
retroauricular lymph node
retrobulbar space
retrocardiac space
retrocaval ureter
retrocecal lymph node
retrococcygeal
  r. air study
retrocrural
  r. node
  r. space
retrodeviation
retroesophageal
retrofacial cells of Broca
retroflexion
retrograde
  r. aortography
  r. arteriogram
  r. cardioangiography

r. catheter
r. cholangiogram
r. cystogram (RC)
r. cystourethrogram
r. cystourethrography
r. pyelogram (RP)
r. pyelography (RP)
r. ureterogram (RUG)
r. urethrogram (RUG)
r. urography
retrography
retrohypopharynx
retroiliac ureter
retroinguinal space
retrolental fibroplasia
retrolisthesis
retromammary
  r. abscess
  r. space
retroperitoneal
  r. abscess
  r. air study
  r. fibrosis
  r. gas
  r. gas insufflation
  r. hemorrhage
  r. lymph node
  r. lymphoma
  r. neoplasm
  r. perforation
  r. pneumogram
  r. pneumography
  r. pneumoradiography
  r. space
retroperitoneum
retropharyngeal
  r. abscess
  r. lymph node
retropulsion
retropyloric node
retrorectal
  r. space
  r. tumor

retrospective
retrosternal
    r. goiter
    r. line
    r. position
    r. space
retrothymic
retrotonsillar abscess
retrotracheal space
retroureter
retrouterine hematoma
retrovascular goiter
return flow hemostatic catheter
Retzius, space of
revascularization phase
reverse
    r. Caldwell position
    r. S-line of Golden
    r. Trendelenburg position
    r. Waters' position
reversed
    r. "3" sign
    r. coarctation of the aorta
    r. Colles' fracture
    r. ductus arteriosus
reversible ischemic
    neurological deficit (RIND)
ReView
Reye's syndrome
Reye-Sheehan syndrome
RF (radiofrequency)
RFA (right femoral artery)
R-G (Radiologist, General)
Rh (rhodium)
rhabdoid
rhabdomyoma
rhabdomyomatosis diffusa
    cordis
rhabdomyosarcoma
RHD (Radiological Health
    Data)
rhenium (Re)
Rheopac

rheostat
rheotachygraphy
Rhese's
    R.'s method
    R.'s position
    R.'s position for the optic
        foramen
    R.'s position for the
        paranasal sinuses
    R.'s prone projection
    R.'s view
rheumarthritis
rheumatalgia
rheumatic
    r. myocarditis
    r. panchondritis
    r. sciatica
    r. sialosis
rheumatism
    palindromic r.
    psychogenic r.
rheumatoid
    r. arthritis (RA)
    r. arthritis diffuse
        idiopathic skeletal
        hyperostosis (RADISH)
    r. factor
    r. myositis
    r. pneumoconiosis
    r. spondylitis
rhinal sulcus
rhinencephalocele
rhinogenous granuloma
rhinotrichophalangeal
    syndrome
rhizomelic
    r. chondrodysplasia
        punctata
    r. spondylosis
rhm (roentgen/hour at 1
    meter)
rhodium (Rh)
rhombic grid

rhomboid
    Michaelis' r.
    r. ligament
rhomboideus
    r. major muscle
    r. minor muscle
rhythmic
RIA (radioimmunoassay)
RIA (right iliac artery)
RIA-Mat Angiotensin
rib
    Luschka's r.
    r. of Zahn
Ribbing's syndrome
Ribbing-Müller syndrome
ribonucleic acid (RNA)
ribose
ribosome
ribosyl
ribothymidine
ribulose
Richet's aneurysm
rickets
rider's
    r.'s bone
    r.'s tendon
ridge
    alveolar r.
    epicondylic r.
    gastrocnemial r.
    interarticular r.
    interosseous r.
    intertrochanteric r.
    mesonephric r.
    petrous r.
    pulmonary r.
    sphenoid r.
    supracondylar r.
    tentorial r.
    trapezoid r.
Riedel's lobe
Riegel's symptom
Rieger's syndrome

right
    r. angle scope
    r. angle test
    r. anterior descending
        (RAD) coronary artery
    r. anterior oblique (RAO)
        projection
    r. atrial enlargement
        (RAE)
    r. atrium (RA)
    r. common carotid artery
        (RCCA)
    r. coronary artery (RCA)
    r. femoral artery (RFA)
    r. iliac artery (RIA)
    r. lateral (RL)
    r. lateral (RL) view
    r. lateral (RLAT) position
    r. lateral (RLAT)
        projection
    r. lower lobe (RLL)
    r. lower quadrant (RLQ)
    r. middle lobe (RML)
    r. occipitotransverse
        (ROT)
    r. parasternal stripe
    r. paratracheal stripe
    r. posterior oblique (RPO)
    r. pulmonary artery (RPA)
    r. renal artery (RRA)
    r. renal vein (RRV)
    r. sacroanterior (RSA)
        scout film
    r. sacroposterior (RSP)
    r. sacrotransverse (RST)
    r. scapuloanterior (RScA)
    r. scapuloposterior (RScP)
    r. subclavian artery
        (RSCA)
    r. subclavian vein (RSCV)
    r. to left (R-L) shunt
    r. upper lobe (RUL)
    r. upper quadrant (RUQ)

r. ventricle (RV)
r. ventricular ejection
fraction (RVEF)
r. ventricular end-diastolic
pressure (RVEDP)
r. ventricular enlargement
(RVE)
r. ventricular hypertrophy
(RVH)
r. ventricular infundibulum
r. ventricular outflow tract
(RVOT)
right-angle method
right-hand rule
right-sided
right-to-left (R-L)
right-to-left shunt
rigid spine
RIHSA (radioiodinated human
serum albumin)
Riley needle
Riley-Day syndrome
Riley-Shwachman syndrome
rim
r. fracture
r. sigmoid
r. sign
RIM (radioisotope medicine)
rima
r. glottidis
r. vestibuli
rima, s.
rimae, pl.
rimae, pl.
rima, s.
rimose, or rimous
rimous, or rimose
RIND (reversible ischemic
neurological deficit)
ring
Albl's r.
anular r.
Cannon's r.

closing r. of Winkler-
Waldeyer
commutator r.
cricoid r.
napkin r. deformity
r. abscess
r. apophysis
r. artifact
r. B chromosome
r. fracture
"r. of bone" concept
r. of Saturn
r. sign
"r." shadow
Schatzki's r.
slip r.s
tendinous r.
tympanic r.
vascular r.
Ring
R. biliary duct drainage set
R. biliary stent set
R. catheter
R. drainage catheter needle
R. intravascular torque
wire guide
R. IV torque guide
R. needle
ring-like
Ring–McLean catheter
Ringer's
R.'s lactate
R.'s solution
rings on CT slices artifact
Riolan's ossicle
ripple
electrical r.
r. sign
r. voltage
RIS (radiology information
system)
RISA (radioiodinated serum
albumin)

RISA cisternogram
risorius muscle
Rivinus' duct
RKG (radiocardiogram)
RKY (roentgen kymography)
RL (Radiation Laboratory)
RL (right lateral) view
R-L (right-to-left) (shunt)
RLAT (right lateral)
RLL (right lower lobe)
RLQ (right lower quadrant)
R-meter
RML (right middle lobe)
RMS (root-mean-square) value
RNA (ribonucleic acid)
RND (radical neck dissection)
Rnt (roentgenologist)
Rnt (roentgenology)
RNV (radionuclide
    venography)
R/O (rule out)
Robb needle
Robengatope I-125, I-131
Robert's pelvis
Robin's
    R.'s anomalad
    R.'s sequence
Robinow-Silverman-Smith
    syndrome
Robinson catheter
Robson's position
Rocher-Sheldon syndrome
rocker deformity
rocker-bottom foot (pes
    convex)
rod
    intramedullary r.
    r. myopathy
rodent ulcer
Rodrigues' aneurysm
Rodriguez-Alvarez catheter
roentgen (R)
    r. absorbed dose (rad)

r. administered dose
    (RAD)
r. equivalent man (rem)
r. equivalent physical
    (rep)
r. kymography (RKY)
r. per hour at 1 meter
    (rhm)
r. ratio
r. ray
r. unit (RU)
Roentgen, Wilhelm Conrad
roentgen-equivalent biological
    (REB)
roentgen-equivalent-man
    period (REMP)
roentgenogram
roentgenography
roentgenologist (Rnt)
roentgenology (Rnt)
roentgenoscopy
Roger Anderson facial fracture
    appliance
ROI (region of interest)
Rokitansky's
    R.'s disease
    R.'s diverticulum
Rokitansky-Aschoff sinuses
rolandic artery
Rolando, fissure of
Rolando's fracture
Romberg's syndrome
roof plate
root
    aortic r.
    r. abscess
    r. of lung
    r. puller's fracture
    r. sleeve fibrosis
root-mean-square (RMS) value
ROS (radiology operations
    system)
rosary bead esophagus

rose bengal
    r. b. scintiscan of liver
    r. b. sodium
Rose's position
Rosen-Castleman-Liebow
    syndrome
Rosen curved safe-T-J wire
    guide
Rosenblum rotating adapter
Rosenmüller's
    R.'s gland
    R.'s node
Rosenthal, basal vein of
Roske-de Toni-Caffey-Smyth
    disease
Ross
    R. catheter
    R. transseptal catheter
Rossi's
    R.'s sphincter
    R.'s syndrome
Rössle-Urbach-Wiethe
    lipoproteinosis
rostrad
rostral plane
rostrate pelvis
rostrum
    r. of corpus callosum
    r. sphenoidale
    sphenoidal r.
ROT (right occipitotransverse)
Rotalix tube
rotary
    r. converter
    r. joint
rotate-only system
rotate-rotate scanning
rotate-stationary
    r.-s. scan
    r.-s. system
rotating
    r. frame of reference
    r. adapter

r. anode
r. anode target
r. frame imaging
rotating-anode
    r.-a. motor
    r.-a. tube
rotation
    organoaxial r.
    r. therapy
    scaphoid r.
rotator cuff tear
rotatores spinae
Rotex needle
Rothene
Rothmund's
    R.'s dystrophy
    R.'s syndrome
Rothmund-Thompson
    syndrome
roto-tomography
rotogram
rotor
Rotor's syndrome
rotoscoliosis
Rotter's node
Rotter-Erb syndrome
rotundum
    foramen r.
round
    r. arthrodesis pin
    r. tip catheter
    r. ulcer
    r. window
Roux-en-Y anastomosis
Roviralta's syndrome
Royal Flush II high-flow thin
    wall catheter
Royer's syndrome
RP (retrograde pyelogram)
RPA (right pulmonary artery)
RPM (rapid processing mode)
RPO (right posterior oblique)
RR (radiation reaction)

RR (radiation response)
RRA (radioreceptor assay)
RRA (right renal artery)
RRV (right renal vein)
RSA (right sacroanterior) scout film
RScA (right scapuloanterior)
RSCA (right subclavian artery)
RScP (right scapuloposterior)
RSCV (right subclavian vein)
RSNA (Radiological Society of North America)
RSP (right sacroposterior)
RST (right sacrotransverse)
RT (radiation therapy)
RT (radiologic technologist)
RT (radium therapy)
RT N(ARRT) (Registered Technologist in Nuclear Medicine Technology)
RT R(AART) (Registered Technologist in Radiation Therapy Technology)
RT$_3$U (resin triiodothyronine uptake)
rTNM (retreatment tumor, nodes, and metastasis)
RTOG (Radiation Therapy Oncology Group)
RTx (radiation therapy)
RU (resin uptake)
RU (roentgen unit)
Ru (ruthenium)
RUBA-tect rubella diagnostic test
Rubacell
rubber catheter
rubella
    r. osteitis
rubidazone (zorubicin) (RBZ)
rubidium chloride (Rb-86)
Rubin's test
Rubinstein-Taybi syndrome

Rubratope
    R. 57 (cyanocobalamin Co 57)
    R. 60
rubroreticular tract
rudimentary trochanter
RUG (retrograde ureterogram)
RUG (retrograde urethrogram)
ruga, s.
    rugae, pl.
rugae, pl.
    ruga, s.
rugal
    r. fold
    r. pattern
Rugar
rugby knee
Rugiero's line
Ruhr's rheumatism
Ruiter-Pompen-Wyers syndrome
RUL (right upper lobe)
rule
    Ampere's r.
    Bell-Thompson r.
    dose r.
    dynamo r.
    Fleming's r.
    left-hand r.
    left-thumb r.
    octet r.
    r. out (R/O)
    right-hand r.
    Simpson's r.
    thumb r.
Runström's
    R.'s projection
    R.'s view (mastoid)
rupture
    aneursymal r.
    bronchial r.
    esophageal r.
    splenic r.

tracheobronchial r.
RUQ (right upper quadrant)
Rusch catheter
Rusch-Foley catheter
Ruschelit catheter
Rush pin
Russell traction
Russell-Silver
    R.-S. dwarf
    R.-S. syndrome
Rustitskii's disease
ruthenium (Ru)
rutherford (rd)
RV (right ventricle)

RV/TLC ratio (residual volume/
    total lung capacity)
RVE (right ventricular
    enlargement)
RVEDP (right ventricular end-
    diastolic volume)
RVEF (right ventricular
    ejection fraction)
RVG (radionuclide
    ventriculography)
RVH (right ventricular
    hypertrophy)
RVOT (right ventricular
    outflow tract)

Ss

S (sacral)
SA (specific activity)
SA (splenic artery)
SA (surface area)
saber
    "s. shin" appearance
saber-sheath trachea
Sabreloc spatula needle
sac
    abdominal s.
    air s.
    alveolar s.
    amniotic s.
    aneurysmal s.
    aortic s.
    chorionic s.
    conjunctival s.
    dental s.
    dural s.
    embryonic s.
    endolymphatic s.
    epiploic s.
    gestational s.
    greater s. of peritoneum
    hernial s.
    Hilton's s.
    jugular lymph s.
    lacrimal s.
    lesser s. of peritoneum
    Lower's s.
    lymph s.
    omental s.
    pericardial s.
    peritoneal s.
    pleural s.
    serous s.
    splenic s.
    thecal s.
    vitelline s.

sacciform kidney
saccular
    s. aneurysm
    s. bronchiectasis
sacculated aneurysm
sacculation
    s. of colon
saccule
    air s.
    alveolar s.
    laryngeal s.
sacra, pl.
    sacrum, s.
sacral (S)
    s. agenesis
    s. canal
    s. cornu
    s. curve
    s. foramen
    s. fusion
    s. hiatus
    s. lymph node
    s. meningoarteritis
    s. meningocele
    s. promontory
    s. spine
    s. vertebra
sacralization
sacroanterior position
sacrococcygeal (SC)
    s. abscess
    s. fusion
    s. joint
    s. teratoma
    s. to inferior pubic point
      (SCIPP)
sacrocoxitis
sacroiliac (SI)
    s. articulation

sacroiliac (SI)—*Continued*
> s. joint (SIJ)
> s. ligament
> s. strain

sacroiliitis
sacrolisthesis
sacrolumbar
sacroperineal
sacroposterior position
sacropromontory
sacrosciatic notch
sacrospinal
sacrospinalis muscle
sacrospinous ligament
sacrotransverse position
sacrotuberous ligament
sacrouterine
sacrovertebral
sacrum
> assimilation s.
> s. anterior position
> s. posterior position
> tilted s.

sacrum, s.
> sacra, pl.

sactosalpinx
SAD (source-to-axis distance)
saddle
> s. deformity of the urinary
> > bladder
> s. joint

Saethre-Chotzen
> acrocephalosyndactyly

Saf-T coils intrauterine device
safelight
sagittal
> s. cuts
> s. groove
> s. orientation
> s. plane
> s. section
> s. sinus
> s. suture

sagittalis

sago
> s. liver
> s. spleen

SAH (subarachnoid
> hemorrhage)

Sahlstedt's line
sail
> s. shadow
> s. sign

Saint's triad
saline
> physiological s.
> s. solution

salivary gland scan
Salmon catheter
salpingeal
salpinges, pl.
> salpinx, s.

salpingitis
> s. isthmica nodosa

salpingocele
salpingocyeses, pl.
> salpingocyesis, s.

salpingocyesis, s.
> salpingocyeses, pl.

salpingography
salpingolithiasis
salpingo-oophorectomy
salpingo-oophoritis
salpingo-oophorocele
salpingo-oothecitis
salpingoperitonitis
salpingopharyngeal
salpingopharyngeus muscle
salpingoplasty
salpingostaphyline
salpingostomy
salpinx
> s. auditiva
> s. uterina

salpinx, s.
> salpinges, pl.

Salpix
saltatory spasm

Salter fracture
Salter-Harris
    S.-H. classification
    S.-H. fracture
Salvioli's syndrome
Salzman, four days technique
  of
SAM (scanning acoustic
  microscope)
samarium
sampling
    s. artifact
    s. rate
Samuel's position
San Joaquin Valley fever
Sanchez-Perez
    S.-P. automatic film
      changer
    S.-P. cassette changer
sand
    intestinal s.
sand-like
    s.-l. appearance
    s.-l. mottling
Sandifer's syndrome
sandpaper gallbladder
"sandwich"
    "s." sign
    "s." vertebrae
Sanfilippo's syndrome
sanguis
sanious
Sansregret modification of
  Chaussé III method
Santorini
    duct of S.
    plexus of S.
Santorini's
    S.'s cartilage
    S.'s ligament
saphenous
    s. artery
    s. vein
    s. vein aortocoronary

      bypass graft
saponaceous
Sappey's ligament
sarcoid
    s. of Boeck
sarcoidosis
    Boeck's s.
    cordis s.
    Schaumann's s.
sarcoma
    ameloblastic s.
    embryonal s.
    Ewing's s.
    Kaposi's s.
    melanotic s.
    neurogenic s.
    osteogenic s.
    parosteal s.
    reticulum cell s.
    s. botryoides
    serocystic s.
    synovial s.
    telangiectatic s.
    Walker's s.
sarcomatous
sartorius muscle
satellite
    s. abscess
    s. lesion
    s. tumor
Saticon (manufacturer)
    S. camera
    S. pick-up tube
    S. vacuum chamber
saturable reactor
saturation
    s. analysis
    s. current
    s. dose
    s. plateau
    s. point
    s. recovery (SR)
    s. recovery image
    s. region

saturation—*Continued*
    s. transfer
    s. tube
    s. voltage
Saturn
    r. of S.
Saturn's ring sign
Satvioni cryptoscope
saucerization
sausage sign
sausaging of a vein
Savac
saw tooth
saw-tooth configuration
SB (small bowel)
SBE (self-breast examination)
SBFT (small bowel follow
    through)
SBO (small bowel obstruction)
SBS (small bowel series)
SC (sacrococcygeal)
Sc (scandium)
SC (sternoclavicular)
SC (sulfur colloid)
scabbard trachea
Scaglietti-Dagnini syndrome
scale
    gray s.
    Hounsfield s.
    Outerbridge s.
scalenus
    s. anterior
    s. anticus syndrome
    s. medius
    s. posterior
    s. syndrome
scaler
scaling circuit
scalloped vertebra
scalp veins
scan
    A-mode (amplitude
      modulation) s.
    A-s. echography

adrenal s.
automatic mode s.
B-mode (brightness
    modulation) s.
B-mode s.
B-s. echography
beta s.
blood pool s.
bone marrow s.
bone s.
brain s.
capillary blocked
    perfusion s.
CAT (computerized axial
    tomography) s.
CAT s.
chlormerodrin s.
cine CT (computed
    tomography) s.
color s.
composite s.
compound s.
contact s.
contiguous s.
continuous s.
    thermograph
CT (computed
    tomography) s.
DISIDA (diisopropyl-
    iminodiacetic acid) s.
dot s.
dual-energy CT (computed
    tomography) s.
dynamic CT (computed
    tomography) s.
enhanced s.
fluorescent s.
full s.
full-line s.
gallbladder s.
gallium s.
gamma s.
General Electric CT/T
    8800 s.

GI bleeding s.
half s.
head s.
hepatobiliary s.
HIDA (hepato-
    iminodiacetic acid) s.
immersion s.
incremented dynamic scan
    (IDS)
incremented s.
indium 111 leukocyte s.
infarct s.
infusion-type s.
inhalation/perfusion lung s.
isotope bone s.
line s.
linear s.
liver s.
liver-spleen (LS) s.
localized image s.
low-dose s.
lung s.
M-mode (motion) s.
mechanical hand s.
Meckel s.
medronate s.
Medx s.
MUGA (multigated
    acquisition) s.
multigated angiographic s.
multigated blood pool s.
multiplanar s.
multislice full line s.
nonenhanced CAT s.
nongated CT s.
nuclear s.
paper dot s.
partial s.
pelvic s.
perfusion lung s.
perfusion s.
PET (positron-emission
    tomography) s.
photo s.

pilot s.
PIPIDA (now called
    DISIDA) s.
placenta blood pool s.
point s.
positron s.
profile s.
PYP (pyrophosphate) s.
radioisotope s.
    r. bone s.
    r. liver/spleen s.
    r. thyroid s.
radionuclide s.
rapid-sequence s.
RBC (red blood cell) s.
rectilinear s.
renal s.
rotate-rotate s.
rotate-stationary s.
s. converter
s. projection radiograph
s. projection radiograph
    systems
s. sequence
s. speed
s. spot
s. time
salivary gland s.
scout view s.
sector s. echocardiography
segmented s.
selective excitation line s.
sensitive point s.
single-energy CT
    (computed tomography)
    s.
single-level dynamic s.
    (SLDS)
single-line s.
single-pass sector s.
spleen s.
stacked s.
survey dynamic s.
technetium brain s.

scan—*Continued*
  technetium
    hepatoiminodiacetic
    acid (TcHIDA) s.
  technetium medronate s.
  technetium stannous
    pyrophosphate s.
  testicular s.
  thallium myocardial s.
  three-phase bone s.
  thyroid s.
  transverse s.
  ultrasound s. (USS)
  venous s.
  VQ or V/Q (ventilation-
    perfusion) s. (Q =
    "quotient")
  water path s. (ultrasound)
  whole-body s. (WBS)
  xenon s.
scan-a-screen
scandium (Sc)
Scanex
scanned
  s. field of view
  s. projection
  s. projection radiography
    (SPR)
scanner
  Aloka linear s.
  AS and E CT s.
  ATL real-time Neurosector
    s.
  Autoscan s.
  beam CT (computed
    tomography) s.
  cardiovascular computed
    tomography (CVCT) s.
  cine CT s.
  crystal s.
  CT (computed
    tomography) body s.
  CTE 100 neurodiagnostic s.
  CVCT (cardiovascular
    computed tomography)

Diasonics Cardiovue
  SectOR s.
DynaPak s.
Elscint Excel 905 s.
EMI (Electrical and
  Musical Industries) s.
EMI 7070 s.
EMI CT 500 s.
gamma-ray s.
gated CT (computed
  tomography) s.
General Electric 8800 s.
General Electric CT/T7 800
  s.
high field strength s.
Imatron s.
"indomitable" s.
Medx s.
millisecond (msec) s.
mobile CT s.
multislice s.
neurodiagnostic s.
nongated CT s.
nuclear s.
Ohio Nuclear Delta 2000 s.
Ohio Nuclear Delta 50 FS
  s.
Ohio Nuclear Delta 50 s.
optic s.
Pfizer 0450 s.
Pfizer 200 FS s.
PHO/CON tomographic
  multiplane s.
photodot s.
Picker Magna s.
Picker Synerview 600 s.
radioisotope s.
real-time s.
rectilinear s.
Siemen Somatom 2 s.
supercam scintillation s.
Synerdyne s.
Technicare Delta 2020 s.
tomographic multiplane s.
Toshiba s.

translate-rotate s.
two-to-five-second s.
ultrafast computed
   tomographic s.
V-360-3 CT s.
Varian CT s.
whole-body s.
scanning
   s. acoustic microscope
     (SAM)
   s. parameters
   s. sequence
   s. technique
scanogram
   s. annotation
   s. resolution
scanography
   slit s.
   spot s.
Scanoscope
scaphocephaly
scaphoid
   s. fracture
   s. necrosis
   s. projection
   s. rotation
   s. scapula
scaphoid-capitate fracture-
  dislocation
scaphoid-lunate dislocation
scaphoid-trapezium fusion
scapholunate
   s. angle
   s. dissociation
scapula (shoulder bone)
   alar s.
   Graves' s.
   s. anterior position
   s. elevata
   s. posterior position
   scaphoid s.
   winged s.
scapular notch
scapuloanterior position
scapuloclavicular joint

scapulohumeral
scapuloposterior position
scar tissue
scarification
scatter
   s. fraction
   s. radiation
   s. suppression
   unmodified s.
scattergram
scattering
   coherent s.
   Compton s.
   elastic s.
   incoherent s.
   inelastic s.
   Rayleigh s.
   Thomson s.
   ultrasound s.
SCBE (single-contrast barium
  enema)
SCH (subdural hematoma)
Schatzki's ring
Schaumann's sarcoidosis
Scheibe's malformation
Scheie's
   S.'s disease
   S.'s syndrome
Scheuermann's
   S.'s disease
   S.'s nodules
Scheuthauer-Marie-Sainton
  syndrome
Schilling's test
schindylesis
schindyletic joint
Schirmer's syndrome
schistosoma
schistosomiasis
   s. japonica
   s. mansoni
Schlatter's syndrome
Schlemm's canal
Schlessinger-Taveras
  syndrome

Schmidel's anastomosis
Schmidt's node
Schmieden's disease
Schmincke tumors
Schmitt's disease
Schmorl's
    S.'s node
    S.'s nodule
Schober's test
Scholte's syndrome
Schonander (manufacturer)
    S. AOT-R changer
    S. film changer
    S. rapid biplane film
      changer
Schoomaker catheter
Schrödinger's equation
Schroetter's syndrome
Schrötter catheter
Schüller's
    S.'s disease
    S.'s method
    S.'s position
    S.'s view
schwannoma
Schwartz introducer
Schwartz-Jampel syndrome
sciatic notch
sciatica
scimitar
    s. shadow
    "s." sign
    s. syndrome
scintiangiogram
scintiangiography
scintigram
scintigraphic
    s. "hot spot"
scintigraphy
    nuclear s.
    renal s.
    thallium perfusion s.
    thyroidal lymph node s.
scintillation
    collimated s. detector

    s. camera
    s. counter
    s. counting technique
    s. detector
    s. probe
    s. spectrometer
    s. well detector
scintiphotography
scintiphotosplenoportogram
scintiphotosplenoportography
scintiscan
scintiview
SCIPP line (sacrococcygeal to
    inferior pubic point)
scirrhoid
scirrhous carcinoma
scissors gait
SCJ (sternoclavicular joint)
sclera, s.
    sclerae, pl.
sclerae, pl.
    sclera, s.
sclerocorneal junction
scleroderma
scleroma
scleromalacia
scleromyxedema
sclerosal
sclerosarcoma
sclerosing
    s. cholangitis
    s. lipogranuloma
    s. lymphosarcoma
    s. myelopathy
    s. nonsuppurative
      osteomyelitis
    s. of varices
    s. osteitis
    s. retroperitonitis
    s. tubular degeneration
sclerosis
    amyotrophic lateral s.
      (ALS)
    anular s.
    cortical s.

diaphyseal s.
end-plate s.
endosteal s.
esophageal s.
metaphyseal s.
multiple s.
parasutural s.
s. fibrosa penis
s. tuberosa
subchondral s.
subendocardial s.
valvular s.
vascular s.
venous s.
ventrolateral s.
sclerotic mastoiditis
scoliosis
congenital s.
idiopathic s.
neuromuscular s.
s-shaped s.
scorbutic
s. position
s. rosary
scotogram
scotography
scout
s. film
s. image
s. radiography
s. tomogram
s. view
SCR (silicon-controlled rectifiers)
screen
fluorescent s.
intensifying s.
s. film
s. lag
s. mottle
s. save feature
s. thickness
screen-film
s. technique
screen-type film

screening mammogram
screw
Basile hip s.
Bigelow s.
Bosworth acromioclavicular s.
Bosworth coracoclavicular s.
Bosworth s.
compression s.
cortical s.
Demuth hip s.
Eggers s.
interfragmentary s.
Johannson lag s.
Kristiansen eyelet lag s.
lag s.
Lippman s.
Lorenzo s.
malleolar s.
McLaughlin navicular s.
Morris biphase s.
olecranon s.
partial thread wood s.
s. joint
Sherman bone s.
transfixion s.
venable s.
virgin hip s.
screw like fracture
scrofula
Scultetus' position
scutiform
scybala
scyballum
scybalous stools
SD (shoulder disarticulation)
SD (skin dose)
Se (selenium)
SE (spin echo)
SE (Starr-Edwards)
Seabright bantam syndrome
seat-belt fracture
seated erect position

sebaceous
    s. adenoma
    s. cyst
Seckel's syndrome
second generation
second-day procedure
second-order beam-hardening
  correction
secondary
    s. curve
    s. diagnosis
    s. effect
    s. electron
    s. emission
    s. filter
    s. fluorescence
    s. fracture
    s. hypertrophic
      osteoarthropathy
    s. osteons
    s. radiation
    s. ray
    s. winding
secreta
secretin
secretion
secreto-inhibitor syndrome
section thickness
sectional
sector scan
sectoring, ultrasound
Sectorscan (manufacturer)
secular equilibrium
SED (skin erythema dose)
seed
    s. calculi
    s. implants
SEG (sonoencephalogram)
SEG (sonoencephalography)
segment
segmental
    s. atelectasis
    s. bronchus
    s. defect
    s. fracture

segmentation artifact
segmentectomy
segmented
    s. intestine
    s. scan
segmentum
Segond's fracture
Seidlitz' powder test
Seip's syndrome
seizure
Seldinger
    S. catheter
    S. needle
Seldinger's
    S.'s catheterization
    S.'s method
    S.'s percutaneous
      technique
    S.'s procedure
    S.'s technique
selective
    s. and superselective
      visceral catheter
    s. angiocardiography
    s. arteriography
    s. catheterization
    s. excitation
    s. irradiation
    s. radiofrequency pulse
    s. venography
    s. visceral aortography
selective excitation
    s. e. irradiation technique
    s. e. line scan
    s. e. projection
      reconstruction imaging
selenium (Se)
    s. 75
    s. rectifier
selenomethionine (Se-75)
Seletz catheter
self-absorption
self-adhesive drape
self-breast examination (SBE)
self-developing film

self-inductance
self-induction
self-quenched counter tube
self-rectification
self-rectified circuit
self-retaining catheter
self-scattering
sella
    dorsum s.
    empty s. syndrome
    s. turcica
    shoe-shaped s.
sellar joint
Semb's classification
semi-Fowler position
semiaxial
    s. anteroposterior
      projection
    s. position
    s. projection
    s. transcranial projection
semicircular canals
semiconductor
    s. chip
    s. detector
semierect
    s. film
    s. position
    s. projection
semiflexion
semihorizontal heart position
  (SHHP)
semiliquid
semilongitudinal
semilunar
    s. cartilage
    s. fold
    s. fossa
    s. notch
    s. space
    s. valve
semimembranosus muscle
seminal
    s. vesicle
    s. vesiculogram

seminiferous tubule dysgenesis
seminoma, s.
    seminomata, pl.
seminomata, pl.
    seminoma, s.
semiprone position
semireclining position
semirecumbent position
semirigid
semispinalis
    s. capitis muscle
    s. cervicis muscle
    s. colli muscle
    s. dorsi muscle
    s. muscle
    s. thoracis muscle
semisupine
semitendinosus muscle
senescent
Sengstaken-Blakemore tube
senile
    s. arteriosclerosis
    s. changes
    s. dementia
    s. emphysema
    s. osteoporosis
Senior's syndrome
senna (compound) powder
senograph
senography
sensiometry
sensitive
    s. line method
    s. plane
    s. plane projection
      reconstruction imaging
    s. point scan
sensitivity
    electrical s.
    line method s.
    plane projection
      reconstruction imaging
      s.
    plane s.
    point s.

s. volume
sensitometer
electroluminescent s.
sensitometry (radiographic film)
Sensor
sensory tract
sentinel
s. loop
s. node
Sephadex
septa, pl.
septum, s.
septal cartilage
septation
septic
s. arthritis
s. shock
septicemic abscess
septomarginal tract
septum
atrioventricular s.
interatrial s.
interventricular s.
nasal s.
s. canalis musculotubarii
s. lucidum
s. pellucidum
s. primum defect
smooth s.
septum, s.
septa, pl.
sequela, s.
sequelae, pl.
sequelae, pl.
sequela, s.
sequence
Carr-Purcell s.
direct mapping s.
Meiboom-Gill s.
Robin's s.
s. time
scanning s.
spin-echo pulse s.

spin-echo s.
voiding s.
sequential
s. film
s. first-pass imaging
s. plane imaging
s. point imaging
s. point method or imaging
sequestration
sequestrum
button s.
Seralute Total T-3 and T-4
serial
s. film
s. image
s. scan
serialoangiocardiogram
serialoangiocardiography
serialograph
series
gallbladder s.
gastrointestinal (GI) s.
radioactive s.
s. circuit
small bowel s. (SBS)
serocystic sarcoma
seroma, s.
seromata, pl.
seromata, pl.
seroma, s.
seropositive nonsyphilitic pneumopathy
serosa, s.
serosae, pl.
serosae, pl.
serosa, s.
serous
s. abscess
s. meningitis
s. otitis media
s. sac
s. tumor
serpentine
s. aneurysm

s. plate
serpiginous
serration
serratus
    s. anterior
    s. magnus
    s. muscle
    s. posterior inferior
    s. posterior superior
serum albumin
service life
sesamoid
    s. index
    s. periostitis
sessile
    s. lesion
    s. polyp
Sethotope (selenomethionine
    Se 75)
Sethre-Chotzen type
    dyscephaly
Settegast
    S. view of the knee
Settegast's
    S.'s method
    S.'s position
setups
seventh or Q-shell
Sever's
    S.'s disease
    S.'s osteonecrosis
SFA (superficial femoral
    artery)
Shadocol
shadow
    acoustic s.
    anular s.
    "bat's-wing" s.
    "butterfly" s.
    calcific s.
    cardiac s.
    "double-bubble" s.
    nipple s.
    "overlap" s.

    psoas s.
    "ring" s.
    s. meal
    s. shield
    sail s.
    scimitar s.
    splenic s.
    triple-line s.
shadowgram
shadowgraphy
shaft
shaggy pericardium
shape
    "baseball bat" s.
    "cricket bat" s.
    "dumbbell" s.
shaped
    barrel-s.
    ovoid-s.
    S-s.
    spheroid-s.
shark jaw biopsy needle
sharp kernel
Sharpey's fibers
Sharrard's
    S.'s kyphectomy
    S.'s operation
Shaver catheter
Shaver's syndrome
Shaver-Ridell syndrome
sheath
    synovial s.
    tendon s.
sheathed
    s. catheter
    s. Chiba needle
Sheehan's syndrome
sheet-like
Shekelton's aneurysm
Sheldon-Ellis syndrome
shelf life
shell
    "s. of bone" appearance
    atomic s.

shell—*Continued*
    valence s.
Shenton's line
shepherd hook visceral
    catheter
shepherd's
    "s.'s crook" deformity
    s.'s fracture
Shepp-Logan filter function
Sherman
    S. "Y" plate
    S. bone plate
    S. bone screw
SHHP (semihorizontal heart
    position)
shield
    abdominal s.
    Dalkon intrauterine device
      (IUD)
    gonadal s.
    lead gonad s.
    phallic s.
    shadow s.
shield-shaped kidney
shift
    left-to-right s.
    midline s.
    paramagnetic s.
    right-to-left s.
shim coil
shimming
shin
Shiner's tube
shirt-stud abscess
shock
    s. lung syndrome
    cardiogenic s.
    hemorrhagic s.
    s. position
    septic s.
shock-wave therapy
shoe-shaped sella
shoemaker chest
Shone's syndrome

Shopfner classification
short
    s. circuit
    s. esophagus
    s. scale contrast
    s. transit time
short-arm Grollman catheter
short-leg gait
short-limbed dwarfism
shotty nodes
shoulder
    s. disarticulation (SD)
    s. girdle
    s. joint
    s. sign
    s. support
shoulder-hand syndrome
shoulder-strap resonance
Shrewsbury mark
shuffling gait
shunt
    arteriovenous s.
    atrioseptal defect s.
    Blalock-Taussig s.
    cardiac s.
    cystoperitoneal s.
    extracardiac s.
    intracardiac s.
    left-to-right s.
    portocaval s.
    right-to-left s.
    s. quantification
    ventriculoperitoneal s.
    Waterston s.
shutters
Shwachman's syndrome
SI (International System)
SI (sacroiliac)
SI unit
sialadenitis
sialadenography
sialoangiography
sialogram
sialography

sialolith
sicca syndrome
sickle cell anemia
sicklemia
SICOR (cardiac catheterization
   recorder)
SID (source-image distance)
side effects
side-arm adapter
sideropenic
   s. dysphagia
   s. syndrome
sideswipe fracture
sidewinder catheter
Siegal-Cattan-Mamou
   syndrome
Siemens (manufacturer)
   S. Lithostar table
   S. Somatoms 2 scanner
   S. system
   S. table
sieve plate irradiation
sievert (Sv)
sigmoid
   s. colon
   s. diverticulum
   s. elevator sign
   s. esophagus
   s. impaction
   s. kidney
   s. lymph node
   s. narrowing
   s. obstruction
   s. sinus
   s. sulcus
   s. volvulus
sigmoid-shaped configuration
sigmoid-vesical fistula
sigmoidoscopy
sign
   abrupt s.
   air bronchogram s.
   air cap s.
   air crescent s.

"air dome" s.
angle s. of scurvy
anterior maxillary bowing
   s.
atrioseptal s.
Babinski's s. (reflex)
batwing s.
beak s.
bent bronchus s.
Bergman's s.
big rib s.
biliary rim s.
"bite" s.
black pleura s.
blister s.
border s.
"bowing" s.
brain stain s.
brain trapped-air s.
brim s.
bronchial meniscus s.
bull's eye s.
button s.
calyceal crescent s.
Carman's meniscus s.
Carman-Kirklin meniscus
   s.
Case's pad s.
cervical prevertebral
   stripe s.
cervicothoracic s.
Chapple's s.
chest-abdomen s.
Chilaiditi's s.
Cole's s.
"crowfoot" s.
cut-off s.
"dagger" s.
Deuel's halo s.
differential density s.
dilated callosal sulcus s.
dilated common duct s.
dimple s.
displaced fat pad s.

sign—*Continued*

Dockray's perirenal "P" s.
double ball s.
"double-bubble" s.
double lesion s.
double track s.
"double wall" s.
"doughnut" s.
draping s.
drawer s.
Duroziez' s. or murmur
Dyke's blistering s.
Dyke's finger s.
eccentric target s.
ellipse s.
epsilon s.
Escudero-Nemenov s.
Ewart's s.
fabella s.
failing lung s.
fat pad s.
"flank stripe" s.
flat waist s.
fleck s.
Fleischner's pointed ileum s.
Fleischner's spearhead s.
"floating mine" s.
"floating tooth" s.
"football" s.
fragmentation s.
Fränkel's s.
free-induction s.
frontopolar s.
Frostberg's s.
gastric air-trapping s.
goblet s.
Golden's "S" s.
gull-wing s.
halo s.
Hamman's s.
hangman's s.
hard palate s.
Hartley's ball s.

hat s.
Haudeck's s.
Hawkins' s.
heel-pad thickness s.
Hefke-Turner s.
Hellmer's s.
high convergence s.
high overlay s.
hilum convergence s.
hilum overlay s.
hook s.
Horner's s.
hypernephroma halo s.
"iceberg" configuration or s.
iliopsoas s.
intestinal string s.
intravascular fetal air s.
"inverted 3" s.
"inverted V" s.
inverted goblet s.
ischial varus s.
jet s.
Kantor's s.
Kernig's s.
Köhler's "teardrop" s.
Kosowicz' s.
Kussmaul's s.
Laugier's s.
Léri's s.
Lhermitte's s.
"lily-pad" s.
Macewen's s.
mass s.
McCort's s.
McMurray's s.
melting s.
meniscus s.
"Mercedes-Benz" s.
metacarpal s.
moon s.
mosaic s.
moulage s.
mustache s.
notch s.

"nubbin" sign
obturator s.
open bronchus s.
Pancoast's s.
pad s. of Case
Parrot's s.
patent bronchus s.
Pelken's s.
pendulous breast s.
perirenal "P" s.
phalangeal s.
"picket fence" s.
pleural meniscus s.
Poppel's s.
positive elbow fat pad s.
positive navicular fat
    stripe s.
positive rim s.
positive stretch s.
pseudopost-Billroth I s.
"pubic" s.
pulmonary meniscus s.
pulmonary notch s.
pulmonary target s.
pyloric string s.
Queckenstedt's s.
rabbit-ear s.
ram's horn s.
Rauber's s.
Remak's s.
renal halo s.
reversed "3" s.
rim s.
ring s.
ripple s.
s. of cane
s. of cervical prevertebral
    stripe
s. of iliac artery
s. of moth-eaten margin of
    the calyces
s. of overhanging margin
    of bone
s. of pyloric tit

s. of widening of the
    tracheal angle
sail s.
"sandwich" s.
Saturn's ring s.
sausage s.
scimitar s.
shoulder s.
sigmoid elevator s.
silhouette s.
"sinking pellet" s.
small intestinal intramural
    air s.
Spalding's s.
spine s.
spinnaker sail s.
squirt s.
stacked-coin s.
starry night s.
steeple s.
Stierlin's s.
stretched bronchus s.
string of beads s.
string s.
subcapsular "C" s.
suprapatellar effusion s.
tacked-down s.
Tager's s.
target s.
teat s.
thick-wall s.
thoracoabdominal s.
thread-and-streaks s.
thumblike s.
thumbprint bronchus s.
thumbprinting s.
Thurston-Holland fracture
    s.
thymic sail s.
thymic spinnaker sail s.
thymic wave s.
tin woodsman s.
trichorhinophalangeal
    (TRP) s.

sign—*Continued*
  "tumbling bullet" s.
  Turner's s.
  upper triangle s.
  "V" s.
  vallecular s.
  van der Swan's s.
  wall s.
  "water-lily" s.
  wedge s.
  Wegelius-Lind s.
  Westermark's s.
  widened Lippes' loop s.
  Wimberger's s.
signal
  s. conducting
  s. intensity
  s. node
signal-to-noise ratio (SNR or
  S/N) ratio
signet
  s. ring
SIJ (sacroiliac joint)
Silastic catheter
silent
  s. disk syndrome
  s. infarction
  s. ischemia
  s. kidney
  s. zone
silhouette
  cardiac s.
  cardiomediastinal s.
    (CMS)
  hilar s.
  s. sigmoid
  s. sign
silicate
silicoarthritis
silicon
  s. rectifier
silicon-controlled rectifiers
  (SCR)
silicone plate

Silitek catheter
silo-filler's disease
silver (Ag)
  metallic s.
  s. bromide (AgBr)
  s. halide
  s. iodide
  s. nitrate
  s. recovery
Silver's syndrome
silver-fork fracture
Silverman's disease
Silverskiöld's syndrome
simian crease
Simmonds'
  S.' cachexia
  S.' syndrome
Simmons
  S. 1 catheter
  S. 2 catheter
  S. 3 catheter
  S. cerebral catheter
  S. Newton Torcon catheter
Simon's
  S.'s foci
  S.'s position
simple
  s. fracture
  s. joint
  s. molecule
  s. skull fracture
Simpson Atherocath catheter
Simpson's rule
Sims' position
simulation
simulator
  Toshiba s.
simultaneous
  s. multifilm tomography
  s. three-dimensional
    measurement
  s. volume imaging
sincalide (Kinevac)
sincipital

sinciput
Sinding-Larsen disease
Sinding-Larsen-Johansson
  syndrome
sine wave
Sinegas classification
singer's node
single-contrast
    s. barium enema
    s. study
single-emulsion film
single-energy CT (computed
  tomography) scanning
single-film
    s. automatic system
    s. triangulation
single-hole collimator
single-level dynamic scanning
  (SLDS)
single-line scan
single-pass
    s. scanning (ultrasound)
    s. sector scan
single-phase
    s. current
    s. generator
    s. system
single-photon
    s. absorptiometry (SPA)
    s. counting system
    s. emission computed
      tomography (SPECT)
    s. emission test
single-pole double-throw
  (spdt)
single-shoulder contrast
  arthrography (SSCA)
single‚slice
    s. line integral projection
      reconstruction
    s. modified KWE direct
      Fourier imaging
    s. projection
      reconstruction

single-stage procedure
single-tube angulation method
Singleton-Merton syndrome
singultation
singultus
sinistrad
"sinking pellet" sign
sinoatrial node
sinobronchial syndrome
sinodural angle of Citelli
Sinografin (meglumine
  diatrizoate 40%, meglumine
  iodipamide 20%)
sinogram
sinography
    cerebral s.
sinospiral
sinus
    cavernous s.
    confluence of s.
    costophrenic s.
    dura mater s.
    ethmoidal s.
    Forssell's s.
    frontal s.
    mastoid s.
    maxillary s.
    occipital s.
    paranasal s.
    petrosal s.
    phrenocostal s.
    piriform s.
    s. arrhythmia
    s. bradycardia
    s. histiocytosis
    s. node
    s. of Morgagni syndrome
    s. of Ridley
    s. pericranii
    s. tract
    s. venosus atrial septal
      defect
    sagittal s.
    sigmoid s.

sinus—*Continued*
    sphenoid s.
    sphenoparietal s.
    straight s.
    tympanic s.
siphon-incisivum line
siphons-carotid
Sipple's syndrome
SIRD (source to image-receptor distance)
Siregraph 2
Siremat
sirenomelia
site
sitting
    s. position
    s. view
situ (in situ)
situs
    s. inversus
    s. perversus
    s. solitus
    s. transversus
six-hole stainless steel plate
six-pulse three-phase generator
Sjögren's syndrome
SK (Sloan-Kettering) (used with chemotherapy)
skeletal
    s. maturation
    s. muscle
    s. pain
    s. traction
skeletography
skeleton
    appendicular s.
    axial s.
    bony s.
Skene catheter
ski
    s. boot fracture
    s. pole fracture
Skiadin

skiagram
skiagraphy
skiameter
skiascopy
Skillern's fracture
skin
    s. depth
    s. dose (SD)
    s. erythema dose (SED)
    s. sparing
skin-to-tumor distance (STD)
Skinner's line
Skiodan
    S. Acacia
skip
    s. areas
    s. tomography
skodaic resonance
SKSD (stretokinase-streptodornase)
skull
    brachycephalic s.
    cloverleaf s.
    contracting s.
    dolichocephalic s.
    hot cross bun s.
    lacunar s.
    map-like s.
    mesocephalic s.
    s. fracture
    s. plate
    Spalteholz s.
    steeple s.
    tower s.
    West's lacunar s.
    West-Engstler's s.
skyline
    s. projection
    s. view
slant-hole collimator
SLAP (superior labral anterior posterior) lesion
SLDS (single-level dynamic scanning)

slice
  CT (computed
  tomography) s.
  s. factor
  s. fracture-dislocation
  s. geometry
  s. number
  s. selection
  s. thickness
sliding hernia
slip rings
slipped capital femoral
  epiphysis
slit scanography
Sloan-Kettering (SK) (used
  with chemotherapy)
slope
  lower ridge s.
slotted plate
slow neutrons
sludge
slug
SMA (sequential multiple
  analyzer)
SMA (superior mesenteric
  artery)
small
  s. bowel (SB)
  s. bowel follow through
    (SBFT)
  s. bowel obstruction (SBO)
  s. bowel series (SBS)
  s. intestinal intramural air
    sign
Smillie nail
Smith-Goyrand fracture
Smith's fracture
Smith-Peterson
  S.-P. arthrodesis pin
  S.-P. concentric hip mold
  S.-P. hip cup
  S.-P. nail
  S.-P. nail with McLaughlin
    bar

S.-P. pin
S.-P. plate
S.-P. vitallium cup
Smith-Peterson-Dooley point
  nail
SMO plate
smoky feature
smooth
  s. muscle
  s. septum
  s.-brain syndrome
SMV (submental vertex)
SMV (superior mesenteric
  vein)
SMX (sulfamethoxazole)
S/N (signal-to-noise ratio)
snail-like retraction of the
  stomach
SNAT (suspected
  nonaccidental trauma)
SNM (Society of Nuclear
  Medicine)
SNMT (Society of Nuclear
  Medicine Technologists)
snowball opacity
"snowstorm" appearance
SNR (signal-to-noise ratio)
snuff-box
  anatomical s.
Soave pull-through procedure
Society of Nuclear Medicine
  (SNM)
Society of Nuclear Medicine
  Technologists (SNMT)
socket joint
SOD (source-to-object
  distance)
sodium
  s. arsenate
  s. bicarbonate
  s. bromide
  s. buniodyl
  s. carbonate
  s. chloride

sodium—*Continued*
- s. chromate
- s. citrate
- s. diatrizoate
- s. diprotrizoate
- s. fluoride
- s. hydroxide
- s. iodide solution
- s. iodipamide
- s. iodohippurate
- s. iodomethamate
- s. iothalamate
- s. ipodate
- s. methiodal
- s. methyglucamine
  diatrizoate
- s. metrizoate
- s. molybdate
- s. pertechnetate Tc
  99m
- s. phosphate
- s. phosphate solution
- s. radioiodide solution
- s. rose bengal
- s. sulfite
- s. sulphate
- s. tartrate
- s. thiosulfate
- s. thorium tartrate
- s. tryopanoate
- s. warfarin

Soemmering's area

soft
- "s." bones
- s. catheter
- s. iron
- s. tissue-negative
  image
- s. x-ray

soft-hand syndrome

soft-tissue
- s.-t. artifact
- s.-t. density
- s.-t. detail
- s.-t. film
- s.-t. shadow
- s.-t. swelling (STS)
- s.-t. technique
- s.-t. view (STV)

solar
- s. energy
- s. plexus
- s. radiation
- s. spectrum

solarization

sole

solenoid coil

soleus muscle

solid
- s. angle
- s. pattern (ultrasound)
- s. structure

solid-state
- s.-s. diode rectifier
- s.-s. physics
- s.-s. rectification

solid-tip catheter

solitary
- s. fibrous dysplasia
- s. focus
- s. lesion
- s. lobar atrophy
- s. myeloma
- s. pulmonary nodule
  (SPN)

Solu-Biloptin

solubilize

soluble

solution
- Carnoy's s.
- cyanocobalamin s.
- diatrizoate sodium s.
- hundredth-normal s.
- hypertonic s.
- ionic s.
- molal s.
- radiocyanocobalamin s.
- radiogold s.

sodium
  s. iodide s.
  s. phosphate s.
  s. radioiodide s.
Solutrast
somatic
  s. cells
somatogram
somatomedin
somatotrophic
Sombracol
Sombradil
somesthetic
Sommer-Foegella method
somnocinematography
sonarography
Sondermann's canal
Sones
  S. catheter
  S. coronary catheter
Sones'
  S.' technique
Sones-Shirey technique
sonoencephalography (SEG)
Sonofluoroscope I
Sonograf DI or EP
sonogram
sonographer
sonographic study
sonography
sonolucent
sonorous
Sontag, Snell, and Anderson
  method
Sontag table
sorbefacient
Sorbol heel
sordes
  s. gastricae
Soriano's syndrome
SOS dilation catheter
Soto's syndrome
Soudat's disease
souffle

source
  s. collimator
source-to-axis distance (SAD)
source-to-image distance (SID)
source-to-image-receptor
  distance (SIRD)
source-to-object distance
  (SOD)
source-to-skin distance (SSD)
source-to-surface distance
  (SSD)
SPA (single-photon
  absorptiometry)
space
  apical s.
  arachnoid s.
  axillary s.
  Bogros' s.
  Bowman's s.
  bregmatic s.
  capsular s.
  cathodal dark s.
  Colles' s.
  complemental s.
  Crookes' s.
  dead s.
  disk or disc s.
  epicerebral s.
  epidural s.
  episcleral s.
  epispinal s.
  epitympanic s.
  extradural s.
  extrapleural s.
  Faraday's dark s.
  H s.
  haversian s.
  Holzknecht's s.
  iliocostal s.
  interarytenoid s.
  intercostal s.
  intercristal s.
  intercrural s.
  interosseous s.

space—*Continued*
    interseptal s.
    intertrabecular s.
    ischiorectal s.
    Kiernan's s.
    Kretschmann's s.
    Larrey's s.
    Lesgraft's s.
    lymph s.
    Magendie's s.
    medullary s.
    meningeal s.
    Mohrenheim's s.
    Obersteiner-Redlich s.
    pararenal s.
    parasinoidal s.
    Parona's s.
    periaxial s.
    perihepatic s.
    perineal s.
    perineuronal s.
    perinuclear s.
    pharyngomaxillary s.
    phrenocostal s.
    physiologic dead s.
    pneumatic s.
    popliteal s.
    pre-epiglottic s.
    presacral s.
    pretracheal s.
    prevascular s.
    prevertebral s.
    prevesical s.
    retrobulbar s.
    retrocardiac s.
    retrocrural s.
    retroinguinal s.
    retromammary s.
    retro-ocular s.
    retroperitoneal s.
    retrorectal s.
    retrosternal s.
    retrotracheal s.
    s. disease
    s. of Retzius
    semilunar s.
    subacromial s.
    subarachnoid s.
    subcarinal s.
    subdural s.
    subepicranial s.
    subhepatic s.
    submaxillary s.
    subphrenic s.
    substernal s.
    subtrapezial s.
    subumbilical s.
    Tenon's s.
    thenar s.
    thiocyanate s.
    thyrohyal s.
    Traube's semilunar s.
    Westberg's s.
    Zang's s.
    zonular s.
space-charge compensator
space-occupying lesion
spade
    s. deformity
    s. hand
Spalding's sign
spallation
Spalteholz skull
span
    liver s.
spark
    s. chamber
    s. coil
    s. gap
spasm
    arterial s.
    coronary s.
    diffuse s.
    esophageal s.
    saltatory s.
spastic
    s. colon
    s. gait

s. ileus
s. paralysis
spasticity
spatial
   s. dose distribution
   s. filter
   s. frequency
   s. information
   s. nonuniformity
   s. resolution
   s. uniformity
   s. vectorcardiography
spatiotemporal resolution
spdt (single-pole double-throw)
specific
   s. activity
   s. gravity
   s. heat
   s. inductive capacity
   s. ionization
   s. radiation
speckled
   s. gastric fundus
   s. spleen
SPECT (single-photon emission computed tomography)
spectacle features
spectra, pl.
   spectrum, s.
spectral analysis
Spectrax pacemaker
spectrograph
   mass s.
spectrometer
   beta-ray s.
   Bragg s.
   gamma-ray s.
   mass s.
   Mossbauer's s.
   scintillation s.
   x-ray s.
spectrometry
   pulse-height s.

spectrophotofluorometer
spectrophotometer
   absorption s.
spectrophotometry
Spectroscaler 4R scintillation camera
spectroscope
spectroscopy
spectrum
   absorption s.
   absorption x-ray s.
   action s.
   characteristic s.
   chromatic s.
   continuous s.
   electromagnetic s.
   emission s. x-ray
   invisible s.
   pulse-height s.
   solar s.
   thermal s.
   x-ray s.
spectrum, s.
   spectra, pl.
Spee's curve
speed
   film s.
   s. factor
   s. of light
   s. of x-rays
Spence, tail of
spermatic
   s. abscess
   s. cord
spermatogenesis
spheno-occipital
   s. joint
   s. suture
spheno-orbital suture
sphenoethmoidal suture
sphenofrontal suture
sphenoid
   s. angle
   s. bone

sphenoid—*Continued*
  s. joint
  s. ridge
  s. rostrum
  s. sinus
  s. strut
  s. wing meningioma
sphenoidal
  s. concha
  s. rostrum
  s. yoke
sphenomalar suture
sphenomandibular ligament
sphenomaxillary suture
sphenopalatine
  s. canal
sphenoparietal sinus
sphenopetrosal suture
sphenopharyngeal
  s. canal
sphenorbital
sphenosalpingostaphylinus
sphenosquamosal
sphenosquamous suture
sphenotemporal suture
sphenoturbinal
sphenovomerine
sphenozygomatic suture
sphere
  s. gap
spherical aberration
spherocytosis
spheroid-shaped
spheroidal
  s. cast
  s. joint
spherophakia-brachymorphia
  syndrome
sphincter
  Balli's s.
  Busi's s.
  Cannon-Bohm s.
  cardioesophageal s.
  Giordano's s.

hepatic s.
Hirsch's s.
Hyrtl's s.
inguinal s.
Kapandjy's s.
Lütkens' s.
Moultier's s.
Nélaton's s.
O'Beirne's s.
palatopharyngeal s.
Payr-Strauss s.
pharyngoesophageal s.
prepyloric s.
pyloric s.
rectal s.
Rossi's s.
s. ani externus muscle
s. ani internus muscle
s. ani muscle
s. oculi
s. of Oddi
s. of pancreatic ampulla
s. oris
s. pylori muscle
s. urethrae
s. urethrae membranaceae
  muscle
s. vaginae muscle
s. vesicae muscle
sphingolipidosis
  cerebral s.
sphingomyelin lipidosis
sphingomyelinosis
sphygmobologram
sphygmocardiogram
sphygmogram
sphygmograph
  Marey's s.
  Vierordt's s.
sphygmography
sphygmoplethysmograph
spicula, pl.
  spiculum, s.
spiculate

spiculation
spicule
spicule-like
spiculum, s.
    spicula, pl.
spider fingers
spigelian
    s. hernia
    s. line
    s. lobe
spill radiography
spillage
spin
    s. coupling
    s. density
spin echo (SE)
spin-echo image
spin-echo relaxation (T2)
spin-echo sequence
spin-lattice constant
spin-lattice relaxation (T1)
    time
spin-lattice relaxation time
    constant
spin-spin
    s. constant
    s. relaxation time
spin-warp imaging
spina
    s. bifida
    s. bifida occulta
    s. luetica
    s. ventosa
spinal
    s. canal
    s. column
    s. cord
    s. dysraphism
    s. epiphysitis
    s. fusion
    s. fusion plate
    s. fusion series
    s. osteochrondritis
    s. osteoporosis

    s. stenosis
spinalis
    s. capitis muscle
    s. cervicis muscle
    s. thoracis muscle
spindle
    s. cell
    s. ureter
spindling
spine
    anterior nasal s.
    "bamboo" s.
    cervical s. (CS)
    Charcot's s.
    coccygeal s.
    iliac s.
    "kissing" s.
    lumbar s.
    lumbosacral s.
    "poker" s.
    s. sign
    sacral s.
    thoracic s.
    thoracolumbar s.
    tibial s.
spinnaker sail sign
spinning
    s. coin motion
    s. top test
    s. top urethra
spinocerebellar tract
spinocervicothalamic tract
spinoglenoid notch
spinogram
spino-olivary tract
spinosum
    foramen s.
spinothalamic tract
spinous
    s. process
    s. tubercle
spinthariscope
spintherometer
spintometer

spiral
- s. canal
- s. fracture
- s. joint
- s. motion
- s. tear
- s. valve

spiral-tip catheter
spirochetal jaundice
Spitz–Holter valve
splanchnic
splayfoot (flatfoot)
spleen
- accessory s.
- cyanotic s.
- floating s.
- lardaceous s.
- porphyry s.
- s. scan
- sago s.
- speckled s.
- wandering s.
- waxy s.

spleen-liver syndrome
splenic
- s. abscess
- s. agenesis syndrome
- s. anemia
- s. angle
- s. arteriography
- s. artery (SA)
- s. cyst
- s. dysfunction
- s. flexure (a bend)
- s. hematoma
- s. hypofunction
- s. infarction
- s. lymph node
- s. needle
- s. rupture
- s. sac
- s. shadow
- s. vein (SV)
- s. venogram

splenium
- s. corporis callosi

splenius
- s. capitis muscle
- s. cervicis muscle
- s. colli muscle

splenogastric omentum
splenography
splenoid
splenomegaly
splenoportal venography
splenoportogram
splenoportography
splenosis
splintered fracture
split sheath catheter
SPN (solitary pulmonary
   nodule)
spondylarthritis ankylopoietica
spondylarthrosis
spondylitis
- ankylosing s.
- paratyphoid s.
- psoriatic s.
- s. deformans
- tuberculous s.

spondyloarthropathy
spondyloenchondrodysplasia
spondyloepiphyseal
- s. dysplasia
- s. dysplasia congenita
- s. dysplasia tarda

spondylohumerofemoral
   hypoplasia
spondylolisthesis
spondylolysis
spondylometaphyseal
   dysplasia
spondylopathia traumatica
spondylorrheostosis
spondyloschisis
spondylosis
- rhizomelic s.
- s. chronica ankylopoietica

s. uncovertebralis
spondylothoracic
spondylotic cervical
   myelopathy
sponge kidney
spongioblastoma
spongy
spontaneous
   s. abortion
   s. fracture
   s. pneumothorax
   s. radiation
spot
   cold s.
   focal s.
   hot s.
   pelvic s.
   s. film
   s. scanography
spot-film
   s. device
   s. radiography
   s. study
   s. view
SPR (scanned projection
   radiography)
SPR (The Society of Pediatric
   Radiologists)
sprain fracture
Sprengel's
   S.'s deformity
   S.'s scapula
spring plate
springwater cyst
sprinter's fracture
spur
   calcaneal s.
spurious
   s. aneurysm
   s. count
   s. finding
   s. meningocele
   s. rib
   s. torticollis

spurring
   arthritis s.
Spurway-Eddowes syndrome
squama, s.
   squamae, pl.
squamae, pl.
   squama, s.
squamosa, s.
   squamosae, pl.
squamosae, pl.
   squamosa, s.
squamo-occipital
squamosomastoid suture
squamosoparietal suture
squamososphenoid suture
squamous
   s. cell carcinoma
   s. cell papilloma
   s. portion
   s. suture
squamozygomatic
squat view
Squibb QC analyzer
SQUID (superconducting
   quantum interference
   device)
Squire catheter
squirt sign
SR (saturation recovery)
SSA (subsegmental atelectasis)
SSCA (single shoulder contrast
   arthrography)
SSD (source-to-skin distance)
SSD (source-to-surface
   distance)
SSFP (steady-state free
   procession)
STA (superficial temporal
   artery)
Stabarium
stable isotope
stacked scan
stacked-coin
   s. effect

stacked-coin—*Continued*
   s. sign
Stafne's
   S.'s cyst
   S.'s mandibular cyst
staghorn
   s. calculus
   s. stone
staging
stain
   tumor s.
stalk
   pituitary s.
stalk-like
standard
   s. catheter needle
   s. curved Safe-T-J wire
      guide
   s. free air ionization
      chamber
   s. straight safety wire
      guide
"standing" waves
Stanescu's dysostosis
Stanford and Wheatstone
   stereoscope
stannosis
stannous
   s. chloride (Sn-113, Sn-
      119m)
   s. diphosphonate
   s. sulfur colloid
   s. pyrophosphate
stapedial joint
stapediovestibular
stapedius muscle
stapes
staphylococcic
Staples osteotomy nail
star
   s. artifact
   s. test pattern
   s. winding
Starr-Edwards (SE)
starry night sign

start test pattern
stasis
   s. gallbaldder
   s. liver
   s. ulcer
statampere
statcoulomb
Statham electromagnetic
   flowmeter
static
   s. column of dye
   s. electricity
   s. image display
   s. magnetic field
   s. marks
   s. renal image
stationary
   s. anode tube
   s. grid
statistical error
statokinetic labyrinth
stator
status
   s. asthmaticus
   s. epilepticus
   s. marmoratus
   s. thymicolymphaticus
   s. vertiginosus
statvolt
Staunig's
   S.'s method
   S.'s position
stave of the thumb
STD (skin-to-tumor distance)
steady-state-free precession
steal syndrome
   subclavian s. s.
steatorrhea
Stecher's
   S.'s method
   S.'s position
steel plate
steep Trendelenburg position
steeple
   s. sign

s. skull
steerhorn stomach
Steffe
  S. plate
  S. screw
Stein's syndrome
Stein-Leventhal
  S.-L. cyst
  S.-L. syndrome
Steiner's syndrome
Steinert's syndrome
Steinmann pin
stellate
  s. clefts
  s. fracture
stem
  brain s.
  s. cell lymphoma
  s. radiation
stenophthalmia
stenoses, pl.
  stenosis, s.
stenosis
  biliary s.
  cerebral aqueduct s.
  foraminal s.
  infundibular subaortic s.
  laryngeal s.
  mitral s. (MS)
  pulmonic s.
  pyloric s.
  renal artery s.
  spinal s.
  subaortic s.
  subglottic s.
  tracheal s.
  tricuspid s.
  tubular s.
stenosis, s.
  stenoses, pl.
Stensen's duct
stent
  antegrade ureteral s.
  biliary s.
  Carey-Coons s.

Coons s.
Cope s.
double-J s.
Druy s.
Mazer s.
Miller double mushroom
  biliary s.
Ring s.
ureteral s.
Stenver's
  S.'s for tips (prone)
    projection
  S.'s method
  S.'s view
  S.'s position
step-down transformer
step-up transformer
step-wedge
stephanion
steppage gait
steradian
stercoraceous abscess
stercoral abscess
stercoroma
stereo right lateral projection
stereocinefluorography
stereofluoroscopy
stereogram
stereophotography
stereoradiogram
stereoradiography
stereoroentgenography
stereoroentgenometry
stereosalpingography
stereoscope
  direct measuring s.
  monocular s.
  Stanford and Wheatstone
    s.
stereoscopic
  s. binoculars
  s. projections
  s. radiographic
  s. view
  s. zonography

stereoscopy
stereoskiagraphy
stereotactic
    s. biopsy
    s. surgery
stereotaxic
    s. brachytherapy
    s. gamma radiation
stereotaxis
stereotropism
stereozonography
Steri-drape
sterile
    s. abscess
    s. drape
Steripaque-BR
Steripaque-V
Stern's position
sterna or sternums, pl.
    sternum, s.
sternal
    s. angle
    s. depression
    s. joint
    s. notch
Sternberg's disease
sternoclavicular (SC)
    s. articulation
    s. joint (SCJ)
    s. ligament
sternocleidomastoid
    s. joint
    s. muscle
sternocleidomastoideus muscle
sternocostal
    s. joint
    s. ligament
    s. triangle
sternohyoid
sternohyoideus
sternomastoid
sternopericardial
sternoscapular
sternothyroideus muscle

sternothyroid
sternotracheal
sternovertebral
sternoxiphoid plane
sternum, s.
    sternums or sterna, pl.
sternums or sterna, pl.
    sternum, s.
steroid
    anabolic s.
Stewart-Hamilton equation
Stewart-Morel syndrome
sthenic habitus
Stickler's syndrome
Stieda-Pellegrini syndrome
Stieda's fracture
Stierlin's sign
stiff-man syndrome
stiffening
stifle joint
Still's
    S.'s disease
    S.'s syndrome
Stiller's rib
stimulation
    faradic s.
stippled
    s. calcification
    s. epiphysis
stippling
stitch abscess
stithe (incus)
Stitt catheter
stockinet or stockinette
stoma, s.
    stomata, pl.
stomach
    cascade s.
    cup-and-spill s.
    eutonic s.
    Holzknecht's s.
    hourglass s.
    hypotonic s.
    infantile s.

Pavlov's s.
s. partition
s. tube
steerhorn s.
upside-down s.
"waterfall" s.
stomal ulcer
stomata, pl.
stoma, s.
stomatognathic
stone
Meckel's s.
milk of calcium s.
staghorn s.
stonebasket catheter
stop bath
stopcock
four-way s.
one-way s.
Osborne precision s.
pin vise s.
s. manifolds
three-way s.
stoss
stosstherapy
Stout's fibromatosis
stove-pipe colon
strabismus of the penis
straddle fracture
straggling
straight
s. catheter
s. guide wire
s. intestine
s. sinus
straight-back syndrome
straight-line artifact
strain fracture
strand-like margins
strandy
strangulation
stratification
stratigraphy
strawberry gallbladder

stray radiation
streak artifact
streaky film
stream
electron s.
Street
S. pin
S. square forearm pin
Street's
S.'s finger joint
streptococcal
s. abscess
s. empyema
streptozocin (SZ) (Zanosar)
stress
s. film
s. fracture
s. incontinence
s. studies
s. ulcer
s. valgus
s. varus
s. view (ankle joint)
stress-induced
stretched bronchus sign
stretokinase-streptodornase
(SKSD)
striated muscle
striation
Strickler's method
stricture
stridor
string
s. galvanometer
s. of beads sign
s. sigmoid
s. sign
s. test
striomesencephalic radiation
striothalamic radiation
strip film
stripe
paratracheal s.
stripped atom

strippled calcification
stroboscopic
stroke volume (SV)
Strom-Zollinger-Ellison
  syndrome
stroma, s.
  stromata, pl.
stromata, pl.
  stroma, s.
strontium (Sr)
  radioactive s.
  s. 78m
  s. 85
  s. 87m
structural noise
structure
  complex s.
  cystic s.
  echo-dense s.
  fluid-filled s.
  mass s.
  multicystic s.
  multiloculated s.
  solid s.
struma suprarenalis cystica
  hemorrhagica
strumous abscess
Strümpell's disease
strut
  sphenoid s.
struvite
Stryker fracture frame
Stryker's notch
STS (soft-tissue swelling)
STS (subtrapezial space)
Stuart's diagrams
stub thumb
study
  aerosol inhalation s.
  air contrast s.
  barium double-contrast s.
  barium meal s.
  blood s.

blood flow s. (BFS)
brain s.
cerebral blood flow s.
cine s.
contrast s.
CT s.
double-contrast s.
dual-contrast s.
dynamic flow s. (DFS)
electrolyte s.
equilibrium gated blood
  pool s. (EGBPS)
equilibrium s.
erythrokinetic s.
eye s.
flow s.
"four-vessel" s.
gallbladder (GB) s.
gastrointestinal tract s.
H reflex s.
horizontal-beam s.
iodized oil s.
isotope s.
kidney s.
liver s.
lumbar flexion and
  extension s.
lung perfusion/ventilation
  (V/Q) s.
magnetic resonance s.
modified barium cookie
  swallow s.
motility s.
multigated blood pool
  (MUGA) s.
perfusion s.
peripheral perfusion s.
perirenal air s.
phonation s.
pulmonary blood flow
  (PBF) s.
quantitative regional lung
  function s.

quantitative tracer s.
rapid-drip s.
redistribution s.
regional ventilation/
  perfusion (V/Q) s.
renal radionuclide s.
retrococcygeal air s.
retroperitoneal air s.
single-contrast s.
sonographic s.
spot-film s.
stress s.
technetium albumin
  (TECA) s.
thyroid s.
tracer s.
ultrasonic s.
ventilation s.
ventilation-perfusion (V/
  Q) imaging s.
videotape s.
wash-out s.
xenon 133 ventilation s.
stump pressure
Sturge-Weber syndrome
STV (soft-tissue view)
stylet
styletted catheter
styloglossus
stylohyoid
stylohyoideus muscle
styloid
  s. bone
  s. process
stylomastoid foramen
stylopharyngeus muscle
STZ (streptozocin) (Zanosar)
subacromial space
subacromial-subdeltoid bursa
subanconeus muscle
subaortic stenosis
subapical
subaponeurotic abscess

subarachnoid
  s. hemorrhage (SAH)
  s. space
subarachnoidal cistern
subareolar abscess
subastragalar
subatomic
subcapital fracture
subcapsular
  s. "C" sign
  s. hematoma
subcarinal
  s. angle
  s. mass
  s. node
  s. space
subchondral
  s. cortex
  s. cyst
  s. osteoporosis
  s. sclerosis
subclavian
  s. catheter
  s. groove
  s. steal syndrome
subclavicular murmur
subclavius
subclinical coarctation of the
  aorta
subcortical
subcostal
  s. groove
  s. line
  s. zone
subcostales muscle
subcostosternal diaphragmatic
  hernia
subcrureus muscle
subcutaneous
  s. abscess
  s. emphysema
  s. fracture
  s. mastectomy

subdeltoid
subdiaphragmatic abscess
subdivided
subdural
   s. abscess
   s. empyema
   s. hematoma (SDH)
   s. hemorrhage
   s. space
subendocardial
   s. infarction
   s. sclerosis
subependymal
subependymoma
subepicranial space
subepidermal
subepiphyseal
   osteochondropathy
subfascial abscess
subfolium
subgaleal abscess
subglenoid dislocation
subglottic
   s. carcinoma
   s. chink
   s. cyst
   s. hemangioma
   s. stenosis
subhepatic
   s. abscess
   s. space
subject
   s. habitus
   s. motion
   s. unsharpness
subject-film distance
sublingual
   s. duct
   s. gland
subluxation
submammary abscess
submandibular
   s. duct

   s. gland
submaxillary
   s. duct
   s. gland
   s. space
submental
   s. lymph node
   s. vertex (SMV) view
submentale
submentovertex position
submentovertical
   s. axial projection
   s. view
submerged segment of the
   esophagus
submucosal fibrosis
suboptimal image
subparietal sulcus
subpectoral abscess
subperiosteal
   s. abscess
   s. cortical hyperostosis
   s. fracture
subphrenic
   s. abscess
   s. space
subpleural cap
subpubic arch
subscapular
   s. abscess
   s. aponeurosis
   s. muscle
subscapularis muscle
subsegmental
   s. atelectasis (SSA)
   s. bronchus
subshell
subspinale
substantia
   s. nigra
substernal
   s. goiter
   s. space

s. thyroid
subtalar
   s. arthritis
   s. joint
subtaloid joint
subtentorial
subtraction
   digital s. angiography
     (DSA)
   film s.
   first-order s.
   photographic s.
   s. angiography
   s. technique
   s. venography
   second-order s.
subtrapezial space (STS)
subtrigonal gland
subtrochanteric
subumbilical space
subungual
   s. epidermoid carcinoma
   s. exostosis
   s. hematoma
   s. keratoacanthoma
subxiphoid
succinic semialdehyde
Sucquet-Hoyer canal
suction
   s. catheter
   s. plate
Sudeck's
   S.'s atrophy
   S.'s porosis
Sudeck-Leriche syndrome
sudoriparous abscess
sugar-icing liver
Sugg catheter
Suit-Fletcher applicator
sulci, pl.
   sulcus, s.
sulculi, pl.
   sulculus, s.

sulculus, s.
   sulculi, pl.
sulcus
   calcaneal s.
   calcarine s.
   callosal s.
   central s.
   cingulate s.
   collateral s.
   frontal lobe s.
   olfactory s.
   postcalcarine s.
   rhinal s.
   s. chiasmatis
   s. for optic chiasm
   s. intermedius
   s. of Reil, circular
   sigmoid s.
   subparietal s.
   superior s.
   suprasplenial s.
sulcus, s.
   sulci, pl.
sulfamethoxazole (SMX)
sulfate
   barium lead s.
   barium s.
   barium strontium s.
sulfatide lipidosis
sulfur
   s. colloid (SC)
sulfuric acid (S-35)
Sulkowitch's test
summit
   s. of the bladder
   s. of the nose
sump ulcer
sunrise view
supercam scintillation
   scanner
superciliary arch
superconducting
   s. magnet

superconducting—*Continued*
  s. quantum interference
    device
superconductive magnet
superficial
  s. abscess
  s. femoral artery (SFA)
  s. temporal artery (STA)
  s. therapy
  s. x-ray (SXR)
superimpose
superimposed artifact
superimposition projection
superior
  s. anastomotic vein
  s. articular process
  s. articulating process
  s. mesenteric
    arteriography
  s. mesenteric artery (SMA)
  s. mesenteric artery
    syndrome
  s. mesenteric vein (SMV)
  s. olive
  s. pulmonary sulcus tumor
  s. radioulnar joint
  s. ramus
  s. straight
  s. sulcus tumor
  s. tendon of Lockwood
  s. vena cava
  s. vena cavagram
supernatant
supernumerary
  s. kidney
  s. nipple
superoinferior
  s. projection
  s. view
superscan
supervascularization
supervoltage
  s. generator
  s. technique

  s. therapy radiation
supinate
supinator
  s. longus muscle
  s. radii brevis muscle
supine
  s. position
  s. projection
supply voltage
suppurative
  s. arthritis
  s. mastoiditis
  s. myositis
  s. pericarditis
supracallosal gyrus
supraciliary
  s. canal
supraclavicular fossa
supraclinoid process
supracondylar
  s. fracture
  s. ridge
supracondyloid process
supracristal ventricular septal
  defect
supradiaphragmatic
  diverticulum
supraglottic carcinoma
supraglottis
suprahepatic abscess
suprahilar
supramesocolic
supraoccipital
supraoptic
  s. canal
supraopticohypophyseal
  tract
supraorbital
  s. border
  s. foramen
  s. groove
  s. margin
  s. notch
  s. projection

suprapatellar
  s. bursa
  s. effusion sign
suprapubic catheter
suprarenal
  s. gland
  s. melasma
suprascapular notch
suprasellar
  s. aneurysm
  s. cistern
  s. cyst
  s. meningioma
supraspinatus
  s. fossa
  s. muscle
supraspinous aponeurosis
suprasplenial sulcus
suprasternal notch
suprasulcus tumor
supra-sylvian region
supratentorial
supratragal notch
supratrochlear
supravalvular
surface
  articular s.
  s. "cuts"
  s. area (SA)
  s. coil
  s. coil method
  s. dose
  s. staples
  s. tension
surgical
  s. changes
  s. head
  s. neck
Surgitek catheter
survey dynamic scanning
Surview
suspected nonaccidental
  trauma (SNAT)
suspended heart syndrome

suspension
suspensorius duodeni
suspensory ligament
suspicion
sustentacula, pl.
  sustentaculum, s.
sustentacular
sustentaculum
  s. lienis
  s. tali
sustentaculum, s.
  sustentacula, pl.
Sutton's angle
Sutton-Babington syndrome
sutural fusion
suture
  arcuate s.
  biparietal s.
  bregmatomastoid s.
  coronal s.
  cranial s.
  cutaneous s.
  dentate s.
  ethmoidomaxillary s.
  frontal s.
  frontoethmoidal s.
  frontomalar s.
  frontomaxillary s.
  frontonasal s.
  frontoparietal s.
  frontosphenoid s.
  frontozygomatic s.
  infraorbital s.
  interendognathic s.
  intermaxillary s.
  internasal s.
  interparietal s.
  jugal s.
  lacrimoconchal s.
  lacrimoethmoidal s.
  lacrimomaxillary s.
  lacrimoturbinal s.
  lambdoidal s.
  longitudinal s.

suture—*Continued*
  malomaxillary s.
  mastoid s.
  mendosal s.
  metopic s.
  nasal s.
  nasofrontal s.
  nasomaxillary s.
  occipitomastoid s.
  occipitoparietal s.
  occipitosphenoidal s.
  opaque s.
  palatine s.
  palatoethmoidal s.
  parietal s.
  parietomastoid s.
  petrobasilar s.
  petrosphenobasilar s.
  petrospheno-occipital s.
  petrosquamous s.
  premaxillary s.
  radiopaque s.
  rhabdoid s.
  s. granuloma
  s. joint
  sagittal s.
  sphenoethmoidal s.
  sphenofrontal s.
  sphenomalar s.
  sphenomaxillary s.
  spheno-occipital s.
  spheno-orbital s.
  sphenopetrosal s.
  sphenosquamous s.
  sphenotemporal s.
  sphenozygomatic s.
  squamosomastoid s.
  squamosoparietal s.
  squamososphenoid s.
  squamous s.
  temporomalar s.
  temporozygomatic s.
  wire s.
  zygomaticofrontal s.
    zygomaticomaxillary s.
    zygomaticotemporal s.
Sv (sievert) unit
SV (splenic vein)
SV (stroke volume)
swallow
  barium s.
  modified barium cookie s.
swallowing
  s. mechanism
  s. motion
Swan-Ganz
  S.-G. catheter
  S.-G. catheter tip
swan-neck deformity
Swanson prosthesis
Swedish line
Sweeley-Klionsky syndrome
Sweet's
  S.'s eye
  S.'s method
swimmer's
  s.'s position
  s.'s projection
  s.'s view
swing-to gait
Swyer-James syndrome
SXR (superficial x-ray)
Syed
  S. implant
  S. template
Syed-Neblitt template
sylvian
  s. cistern
  s. fissure
  s. point
  s. triangle
  s. vessels group
Sylvius
  aqueduct of S.
  fissure of S.
  valve of S.
symbol
symbrachydactyly

Symmers' syndrome
symmetric
  s. asphyxia
  s. changes
  s. gangrene
  s. involvement
  s. keratodermia of the
    extremities
symmetrical-unsymmetrical
  movement
Symonds' syndrome
sympathetic abscess
sympathoblastoma, s.
  sympathoblastomata, pl.
sympathoblastomata, pl.
  sympathoblastoma, s.
symphalangism-surdity
  syndrome
symphyseal
symphyses, pl.
  symphysis, s.
symphysis
  mandibular s.
  s. diastasis
  s. menti
  s. pubis
symphysis, s.
  symphyses, pl.
symptom
symptomatic
symptomatology
synarthrodial joint
synarthrosis
synchiotron
synchondroses, pl.
  synchondrosis, s.
synchondrodial joint
synchondrosis, s.
  synchondroses, pl.
synchrocyclotron
synchronism
synchronization
synchronizer
synchronizing pulse

synchronous
  s. motor
  s. timer
synchrotron
syncopal
  s. episode
syncope
  near s.
syncytial
syncytium
  venous epidural s.
syndactyly
syndesmitis ossificans
syndesmodial joint
syndesmophyte
syndesmophytic
syndesmosis
syndrome
  13 Q s.
  Aarskog-Scott s.
  Abt-Letterer-Siwe s.
  acquired
    immunodeficiency s.
    (AIDS)
  acrocallosal s.
  acute disk s.
  acute radiation s. (ARS)
  Adair-Dighton s.
  Adson's s.
  adult respiratory distress
    s. (ARDS)
  aglossia-adactyly s.
  Aicardi's s.
  Albright's s.
  Albright-Hadorn s.
  Albright-McCune-
    Sternberg s.
  Aldrich's s.
  Allemann's s.
  Alport's s.
  angiosteohypertrophic s.
  Anglemann's s.
  Anton's s.
  antral remnant s.

syndrome—*Continued*
  aortic arch s.
  aortic bifurcation s.
  Apert's s.
  argentaffinoma s.
  Arrillaga-Ayerza s.
  arthrogryposis s. in the
    Eskimo
  Asherman's s.
  aspiration s.
  Ayerza's s.
  Ayerza-Arrillaga s.
  Baastrup's s.
  Baber's s.
  Babinski-Fröhlich s.
  Bakwin-Eiger s.
  Bakwin-Krida s.
  Bamatter's s.
  Banti's s.
  Bard-Pic s.
  Barrett's s.
  Bársony-Polgár s.
  Bársony-Teschendorf s.
  Bartenwerfer's s.
  Bartholin-Patau s.
  Bartter's s.
  basal cell nevus s.
  Bass s.
  Bassen-Kornzweig s.
  battered-baby s.
  battered-child s.
  Beckwith's s.
  Beckwith-Wiedemann s.
  Berardinelli's
    lipodystrophy s.
  Bernheim's s.
  Berry's s.
  Besnier-Boeck-Schaumann
    s.
  Besnier-Tennesson s.
  Beuren's s.
  Bezold's s.
  Biemond's s.

  bilateral polycystic ovarian
    s.
  Biorck-Thorson s.
  bird-fancier's lung s.
  black liver-jaundice s.
  Bland-White-Garland s.
  Blegvad-Haxthausen s.
  blind loop s.
  Bloom's s.
  Bloom-German s.
  Blount's s.
  Blount-Barber s.
  blue sclera s.
  "bobble-head doll" s.
  body cast s.
  Boerhaave's s.
  Borries' s.
  Bourneville's s.
  Bourneville-Brissaud s.
  Boyd-Stearns s.
  Brachman-de Lange s.
  Brailsford-Morquio s.
  branchial arch s.
  Brauer's s.
  Bret's s.
  Bridges and Good s.
  broad thumb-hallux s.
  Brock's s.
  brown-spot s.
  Brunauer's s.
  "bubbly lung" s.
  Budd-Chiari s.
  Büdlinger-Ludloff-Läwen

  Burke's s.
  busulfan lung s.
  C s. of multiple congenital
    anomalies
  Caffey's pseudo-Hurler's s.
  Caffey's s.
  Caffey-Kempe s.
  Caffey-Silverman s.
  Cairns' s.

Calvé-Perthes-Legg s.
Camurati-Englemann s.
Caplan's s.
Caplan-Colinet s.
carcinoid s.
cardiocutaneous s.
cardiomelic s.
cardiotomy s.
cardiovasorenal s.
Caroli's s.
carpal tunnel s.
Carpenter's s.
cartilage-hair hypoplasia
    s.
"cast" s.
cauda equina s.
cerebrohepatorenal
    (CHRS) s.
cervical rib s.
cervico-oculo-acusticus s.
Chaufford-Ramon s.
Chaufford-Still s.
Chédiak-Higashi s.
Chilaiditi's s.
Christian's brachydactyly
    s.
click-murmur s.
Cockayne's s.
Costen's s.
Cowden's s.
cri-du-chat s.
Cushing's s.
Dameshek's s.
Dandy-Walker s.
Danlos' s.
De Martini-Balestera s.
de Morsier's s.
De Toni-Caffey s.
deafness-
    onychodystrophy-
    osteodystrophy
    retardation s. (DOOR)
Debré-Sémélaigne s.

Déjérine-Sottas.s.
Demons-Meigs s.
Denny-Brown's s.
Dickinson's s.
Dietrich's s.
digitofaciomental
    retardation s.
Dimitri-Sturge-Weber s.
Donohue's s.
Down's s.
Dressler's s.
Dreyfus' s.
"drowned newborn" s.
Dubin-Johnson s.
Dubovitz' s.
Dudley-Klingenstein s.
dumping s.
duodenal stasis s.
Durand-Zunin s.
Dyggve-Melchior-Clausen
    s.
Dyke-Davidoff s.
E s.
Eagle's s.
earth-eating s.
Eaton-Lambert s.
ectrodactyly-ectodermal
    dysplasia-clefting (EEC)
    s.
ectromelia-ichthyosis s.
Eddowes' s.
Edwards' s.
Ehlers-Danlos s.
Ekman-Lobstein s.
Ellis-van Creveld s.
empty-sella s.
Engel-von Recklinghausen
    s.
Engelmann's s.
epibronchial right
    pulmonary artery s.
Erdheim's s.
Erlacher-Blount s.

syndrome—*Continued*
  Evans-Lloyd-Thomas s.
  exomphalos-macroglossia-
    gigantism s.
  extremity
    osteochondrodystrophy
    s.
  F s.
  Fabry's s.
  Fabry-Anderson s.
  faciodigitogenital s.
  Fanconi's s.
  Fanconi-Albertini-
    Zellweger s.
  Fanconi-De Toni-Debré s.
  Fanconi-Hegglin s.
  Farber-Uzman s.
  Felty's s.
  female pseudo-Turner's s.
  femur-fibula-ulna (FFU) s.
  fetal alcohol s.
  fetal Dilantin s.
  fetal folic acid antagonist
    s.
  fetal hydantoin s.
  Fiessinger-Leroy s.
  first arch s.
  Fitz' s.
  floppy valve s.
  flush s.
  Fölling's s.
  Fong's s.
  Forestier and Rotés-Querol
    s.
  forme fruste of Hurler's s.
  Foster-Kennedy s.
  Fraley's s.
  Franceschetti's s.
  François' s.
  François-Haustrate s.
  Freeman-Sheldon s.
  Friedrich's s.
  Fröhlich's obesity s.
  Fuller-Albright s.

  Furst-Ostrum s.
  G s.
  Gardner's s.
  Gardner-Bosch s.
  gargoyle s.
  gastric remnant s.
  gastrocardiac s.
  Gaucher-Schlagenhaufer s.
  Gee-Herter-Heubner s.
  geophagia-dwarfism-
    hypogonadism s.
  Giedion's s.
  Gillespie's s.
  Glanzmann-Riniker s.
  Golden-Kantor s.
  Goldenhar's s.
  Goldschneider's s.
  Goltz-Gorlin s.
  gonadal dysgenesis s.
  Goodpasture's s.
  Gorham's s.
  Gorlin-Chaudhry-Moss s.
  Gorlin-Goltz s.
  Gorlin-Psaume s.
  Gougerot-Houwer-Sjögren
    s.
  Gradenigo's s.
  Graham-Steell s.
  Grebe's s.
  Greig's s.
  Gringolo's s.
  Grisel's s.
  Grönblad-Strandberg s.
  Grönblad-Strandberg-
    Touraine s.
  Guérin-Stern syndrome
  Guillain-Barré s.
  gynecomastia-
    aspermatogenesis s.
  Haferkamp's s.
  Haglund-Läwen-Fründ s.
  Hallermann-Streiff-
    François s.
  Hamman-Rich s.

hand-foot s.
hand-foot-genital s.
hand-foot-uterus s.
Hand-Schüller-Christian s.
Hanhart's s.
"happy puppet" s.
Hare's s.
Harkavy's s.
Haven's s.
Hedinger's s.
Heiner's s.
Helmholtz-Harrington s.
hemolytic-uremic s.
Henderson-Jones s.
hereditary extremity
   malformation s.
hereditary hematuria-
   nephropathy-deafness s.
Herrick's s.
Hertwig-Weyers s.
Heubner-Herter s.
Hicks' s.
Hippel-Czermack s.
Hirsch's s.
Hoffa-Kastert s.
Holt-Oram s.
Holtermüller-Wiedemann
   s.
HOOD (hereditary
   onycho-osteodysplasia)
   s.
Horner's s.
Hozay's s.
Hughes-Stovin s.
Hultkrantz' s.
Hünermann's s.
Hunter's s.
Hunter-Hurler s.
Hurler's s.
Hutchinson-Gilford s.
Hutchinson-Weber-Peutz
   s.
Hutinel-Pick s.
hydantoin s.

hydrometrocolpos-
   polydactyly s.
hyperlucent lung s.
hypocalcemic convulsions-
   dwarfism s.
hypophysial or
   hypophyseal s.
hypophysiothalamic s.
hypopituitarism s.
hypothalamic
   hamartoblastoma s.
hypothenar hammer s.
iatrogenic afferent loop s.
icteric-hepatic
   pigmentation s.
inspissated milk s.
intestinal carcinoid s.
inverted Marfan's s.
Ivemark's s.
Jaffe-Lichtenstein s.
Jaffe-Lichtenstein-
   Uehlinger s.
Jahnke's s.
Janus' s.
Jefferson's s.
jejunal s.
Johnie McL's s.
jugular foramen s.
Kalischer's s.
Kartagener's s.
Kashin-Beck s.
Kast's s.
Kawasaki's s.
Kaznelson's s.
Kearns-Sayre s.
Kenney-Caffey s.
"kinky-hair" s.
kleeblattschädel s.
Klein-Waardenburg s.
Klinefelter's s.
Klinefelter-Reifenstein-
   Albright s.
Klippel-Feil s.
Klippel-Feldstein s.

syndrome—*Continued*
   Klippel-Trenaunay-Weber
      s.
   Klüver-Bucy-Terzian s.
   Kniest's s.
   Kocher-Debré-Sémélaigne
      s.
   Köhler-Stieda-Pellegrini s.
   Krabbe's s.
   Kundrat's s.
   lacrimo-auriculo-dento-
      digital s.
   Ladd's s.
   Ladd-Gross s.
   Langdon Down's s.
   Lannelongue-Osgood-
      Schlatter s.
   Lannois-Gradenigo s.
   Larsen's s.
   Larsen-Johansson s.
   late Hurler's s.
   Launois-Cléret s.
   Laurence-Moon-Biedl s.
   Laurence-Moon-Biedl-
      Bardet s.
   Lawford's s.
   Lawrence-Seip s.
   "lazy leukocyte" s.
   Legg-Calvé-Perthes s.
   Lejeune's s.
   lentiginopolypose
      digestive s.
   lentiginosa profusa s.
   Lenz' s.
   leopard s.
   Léri-Joanny s.
   Léri-Weill s.
   Leriche's s.
   Lesch-Nyhan s.
   Letterer-Siwe s.
   Lévi's s.
   Lightwood's s.
   Lightwood-Albright s.
   lissencephaly s.
   Löffler's or Loeffler's s.

   Löfgren's s.
   Looser-Debray-Milkman
      s.
   Lorain-Lévi s.
   Lowe's s.
   Lowe-Terrey-MacLachlan
      s.
   Lutembacher's s.
   luxury perfusion s.
   MacLeod's s.
   macroglossia-omphalocele
      s.
   Maffucci's s.
   malignant malnutrition s.
   Mallory-Weiss s.
   Mankowsky's s.
   Marchesani's s.
   Marfan's s.
   Marie's s.
   Marie-Bamberger s.
   Marie-Léri s.
   Maroteaux-Lamy s.
   Marshall's s.
   Martorell-Fabré s.
   McCune-Albright s.
   meconium aspiration s.
      (MAS)
   meconium plug s.
   Meekeren-Ehlers-Danlos
      s.
   Meigs' s.
   Meigs-Cass s.
   Melnick-Needles s.
   Mendelson's s.
   Menkes' "kinky-hair" s.
   metacarpotalar s.
   metastatic carcinoid s.
   Meyenburg-Altherr-
      Uehlinger s.
   Meyer-Schwickerath and
      Weyers s.
   Michotte's s.
   micrognathia-glossoptosis
      s.
   microphthalmos s.

middle lobe s.
Mikulicz' s.
milk-alkali s.
milk-allergy s.
milk-drinker's s.
milk-poisoning s.
Milkman's s.
Milkman-Looser s.
Miller's s.
Milles' s.
Mirizzi's s.
mirror image lung s.
MMM s.
Möbius' s.
Moersch-Woltmann s.
Mohr's s.
Morgagni-Stewart-Morel
  s.
Morgagni-Turner-Albright
  s.
Morquio's s.
Morton's s.
Mosse's s.
Mounier-Kuhn s.
Müller-Weiss s.
multiple enchondromata s.
multiple hamartoma s.
multiple lentigines s.
Münchmeyer's s.
Murk-Jansen s.
mushroom worker's s.
Naffziger's s.
Nager-de Reynier s.
nail-patella s.
narrow lumbar spinal
  canal s.
Nelson's s.
Neuhauser-Berenberg s.
nevoid basal cell
  carcinoma s.
Niemann-Pick s.
Nierhoff-Hübner s.
Nievergelt's s.
Nievergelt-Erb s.
Nievergelt-Pearlman s.

Noack's s.
Nonne's s.
Nonne-Milroy-Meige s.
Noonan's s.
Obrinsky's s.
"obui-himo" s.
oculo-urethro-articular s.
oculocerebrorenal s.
oculodentodigital s.
oligodactylia s.
Ollier's s.
Ollier-Trenaunay-Klippel
  s.
organic brain s.
Ormond's s.
orofaciodigital (OFD) s. I
orofaciodigital (OFD) s. II
orogenital s.
Ortner's s.
Osgood-Schlatter s.
Osler's s.
osteodermapathic
  hyperostosis s.
osteohypertrophic
  varicose nevus s.
osteoporosis-osteomalacia
  s.
Österreicher-Turner s.
otopalatodigital (OPD) s.
Otto's s.
ovarian ascites-pleural
  effusion s.
ovarian short-stature s.
Paget-Schroetter s.
painful
  apicocostovertebral s.
Pancoast's s.
pancreas-blood-bone s.
pancreatic malignancy s.
pancytopenia-dysmelia s.
Papillon-Léage and
  Psaume s.
Papillon-Lefèvre s.
parent-infant traumatic
  stress (PITS) s.

syndrome—*Continued*
Parkes Weber s.
Parrot-Kaufmann s.
Parry-Romberg s.
Patau's s.
Paterson-Kelly s.
pectoral aplasia-
dysdactyly s.
Pendred's s.
peritubal s.
persistent fetal circulation
s.
Peutz-Jeghers s.
Pfaundler-Hurler s.
Pfeiffer's s.
phalangeal microgeodic s.
phrenopyloric s.
pickwickian s.
PIE (pulmonary infiltrate
with eosinophilia) s.
"pierre de la peau" s.
Pierre-Marie-Bamberger
s.
Pierre Robin's s.
PITS (parent-infant
traumatic stress) s.
Plummer-Vinson s.
popliteal pterygium s.
Porak-Durante s.
postcholecystectomy s.
postcommissurotomy s.
posterior bowing s.
postgastrectomy s.
postmyocardial infarction
s.
postpericardiotomy s.
postprandial s.
Potter's s.
Prader-Labhart-Willi-
Fanconi s.
progeria s.
progeria-like s.
proximal femoral focal
deficiency (PFFD) s.

prune-belly s.
pseudo-Hurler's s.
pseudo-Turner's s.
pseudoacromegalic s.
pterygium s.
ptosis-epicanthus s.
pulmonary renal s.
pulmonary venolumbar s.
Putti's s.
quadruple s.
Raeder-Harbitz s.
Raynaud's s. of the upper
limb
reflex sympathetic
dystrophy s.
Reichel-Jones-Henderson
s.
Rendu-Osler s.
Rendu-Osler-Weber s.
renofacial s.
respiratory distress s.
(RDS)
retained gastric antrum s.
(RGAS)
Reye's s.
Reye-Sheehan s.
rhinotrichophalangeal s.
Ribbing's s.
Ribbing-Müller s.
Rieger's s.
Riley-Day s.
Riley-Shwachman s.
Robinow-Silverman-Smith
s.
Rocher-Sheldon s.
Romberg's s.
Rosen-Castleman-Liebow
s.
Rossi's s.
Rothmund's s.
Rothmund-Thompson s.
Rotor's s.
Rotter-Erb s.
Roviralta's s.

Royer's s.
Rubinstein-Taybi s.
Ruiter-Pompen-Wyers s.
Russell-Silver s.
s. de Profichet
s. of the apex of the
  petrous bone
s. of the first branchial
  arch
Salvioli's s.
Sandifer's s.
Sanfilippo's s.
Scaglietti-Dagnini s.
scalenus anticus s.
scalenus s.
Scheie's s.
Scheuthauer-Marie-Sainton
  s.
Schirmer's s.
Schlatter's s.
Schlessinger-Taveras s.
Scholte's s.
Schroetter's s.
Schwartz-Jampel s.
scimitar s.
Seabright bantam s.
Seckel's s.
secreto-inhibitor s.
Seip's s.
Senior's s.
Shaver's s.
Shaver-Ridell s.
Sheehan's s.
Sheldon-Ellis s.
shock lung s.
Shone's s.
shoulder-hand s.
Shwachman's s.
sicca s.
sideropenic s.
Siegal-Cattan-Mamou s.
silent disk s.
Silver's s.
Silverskiöld's s.

Simmonds' s.
Sinding-Larsen-Johansson
  s.
Singleton-Merton s.
sinobronchial s.
sinus of Morgagni s.
Sipple's s.
Sjögren's s.
smooth-brain s.
soft-hand s.
Soriano's s.
Sotos' s.
spherophakia-
  brachymorphia s.
spleen-liver s.
splenic agenesis s.
Spurway-Eddowes s.
steal s.
Stein's s.
Stein-Leventhal s.
Steiner's s.
Steinert's s.
Stewart-Morel s.
Stickler's s.
Stieda-Pellegrini s.
stiff-man s.
Still's s.
straight-back s.
Strom-Zollinger-Ellison s.
Sturge-Weber s.
subclavian steal s.
Sudeck-Leriche s.
superior mesenteric artery
  (SMA) s.
suspended heart s.
Sutton-Babington s.
Sweeley-Klionsky s.
Swyer-James s.
Symmers' s.
Symonds' s.
symphalangism-surdity s.
Tabatznick's s.
Takayasu's s.
Takayasu-Onishi s.

syndrome—*Continued*
  Taussig-Bing s.
  Taussig-Snellen-Albers s.
  Taybi's s.
  telangiectasia-
    pigmentation-cataract s.
  temporal s.
  temporomandibular joint
    s.
  Terry's s.
  tethered cord s.
  Teutschländer's s.
  Thévenard's s.
  Thibierge-Weissenbach s.
  Thomas' s.
  Thompson's s.
  thoracic outlet s.
  thoracogenous rheumatic
    s.
  Thorson-Biörk s.
  thrombocytopenia-absent
    radius s.
  Tietze's s.
  Tobias' s.
  Tolosa-Hunt s.
  Touraine-Solente-Golé s.
  Treacher Collins' s.
  trisomy 8 mosaicism s.
  Troell-Junet s.
  Trotter's s.
  Turcot's s.
  Turner's s.
  Turner-Fong s.
  Turner-Kieser s.
  Turner-like s.
  Turpin's s.
  ulcerogenic tumor of the
    pancreas s.
  Ullrich and Fremerey-
    Dohna s.
  Ullrich-Turner s.
  Unna-Thost s.
  upper limb cardiovascular
    s.
  van Bogaert-Hozay s.

  van Bogaert-Nyssen-
    Pfeiffer s.
  van Buchem's s.
  van Neck-Odelberg s.
  venolobar s.
  Verbrycke's s.
  Verner-Morrison s.
  Vernet's s.
  vertebral s.
  Vesell's s.
  Virchow-Seckel s.
  von Gierke's s.
  Waardenburg's
    acrocephalosyndactyly
    s.
  Waardenburg's s.
  Waelsch's s.
  Weber's s.
  Weber-Dimitri s.
  Weill-Marchesani s.
  Weinberg-Himelfarb s.
  Weingarten's s.
  Weismann-Netter s.
  Wermer's s.
  Werner's s.
  Westphal-Strümpell s.
  Weyers-Thier s.
  whistling face s.
  Wiedemann's s.
  Wiedemann-Beckwith s.
  Wilkie's s.
  Williams' elfin facies s.
  Williams-Campbell s.
  Wilson's s.
  Wilson-Mikity s.
  Winchester-Grossman s.
  WL symphalangism-
    brachydactyly s.
  Wolff-Parkinson-White s.
  WT s.
  Wyburn-Mason s.
  XO s.
  XX and XY Turner
    phenotype s.
  XXXXY s.

XXY s.
young female arteritis s.
Youssef's s.
Zellweger's s.
Zellweger-Bowan s.
Zollinger-Ellison s.
Zwahlen's s.
Synerdyne scanner
synostosis
    radioulnar s.
synovia (the fluid)
synovial
    s. capsule
    s. chondromatosis
    s. cyst
    s. fluid
    s. gland
    s. joint
    s. margin
    s. membrane
    s. osteochondromatosis
    s. sac
    s. sarcoma
    s. sheath
    s. thickening
synovioblast
synovioma
synoviosarcoma
synovitis
    tuberculous s.
    villonodular s.
synovium (the membrane)
synpolydactyly
Syntetragnost
synthes prosthesis
syntheses, pl.
    synthesis, s.
synthesis, s.
    syntheses, pl.
syphilitic
    s. abscess
    s. aneurysm
    s. arthritis
    s. lesion
    s. meningoencephalitis

s. node
s. osteitis of the newborn
s. osteochondritis
syringoadenoma
syringocarcinoma
syringocystadenoma
syringocystoma
syringoencephalomyelia
syringomyelia
system
    acquisition s.
    Aus-tect test s.
    AutoLogic 100 gamma
        counting s.
    AutoLogic 50 gamma
        counting s.
    automatic processing s.
    British engineering s.
    calyceal s.
    capacitor discharge s.
    catenary s.
    centimeter-gram-second
        (cgs or CGS) s.
    collecting s.
    constant potential s.
    conventional single-phase
        s.
    CT/T computed
        tomography s.
    "cow" s.
    data acquisition s. (DAS)
    data reduction s.
    daylight s.
    dryer s.
    electron transmitter s.
    Elscint s.
    field emission x-ray s.
    Galen's s.
    gamma-counting s.
    gradient s.
    Hakim valve s.
    Holter valve s.
    image intensifier s.
    International 10-20 s.
    Jewett-Marshall s.

system—*Continued*
  linear compartmental s.
  linear s.
  liquid scintillation s.
  Logic 101, 111, and 121
    gamma counting s.
  mammillary s.
  Manchester Dosage s.
  mechanical life support s.
  meter-kilogram-second s.
  metric s.
  mobile x-ray s.
  MR MAX (magnetic
    resonance imaging
    system)
  Orbitome tomographic s.
  Paterson-Parker Dosage s.
  Pfizer whole-body CT s.
  Philips s.
  Picker Pace-1 gamma-
    counting s.
  Picker s.
  Picture Archiving and
    Communication s.
    (PACS)
  Puder-Hayer valve s.
  rectifying s.
  remote control diagnostic
    s.
  reticuloendothelial s.
    (RES)
  rotate-only s.

  rotate-stationary s.
  scan projection radiograph
    s.
  Siemens s.
  single-film automatic s.
  single-phase s.
  single-photon counting s.
  Thomson-CGR s.
  three-compartment s.
  three-phase s.
  three-wire s.
  Tomolex tomographic s.
  transport s.
  tube-detector s.
  two-compartment s.
  vacuum cassette s.
  vertebrobasilar s.
  whole-body proton
    magnetic resonance
    imaging s.
systemic
  s. chondromalacia
  s. elastodystrophy
  s. elastorrhexia
  s. idiopathic fibrosis
  s. myelopathy
systole
systolic
  s. murmur
  s. prolapse
SZ (streptozocin)

Tt

T1 (longitudinal or spin-lattice relaxation time constant)
T1 (spin-lattice relaxation)
T1 weighted
T1-weighted coronal image
T1-weighted sagittal image
T_2 (spin-echo relaxation)
T2 (transverse or spin-spin relaxation time constant)
T2 weighted
T3 (1-3,5,3'-triiodothyronine)
T-3 red cell uptake estimate
T4 (1-3,5,3', 5'-tetraiodothyronine)
T4 (thyroxine)
T-1824 (Evans blue)
T (tesla)
T (thoracic)
Tabatznick's syndrome
tabes dorsalis
tabetic
    t. gait
    t. osteoarthropathy
    t. spondylitis
table
    biplane t.
    Buckey t.
    free-floating cradle t.
    Siemens Lithostar t.
    Sontag t.
    t. incrementation
    tilted t.
    x-ray t.
tables
    t. of Bayley and Pinneau
    t. of Caffey
    t. of Ghantus
    t. of Maresh

tachycardia
tachypnea
tacked-down sign
TAD (total administered dose)
taenia
    t. chorioidea
    t. cinerea
    t. coli
    t. fimbriae
    t. hippocampi
    t. libera
    t. mesocolica
    t. omentalis
    t. pontis
    t. saginata
    t. terminalis
    t. thalami
    t. ventriculi tertii
taenia, s.
    taeniae, pl.
taeniae, pl.
    taenia, s.
Tager's sign
tagged atom
tagging
    radioactive t.
tail-on detector (TOD)
Taillefer, valve of
tailored excitation
tainted view
Takayasu's
    T.'s arteritis
    T.'s syndrome
Takayasu-Onishi syndrome
talcosis
Taldt fusion fascia
tali, pl.
    talus, s.

talipes
    t. calcaneovalgus
    t. calcaneovarus
    t. calcaneus
    t. cavovalgus
    t. cavus
    t. equinovalgus
    t. equinovarus (clubfoot)
    t. equinus
    t. planovalgus
    t. valgus
    t. varus
talipomanus (clubhand)
talocalcaneal
    t. angle
    t. joint
    t. ligament
talocalcaneonavicular joint
talocrural
talofibular
    t. joint
    t. ligament
talonavicular
    t. joint
    t. ligament
talotibial joint
talus (astragalus)
talus, s.
    tali, pl.
tamaxifen (PFT)
  (phenylalanine mustard
  [melphalan] fluorouracil)
tam-o-shanter skull
tamponade
tandem and ovoids (T&O)
tangential
    t. portals
    t. projection
    t. view
TANI (total axial [lymph]node
  irradiation)
Tanner-Whitehouse-Healy
    T.-W.-H. assessment
    T.-W.-H. method

tannic acid
tantalum (Ta)
    t. bronchogram
    t. plate form
    t. wire mesh
tap
tapered movable
    t. m. core curved wire
      guide
    t. m. core straight wire
      guide
target
    rotating anode t.
    t. angle
    t. reconstruction
    t. resolution
    t. sign
target-film distance (TFD)
target-oval cell anemia
target-skin distance (TSD)
target-to-nontarget ratio
target-type reconstruction
targeted
    t. field of view
    t. reconstruction
Tarrant's
    T.'s method
    T.'s position
tarsal
    t. arch
    t. joint
    t. plate
    t. scaphoiditis
    t. tunnel
tarsalia
tarsi, pl.
    tarsus, s.
tarsoepiphyseal aclasis
tarsomegaly
tarsometatarsal joint
tarsophalangeal
tarsophyma
tarsoptosis
tarsotarsal

tarsotibial
tarsus (talus, calcaneus,
   navicular, cuneiform, and
   cuboid)
tarsus, s.
   tarsi, pl.
taste blindness
tattoo
Tauber catheter
Taussig-Bing
   T.-B. anomaly
   T.-B. complex
   T.-B. syndrome
Taussig-Snellen-Albers
   syndrome
tautography
Taveras hydraulic injector
Tay-Sachs disease
Taybi's syndrome
Taylor-Haughton lines
Taylor's
   T.'s method
   T.'s position
Tb (terbium)
TBG (thyroxin-binding
   globulin)
TBI (total body irradiation)
TCA (transluminal coronary
   angioplasty)
TD (total dose)
TD (treating distance)
TDF (tumor dose fractionation)
TE (echo time)
TE (time echo)
TE (tracheoesophageal)
TEA (thromboendarterectomy)
teacher's node
teardrop
   t. distance
   t. fracture
   t. heart
teat
   t. markers

t. sign
thebesian valve
TECA (technetium albumin
   study)
Techne-Coll kit
TechneScan
   T. gluceptate
   T. MAA
technetium (Tc)
   t. hepatoiminodiacetic acid
      (scan) (TcHIDA)
   t. sulfur colloid (TSC)
   t. albumin study (TECA)
   t. brain scan
   t. medronate (scan)
   t. stannous pyrophosphate
      scan (TSPP)
   Tc 99m
      Tc 99m 2,3
         dimercaptosuccinic
         acid
      Tc 99m aggregated
         albumin
      Tc 99m antimony
      Tc 99m autologous
         red cells
      Tc 99m BIDA
      Tc 99m blood-pool
         study
      Tc 99m ceretec (Hg-
         197, Hg-203)
      Tc 99m
         diethylenetriamine
         penta-acetic acid
      Tc 99m
         dimercaptosuccinic
         (DISIDA) scan
      Tc 99m
         dimethylacetanilide
         iminodiacetic acid
         (HIDA)
      Tc 99m disofenin
         (DISIDA) scan

Tc 99m DISDA
(diisopropylacetanilideimino
diacetic acid or
disofenin)
Tc 99m DMSA
(dimercaptosuccinate
acid)
Tc 99m DTPA
(diethylenetriaminepenta-
acetic acid)
Tc 99m etidronate
sodium kit
Tc 99m ferric
hydroxide
Tc 99m fibriscint
Tc 99m generator
Tc 99m GHP
(glucoheptonate)
Tc 99m HAM
perfusion scan
Tc 99m HDP
(hydroxydiphosphonate)
Tc 99m hepatolite
Tc 99m HIDA
(dimethyl
acetanilidoiminodiacetic
acid)
Tc 99m HSA
Tc 99m
hydroxydiphosphonate
(HDP)
Tc 99m IDA
(iminodiacetic acid)
Tc 99m
imidodiphosphonate
Tc 99m labeled heat
denatured RBCs
Tc 99m labeled RBCs
Tc 99m lung aggregate
Tc 99m MAA
(macroaggregated
albumin)
Tc 99m MDP

(methylene
diphosphonate)
Tc 99m medronate
sodium kit
Tc 99m methylene
diphosphonate
(MDP)
Tc 99m microlite
Tc 99m microspheres
Tc 99m osteolite
Tc 99m osteoscan
(HDP)
Tc 99m pentetate
sodium kit
Tc 99m pertechnetate
Tc 99m phosphate
Tc 99m phosphate
uptake
Tc 99m PIPIDA (P-
isopropylacetanilido-
iminodiacetic acid)
Tc 99m PYP
(pyrophosphate)
Tc 99m
pyridoxylideneglutamate
Tc 99m
radiopharmaceutical
Tc 99m serum
Tc 99m serum
albumin kit
Tc 99m sodium
pertechnetate
Tc 99m stannous
pyrophosphate
Tc 99m stannous
pyrophosphate/
polyphosphate kit
Tc 99m sulfur colloid
Technicare Delta 2020
scanner
technique
afterloading t.
air-gap t.

technique—*Continued*
  algebraic reconstruction t.
  Andren-von Rosen t.
  autoradiographic t.
  background subtraction t.
  bone window t.
  chromatographic-
    fluorometric t.
  Colcher-Sussman t.
  compression t.
  contact t.
  Corbin t.
  CR 51-labeled red cell t.
  Doppler t.
  drip-infusion t.
  Egan t.
  elution t.
  Flocks t.
  flushing t.
  four days t. of Salzman
  gap t.
  high-detail t.
  immersion t.
  interleaving ray data
    samples t.
  Judkins' t.
  Klein's t.
  Madden t.
  manual t.
  Maquet t.
  Mohs' t.
  occlusal film t.
  Orr-Loygue t.
  plain film t.
  radiographic t.
  Rashkind's t.
  scanning t.
  scintillation counting t.
  screen-film t.
  Seldinger t.
  Seldinger percutaneous t.
  selective excitation
    irradiation t.
  soft-tissue t.
  Sones t.
  Sones–Shirey t.
  subtraction t.
  supervoltage t.
  t. of Waterhouse
  three-dimensional t.
  time-dependent gradient t.
  time-motion (TM) t.
  tine t.
  tissue t.
  Welin t.
tectocerebellar tract
tectum
  t. of mesencephalon
TECV (traumatic epiphyseal
  coxa vera)
TED (threshold erythema
  dose)
teeter-totter phenomenon
Teevan's law
TEF (tracheoesophageal
  fistula)
Tefcor
  T. movable core curved
    wire guide
  T. movable core straight
    wire guide
Teflon
  T. catheter
  T. plate
  T. sheath needle sets
tegmen
  t. antri
  t. mastoideum
  t. tympani
  t. ventriculi quarti
tegmen, s.
  tegmina, pl.
tegmenta, pl.
  tegmentum, s.
tegmental tract
tegmentospinal tract
tegmentum
  hypothalamic t.

subthalamic t.
t. auris
t. of pons
t. rhombencephali
tegmentum, s.
tegmenta, pl.
tegmina, pl.
tegmen, s.
telangiectasia-pigmentation-cataract syndrome
telangiectatic
t. osteosarcoma
t. sarcoma
Telebrix
telecardiogram
telecardiography
telecobalt
telecord
telecurietherapy
teledetos paper
telefluoroscopy
telemetry
telencephalon
teleoroentgenogram
teleoroentgenography
Telepaque (iopanoic acid)
teleradiography
teleradium treatment
teleroentgenogram
teleroentgenography
teleroentgentherapy
teletherapy
Teletrol
tellurium (Te)
telophase
telradium
temperature
electrical t.
t. control device
t. effect on screen speed
template
Syed t.
Syed-Neblitt t.
Temple University plate

Templeton and Zim carpal tunnel projection
temporal
t. aponeurosis
t. fossa
t. gyrus
t. horn
t. lobe
t. process
t. resolution
t. syndrome
temporalis
temporoauricular
temporofacial
temporofrontal
temporohyoid
temporomalar suture
temporomandibular (TM)
t. articulation
t. fossa
t. joint (TMJ)
temporomaxillary
temporo-occipital
temporoparietal
temporopontile tract
temporosphenoid
temporosquamous
temporozygomatic suture
ten-degree off-lateral position
Tenckhoff catheter
tendinitis (also tendonitis)
calcific t.
tendinotrochanteric ligament
tendinous
t. attachment
t. ring
t. sprain
t. strain
tendofascitis calcarea
tendon
Achilles t.
bowed t.
calcaneal t.
central t.

tendon—*Continued*
  common t.
  conjoined t.
  cordiform t.
  coronary t.
  cricoesophageal t.
  extensor t.
  flexor carpi radialis t.
  flexor digitorum profundus
      t.
  flexor digitorum sublimis t.
  Gerlach's t.
  hamstring t.
  Hector's t. {
  membranaceous t.
  palmaris longus t.
  patellar t.
  riders' t.
  superior t. of Lockwood
  supraspinatus t.
  t. of Zinn
  t. sheath
  "trefoil" t.
tennis
  t. elbow
  t. thumb
  t. wrist
tenogram
tenography
Tenon, interfascial space of
Tenon's
  T.'s capsule
  T.'s fascia
  T.'s space
tenosynovial
tenosynovitis
tensile
  t. strength
  t. stress
tension band wiring
tensor
  t. fasciae femoris muscle
  t. fasciae latae muscle
  t. palati muscle

  t. tarsi muscle
  t. tympani muscle
  t. veli palatini muscle
tenth value layer (TVL)
tenting of diaphragm
tentoria
  t. cerebelli
tentoria, pl.
  tentorium, s.
tentorial
  t. incisura
  t. notch
  t. ridge
tentorium
  t. cerebelli
  t. of hypophysis
tentorium, s.
  tentoria, pl.
teracurie
teratoblastoma
teratocarcinoma
teratogenetic
teratogenic
teratogenous
teratoma
  calvarial t.
  ovarian t.
  sacrococcygeal t.
  testicular t.
teratoma, s.
  teratomas or teratomata,
      pl.
teratomas or teratomata, pl.
  teratoma, s.
teratomatous
terbium (Tb)
teres
  t. major muscle
  t. minor muscle
Teridax
terminal
  t. aortic thrombosis
  t. bronchiole
  t. cistern

t. ileitis
t. ileum (TI)
t. phalanx
t. ventricle
terminalis
terrestrial radiation
Terry's syndrome
Terson's disease
tertiary
    t. contractions
    t. motion
    t. pattern
tesla (T)
test
    125I-fibrogen uptake t.
    14C-lactose breath t.
    14C-glycocholic acid t.
    alkaline phosphatase t.
    bile salt breath t.
    chlormerodrin
       accumulation t. (CAT)
    cholescintigraphy
       radionuclide t.
    Cybex t.
    Dicopac t.
    "duck waddle" t.
    exercise tolerance t. (ETT)
    fat-absorption t.
    gastrointestinal blood loss
       t.
    gastrointestinal protein
       loss t.
    Graham's t.
    hepatic t. of Glass
    Hitzenberger's sniff t.
    limulus lysate t.
    Monospot t.
    Murphy-Pattee t.
    perchlorate discharge t.
    positive washout t.
    radioallergosorbent t.
       (RAST)
    radioimmunoprecipitation
       t.

radioiodine t.
regional lung function t.
Rubin's t.
Schilling's t.
Schober's t.
Seidlitz' powder t.
single-photon emission t.
"spinning top" t.
star t. pattern
string t.
Sulkowitch's t.
t. scan
t. sonography
Tetrasorb-125 t.
thallium stress t.
thyroid function t. (TFT)
thyroid stimulating
    hormone (TSH) t.
tilt t.
tine t.
tracer t.
triiodothyronine red cell
    uptake t.
triiodothyronine resin t.
UTI-tect bacteriuria
    diagnostic t.
Voluter t. (V-test)
wash-out t.
water siphonage t.
Wisconsin timing and mA.s
    t. tool
testicular
    t. scan
    t. teratoma
    t. torsion
testosterone
    t. propionate
Tesuloid (technetium Tc 99m
   sulfur colloid)
tetany
tethered cord syndrome
tetrabromophenolphthalein
tetrafluoroborate
tetragonus

tetraiodophenolphthalein
tetraiodothyronine
tetralogy of Fallot (TOF)
Tetrasorb-125 test
Teufel's
    T.'s method
    T.'s position
Teutschländer's syndrome
Texas catheter
textile drape
T-fracture
TFD (target-film distance)
TFT (thyroid function test)
TGC (time gain compensation)
Th (thorium)
THA (total hip arthroplasty)
thalami, pl.
    thalamus, s.
thalamic radiation
thalamocortical
    t. projection
    t. tract
thalamoperforate
thalamotegmental
thalamus, s.
    thalami, pl.
thalassemia
    t. major
    t. minor
thalidomide embryopathy
thallium (Tl)
    t. 201 imaging
    t. 201 stress testing
    t. chloride (Tl-201)
    t. myocardial scan
    t. nitrate (Tl-204)
    t. perfusion scintigraphy
    t. stress test
thallous chloride (Tl-201)
thanatophoric dwarfism
The American Board of
    Radiology (ABR)
The American Club of
    Therapeutic Radiologists
    (ACTR)

The Association of University
    Radiologists (AUR)
The Bureau of Radiological
    Health
The Canadian Society of
    Radiological Technicians
    (CSRT)
The InterAmerican College of
    Radiology (IACR)
The Society of Pediatric
    Radiologists (SPR)
thebesian
    t. valve
    t. veins
theca
    t. lutein cyst
theca, s.
    thecae, pl.
thecae, pl.
    theca, s.
thecal
    t. abscess
    t. sac
thecoma
thecostegnosis
Theile's canal or gland
thelarche
thelium
thenar
    t. crease
    t. eminence
    t. space
theorem
    Bayes' t.
    dose reciprocity t.
theory
    atomic t.
    Bohr's t.
    Culiner's t.
    electron t.
    Fermi's t.
    Hutch's t.
    Maxwell's t. of radiation
    neuron t.
    Planck's quantum t.

quantum t.
resonance t.
Traube's t.
undulating t.
wave t.
therapeutic
t. embolization
t. radiology (TR)
t. radiology implant
therapy
beam t.
blood disease t.
cancer t.
deep roentgen-ray t.
filter t.
fixed-field t.
fluoride t.
grid or sieve t.
heat particle t.
high-voltage roentgen t.
immunosuppressive t.
interstitial t.
intracavitary t.
intraoperative electron
beam t. (IOEBT)
intraoperative radiation t.
(IORT)
irradiation t.
light t.
megavolt t.
nucleotherapy
Phillips' contact t. unit
radiation t. (RT or RTx)
radiation t. oncology group
(RTOG)
radiotherapy (XRT)
radium beam t.
radium t. (RT)
rotation t.
shock-wave t.
superficial t.
supervoltage t. radiation
t. quality
t. tube
thyroid t.

x-ray t. (XRT)
TheraSeed implant
Theratron-80 machine
thermal
t. conductivity
t. energy
t. equilibrium
t. luminescent dosimetry
(TLD)
t. neutrons
t. radiation
t. spectrum
thermionic
t. emission
t. rectifier
t. vacuum tube
thermistor
thermistor-plethysmography
thermodilution
thermodynamic
thermoelectron
thermogram
thermograph
continuous scan t.
thermography
thermoluminescent dosimeter
(TLD)
thermoluminescent dose
thermomastography
thermonuclear
t. reaction
thermoplacentography
thermoradiotherapy
thesaurismosis lipoidica
hereditaria
theta wave
Thévenard's syndrome
thiazide
Thibierge-Weissenbach
syndrome
thick-layer autoradiography
thick-septa collimator
thick-wall sign
Thiemann-Fleischner disease
Thiemann's disease

thiethylperazine maleate
thigh joint
thin-layer
    t. chromatography (TLC)
    t. radiochromatography
      (TLRC)
thin-section cut
thin-septa collimator
thin-slice
thiocyanate space
thiosemicarbazide
thiosemicarbazone
thiosulfate
third
    t. generation
    t. mogul
    t. ventricle tumor
Thixokon
ThO_2 (thorium dioxide)
Thomas' syndrome
Thompson
    (F. R.) T. prosthesis
    T. catheter
    T. finger joint
    T. tibial plate
Thompson's syndrome
Thoms'
    T.'s method
    T.'s position
Thomson
    T. fracture frame
    T. scattering
Thomson-CGR system
thoracentesis
thoracic (T)
    t. aneurysm
    t. aorta
    t. aortic dissection
    t. aortography
    t. cage
    t. calcification
    t. curve
    t. dehiscence
    t. duct

    t. inlet
    t. kidney
    t. myelography
    t. outlet syndrome
    t. plane
    t. spine
    t. vertebra
    t. viscera
thoracoabdominal sign
thoracodorsal
thoracogenous rheumatic
    syndrome
thoracolumbar
    t. curve
    t. fracture
    t. spine
thoracopagus
thoracopelvophalangeal
    dystrophy
thoracoplasty
thoracostomy
thoracotomy
Thoraeus filter
Thoraflex catheter
Thoramat
thorax
    barrel-shaped t.
    Peyrot's t.
    pyriform t.
thoriagram
thorinated tungsten filament
thorium (Th)
    radioactive t.
    t. dioxide (ThO2)
    t. nitrate
    t. tartrate
    t. X
Thornton
    T. "T" bolt
    T. nail
    T. plate
Thornwaldt's cyst
Thorotrast
Thorpe plastic lens

Thorson-Biork syndrome
thousand (kilo)
thousand electron volts (KeV
   or kev)
THP (transhepatic
   portography)
THR (total hip replacement)
thread galvanometer
thread-and-streaks sign
thread-like
three-compartment system
three-dimensional
   t. echo planar imaging
   t. Fourier imaging
   t. Fourier transform
      (3DFT)
   t. KWE direct Fourier
      imaging
   t. physiologic flow pattern
   t. projection
      reconstruction imaging
   t. technique
three-phase
   t. bone scan
   t. circuit
   t. current
   t. generator
   t. system
three-point gait
three-vessel angiography
three-way
   t. catheter
   t. stopcock
three-wire system
thresher's
   t.'s disease
   t.'s lung
threshold
   alpha t.
   t. dose
   t. erythema dose (TED)
thrombi, pl.
   thrombus, s.
thromboangiitis obliterans

thrombocytopenia
   hypoplastic t.
   t.-absent radius syndrome
thrombocytosis
thromboembolus
thromboendarterectomy (TEA)
thrombophlebitis
thrombosis
   catheter-induced t.
   cerebral t.
   coronary t.
   deep vein t. (DVT)
   mesenteric t.
   pulmonary t.
   umbilical t.
   venous t. (VT)
thrombotic
   t. hemorrhoids
   t. infarction
   t. thrombocytopenic
      purpura (TTP)
thrombus
   calcified t.
   intracardiac t.
   obstructive t.
   occluding t.
   organized t.
   t. calcification
thrombus, s.
   thrombi, pl.
through
   t. joint
   t. transmission (echos)
throughput
thulium (Tm)
   t. chloride (Tm-170)
thumb
   bifid t.
   gamekeeper's t.
   hitchhiker's t.
   murderer's t.
   Potter's t.
   stub t.
   t.-printing of the bowel

thumb—*Continued*
t. rule
tennis t.
triphalangeal t.
thumblike sign
thumbprint bronchus sign
thumbprinting sign
"thunderclap" headache
Thurston-Holland fracture sign
thymic
t. abscess
t. alymphoplasia
t. artery
t. sail sign
t. spinnaker sail sign
t. wave sign
thymidine
thymolipoma
thymoma
thymus gland
Thypinone (protirelin)
thyratron
thyreoarytenoideus muscle
thyreoepiglotticus muscle
thyreohyoideus muscle
Thyrimeter
thyroarytenoid
thyroglossal
t. duct cyst
t. fistula
thyrohyal space
thyrohyoid
t. membrane
thyroid
ectopic t.
intrathoracic t.
substernal t.
t. acropachy
t. adenoma
t. carcinoma
t. cartilage
t. cyst
t. function test (TFT)
t. gland uptake
t. neoplasia

t. nodule
t. radioisotope assay
(TyRIA)
t. scan
t. stimulating hormone
(TSH)
t. stimulating
immunoglobulin (TSI)
t. storm
t. studies
t. therapy
t. uptake
thyrotoxic t.
thyroidal lymph node
scintigraphy
thyroiditis
de Quervain's t.
focal t.
Hashimoto's t.
lymphocytic t.
thyrolaryngeal fascia
Thyrolute
Thyrostat-3
thyrotoxicosis
thyrotrophic
thyrotropin (thyrotrophic
hormone)
thyrotropin-releasing hormone
(TRH)
thyroxine-binding globulin
(TBG)
thyroxine (T_4)
Thyrx timer
Thytropar (thyrotropin from
bovine anterior pituitary
glands)
TI (inversion time)
TI (terminal ileum)
Ti (titanium)
TIA (transient ischemic attack)
TIBC (total iron-binding
capacity)
tibia (shin)
saber t.
t. valga

t. vera
tibia, s.
    tibiae, pl.
tibiae, pl.
    tibia, s.
tibial
    proximal t.
    t. condylar fracture
    t. malleolus
    t. plafond fracture
    t. plateau
    t. pseudoarthrosis or
        pseudarthrosis
    t. shaft fracture
    t. spine
    t. tubercle
    t. tuberosity
tibialis
    t. anterior muscle
    t. posterior muscle
tibiocalcanean
tibiofemoral fossa
tibiofibular
    t. articulation
    t. joint
tibionavicular
tibioperoneal diaphyseal
    toxopachyostosis
tibiotarsal
Tiemann catheter
Tiemann-Coudé catheter
Tietze's syndrome
Tillaux's fracture
Tillaux-Kleiger fracture
tilt test
tilted
    t. sacrum
    t. table
time
    bowel transit t.
    compensated gain t.
    doubling t.
    exposure t.
    gain compensation t.
    proton relaxation t.

recovery t.
renal transit t.
spin-lattice relaxation t.
spin-spin relaxation t.
t. density curve
t. density plotting
t. echo (TE)
t. gain compensation
    (TGC)
t. recovery (TR)
t. sharing
"tincture of t." (watchful
    waiting)
transverse relaxation t.
time-dependent gradient
    technique
time-motion (TM) technique
time-temperature chart
time-temperature developing
    manual
timer
    fluoroscopic t.
    impulse t.
    photoelectric t.
    Thyrx t.
tin (Sn)
    t.-113 (Sn-113)
    t.-119m (Sn-119m)
tin woodsman sign
tine
    t. technique
    t. test
tinnitus
tip
    feeding tube t.
    Swan-Ganz catheter t.
    t. angle
tip-deflecting catheter
tissue
    adipose t.
    connective t.
    fibrous t.
    glandular t.
    granulation t.
    pathologic t.

tissue—*Continued*
    scar t.
    soft t.
    t. characterization
    t. discrimination
    t. dose
    t. polypeptide antigen
      (TPA)
    t. technique
    t. tolerance dose (TTD)
tissue-equivalent detector
tissue plasminogen activator
  (TPA)
titanium (Ti)
    t. dioxide 47 (Ti-47)
titer
Titterington's
    T.'s position
    T.'s semiaxial position
    T.'s view
TKA (total knee arthroplasty)
TKR (total knee replacement)
Tl (thallium)
TLA (translumbar aortogram)
TLA (transluminal angioplasty)
TLC (thin-layer
  chromatography)
TLD (thermoluminescent
  dosimeter)
TLD (tumor lethal dose)
TLI (total lymphoid
  irradiation)
TLRC (thin-layer
  radiochromatography)
TM (temporomandibular)
TM (time-motion)
TM (time-motion) technique
TM (tympanic membrane)
TMJ (temporomandibular
  joint)
TM-mode
TMNG (toxic multinodular
  goiter)
TMP (trimethoprim)

TMR (topical magnetic
  resonance)
TNF (tumor necrosis factor)
T&O (tandem and ovoids)
TOA (tubo-ovarian abscess)
Tobias' syndrome
TOD (tail-on detector)
Todd's
    T.'s cirrhosis
    T.'s paresis
    T.'s standards
toddler's fracture
toe
    claw t.
    great t.
    hammer t.
    mallet t.
    Morton's t.
    pigeon t.
toe-touch maneuver
TOF (tetralogy of Fallot)
Tokut-ze disease
tolazoline hydrochloride
Toldt, white line of
tolerance dose
tolmetin
Tolosa-Hunt syndrome
tolpovidone
toluidine blue
Tomac catheter
tomoangiography
TomoCat
tomogram
tomograph
    hypocycloidal t.
    ultrasonic t.
tomographic
    t. cut
    t. image
    t. multiplane scanner
    t. principle
tomography
    analog computer t.
    axial computed t. (ACT)

axial transverse t.
circular t.
computed axial t. (CAT)
computed t. (CT)
computer assisted t. (CAT)
computerized axial t.
   (CAT)
computerized transaxial t.
   (CTAT)
emission computed t.
focal plane t.
hypercycloidal t.
hypocycloidal t.
linear t.
longitudinal section t.
metrizamide-assisted
   computed t.
narrow-angle t.
Orbitome t.
panoramic t.
plesiosectional t.
pluridirectional t. (PT)
polycycloidal t.
positron emission t. (PET)
positron emission
   transverse t. (PETT)
quantitative computed t.
radionuclide emission t.
rotational t.
simultaneous multifilm t.
single-photon emission t.
   (SPECT)
skip t.
Tomolex t.
transmission computer-
   assisted t.
transversal t.
ultrasonic t.
wide-angle t.
tomolaryngography
Tomolex tomographic system
tomos
tomoscan
tomoscanner

tomoscopy
tongue
   t. fracture
   t. of tissue
tonicity
tonsil
   cerebellar t.
   faucial t.
   Luschka's t.
   palatine t.
   t. position
tonsillar capsule
tonus
tophaceous
   t. gout
tophus
topical magnetic resonance
   (TMR)
topograph
topographical
toposcopic catheter
Torcon balloon embolization
   catheter
torcula
torcular Herophili
Torg's classification
Tornwaldt's abscess
Torq-Flex guide
torr
torricellian vacuum
torsed cystic pedicle
torsion
   femoral t.
   lobar t.
   negative t.
   positive t.
   t. fracture
   testicular t.
torticollis
   congenital t.
   labyrinthine t.
   spurious t.
   t. atlanto-epistrophealis
   t. nasopharyngiene

tortuosity
tortuous
torus
    t. fracture
    t. mandibularis
    t. palatinus
Toshiba (manufacturer)
    T. scanner
    T. simulator
total
    t. administered dose
        (TAD)
    t. axial (lymph) node
        irradiation (TANI)
    t. body irradiation (TBI)
    t. body surface area
    t. dose (TD)
    t. filtration
    t. hip arthroplasty (THA)
    t. hip replacement (THR)
    t. iron-binding capacity
        (TIBC)
    t. joint replacement
    t. knee arthroplasty (TKA)
    t. knee replacement (TKR)
    t. lymphoid irradiation
        (TLI)
    t. renal blood flow (TRBF)
    t. shoulder replacement
        (TSR)
Touraine-Solente-Golé
    syndrome
tourniquet
tower skull
tower-shaped skull
Towne-Chamberlain
    T.-C. position
    T.-C. projection
Towne's
    T.'s flexion
    T.'s position
    T.'s view
Townsend's avalanche
toxic
    t. fluid

t. gastritis
t. hydrocephalus
t. multinodular goiter
    (TMNG)
t. myocarditis
toxigenic periostitis ossificans
toxopachy
TPA (tissue plasminogen
    activactor)
TPA (tissue polypeptide
    antigen)
TR (repetition time)
TR (therapeutic radiology)
TR (time recovery)
trabecula, s.
    trabeculae, pl.
trabeculae, pl.
    trabecula, s.
trabeculation
tracer
    isotopic t.
    t. microspheres
    t. study
    t. test
    tumor t.
trachea
    saber-sheath t.
    scabbard t.
tracheal
    t. amyloidosis
    t. band
    t. bronchus
    t. "button"
    t. catheter
    t. deviation
    t. dilatation
    t. diverticulum
    t. duplication
    t. fistula
    t. intubation
    t. lymph node
    t. perforation
    t. "spill"
    t. stenosis
    t. tube

t. web
trachelokyphosis
trachelomastoid
tracheobronchial
t. hemorrhage
t. rupture
t. tree
tracheobronchiectasis
tracheobronchiomegaly
tracheobronchitis
tracheobronchography
tracheobronchomalacia
tracheobronchopathia
  osteochondroplastica
tracheobronchoscopy
tracheoesophageal (TE)
t. fistula (TEF)
tracheoesophagus
tracheoinnominate fistula
tracheolaryngeal
tracheomalacia
tracheopathia
t. malacia
t. osteoplastica
tracheopharyngeal
tracheostenosis
tracheostomy
tracheotomy
trachiectasis
tract
alimentary t.
biliary t.
bulbar t.
bulbospinal t.
cerebellar t.
cerebellorubrospinal t.
cerebellospinal t.
cerebellotegmental t.
cerebellothalamic t.
cerebrospinal t.
cornucommissural t.
corticobulbar t.
corticocerebellar t.
corticopontile t.
corticorubral t.

corticospinal t.
corticothalamic t.
digestive t.
extracorticospinal t.
extrapyramidal t.
fistulous t.
foraminous spiral t.
frontopontine t.
gastrointestinal t.
geniculocalcarine tract
geniculotemporal tract
genitourinary (GU) t.
hypothalamicohypophyseal
  t.
iliopubic t.
iliotibial t.
intestinal t.
mamillotegmental t.
olfactory t.
olivocerebellar t.
olivospinal t.
optic t.
pyramidal t.
respiratory t.
rubroreticular t.
sensory t.
septomarginal t.
spinocerebellar t.
spinocervicothalamic t.
spino-olivary t.
spinothalamic t.
supraopticohypophyseal t.
tectocerebellar t.
tegmental t.
tegmentospinal t.
temporopontile t.
thalamocortical t.
urinary t.
uveal t.
ventricular outflow t.
vestibulocerebellar t.
vestibulospinal t.
traction
Bryant's t.
Buck's t.

traction—*Continued*
    Cotrel's t.
    Crutchfield's skeletal t.
    halo t.
    halopelvic t.
    halter t.
    Russell's t.
    skeletal t.
tragacanth
tragicus muscle
tragus
trajectory
TRAM (transverse rectus
  abdominis myocutaneous)
transabdominal
    t. (A-P) projection
    t. cholangiography
    t. position
transacral
transaxillary position
transbrachial arch aortogram
transcervical fracture
transcondylar fracture
transcranial position
transducer
    3.5 MHz t.
    t. angulation
    t. aspiration
    transrectal t.
    transvaginal t.
transduodenal
    t. fiberscopic duct
      injection
    t. method
transependymal
transfacial projection
transfalcine
transferrin
transfiberscopic duct injection
transfixing
transfixion screw
transformer
    air-core t.
    closed-core t.

Coolidge t.
distribution t.
"doughnut" t.
filament t.
high-voltage t.
iron-core t.
open-core t.
ratio t.
shell-type t.
step-down t.
step-up t.
t. coil
t. equation
t. law
t. loss
t. oil
transfusion
transglottic carcinoma
transglottis
transhepatic
    t. cholangiogram
    t. cholangiography
    t. obstruction
    t. portography (THP)
transhepatogram
transhepatography
transient
    t. equilibrium
    t. ischemic attack (TIA)
    t. myocardial ischemia
    t. respiratory distress of
      the newborn (TRDN)
    t. response resonance
    t. tachypnea of the
      newborn (TTN)
transillumination
transition
    beta t.
    isomeric t.
transitional cell carcinoma
    t. stage A
    t. stage B1
    t. stage B2
    t. stage C

t. stage D1
t. stage D2
transitor-transitor logic (TTL)
translate-rotate scanner
translateral projection
translation
translocation
translucent
translumbar
t. aortic catheter needle
t. aortogram (TLA)
t. aortography
transluminal
t. angioplasty (TLA)
t. coronary angioplasty (TCA)
transmission computer-assisted tomography (TCAT)
transmitted
transmural infarction
transmutation
transonance
transoral projection
transorbital position
transparent
transplantation
transport
t. case
t. feeder
t. system
transposition
t. of great vessels
transpyloric line
transradiant
transrectal transducer
transscaphoid perilunate dislocation
transsegmental
transseptal catheter
transsphenoidal
transsternal
transtabular AP/PA projection
transtentorial

transthoracic
t. catheter
t. position
t. projection
transtracheal
transtubercular
t. line
t. plane
transudate
transurethral
transvaginal transducer
transvenous pacemaker catheter
transventricular
transveral tomography
transversalis
t. abdominis
t. colli
t. fascia
transversaria
transverse (X)
t. arch
t. colon
t. crural ligament
t. deficiency
t. facial fracture
t. fissure
t. foramen
t. fracture
t. ligament
t. ligament of atlas
t. line
t. lines of Park
t. magnetization
t. maxillary fracture
t. mesocolon
t. muscle
t. myelopathy
t. or spin-spin relaxation time constant (T2)
t. orientation
t. plane
t. process
t. relaxation time

transverse (X)—*Continued*
  t. scanning
  t. section imaging
  t. sinus
  t. sulcus
  t. time constant
  t. tubercle
transversus
  t. abdominis muscle
  t. auriculae muscle
  t. pedis muscle
  t. perinei profundus
    muscle
  t. perinei superficialis
    muscle
  t. rectus abdominis muscle
  t. thoracis muscle
transvesical
trapezia or trapeziums, pl.
  trapezium, s.
trapezioscaphoid
trapezium, s.
  trapeziums or trapezia, pl.
trapezium-trapezoid fusion
trapeziums or trapezia, pl.
  trapezium, s.
trapezius muscle
trapezoid
  t. ligament
  t. ridge
trapezoideum
Trattner catheter
Traube's
  T.'s semilunar space
  T.'s theory
traumatic
  t. amputation
  t. aneurysm
  t. clinodactyly
  t. epiphyseal coxa vera
    (TECV)
  t. myelopathy
  t. pneumonia
  t. thrombosis of the
    axillary vein

traversing
tray
  Bucky t.
TRBF (total renal blood flow)
TRDN (transient respiratory
  distress of the newborn)
Treacher Collins' syndrome
treadmill
treating distance (TD)
treatment
  eventration t.
  Finsen's t.
  Goeckerman's t.
  palliative t.
  teleradium t.
tree
  bronchial t.
  tracheobronchial t.
trefoil
  "t." appearance
  t. bulb
  t. deformity
  t. skull
  t. tendon
Treitz'
  T.' angle
  T.' ligament
tremolite talc
Trendelenburg's
  T.'s gait
  T.'s position
trephine holes
tretinoin (Retin-A)
Trevor's disease
TRH (thyrotropin-releasing
  hormone)
Triabrodil
triaditis
trial fracture frame
triangle
  aortic t.
  Codman's t.
  femoral t.
  Hesselbach's t.
  Pawlik's t.

sternocostal t.
sylvian t.
"tell-tale" t.
t. of Calot
t. of Lanier
triangular
    t. cartilage
    t. head
triangularis sterni muscle
triangulation
tributary
triceps
    t. brachii muscle
    t. surae muscle
    t. tendon
trichloroacetic acid
trichorhinophalangeal (TRP)
  sign
tricrotic wave
tricuspid
    t. atresia
    t. murmur
    t. regurgitation
    t. stenosis
    t. valve
    t. vertebra
Tridrate
triethylenemelamine
trifid stomach
triflanged nail
trifurcation
trigeminal
    t. groove
    t. neuralgia
    t. neuroma
trigemino-
  encephaloangiomatosis
trigger
    t. finger
    t. finger deformity
    webbed t. fingers
trigonal
trigone
trigonocephaly
trigonum parietale

triiodinated
    t. benzene ring
    t. benzoic acid
    t. molecules
triiodobenzoic acid
triiodoethionic acid
triiodothyronine
    t. red cell uptake test
    t. resin test
Triiodyl
trilogy of Fallot
Trilute 125I uptake rest
trimalleolar fracture
trimethoprim (TMP)
    t. sulfa
triode tube
triolein (I-131)
triolein (glyceral triloeate)
Triolium
Triomet
Triopac
Triosil (sodium metrizoate)
Triosorb
    T. 131 T3 diagnostic kit
    T. M-125 T3 diagnostic kit
tripartite
triphalangeal thumb
Triphasix generator
triphenyl tetrazolium chloride
triphosphate
triplane fracture
triple
    t. arthrodesis
    t. lumen catheter
    t. vessel disease
triple-line shadows
triple-voiding cystogram (TVC)
tripod position
triquetral
    t. bone
triquetrum
triquetrum-hamate fusion
triquetrum-lunate fusion
triradiation
trismus

trisomy
  t. 8 mosaicism syndrome
  t. 9p
  t. 13-15
  t. 16-18
  t. 18
  t. 20
  t. 21
  t. 22
  t. D1
  t. E
  t. G
trispiral
tritiated water
triticeous node
tritium
triton
Triurol
Trixobar
trocar
  t. catheter
  t. needle
trochanter
  greater t.
  lesser t.
  rudimentary t.
  t. tertius
trochanteric
  t. bursa
  t. bursitis
  t. fixation device
  t. fossa
  t. fracture
  t. plate
trochlear
  t. nerve
  t. notch
  t. surface
trochocephaly
trochoid joint
Troell-Junet syndrome
Troisier's node
Trolard's vein
trophic fracture
trophoblastic

trophoneurosis
trophopathia myelodysplastica
tropical
  t. eosinophilia
  t. eosinophilic asthma
  t. pulmonary eosinophilia
  t. ulcer osteoma
tropism
Trotter's syndrome
trough line
TRP (trichorhinophalangeal)
TruCut needle
true
  t. aneurysm
  t. conjugate
  t. double-sellar floor
  t. lateral view
  t. opening of Moniz'
    siphon
  t. vocal cord (TVC)
Truemmerfeld's zone
Trueta's phenomenon
truncus arteriosus communis
trunk
T-shaped fracture
TSC (technetium sulfur
  colloid)
TSD (target-skin distance)
TSH (thyroid stimulating
  hormone)
TSI (thyroid stimulating
  immunoglobulin)
TSPP (technetium stannous
  pyrophosphate)
TSR (total shoulder
  replacement)
TTD (tissue tolerance dose)
TTL (transitor-transitor logic)
TTN (transient tachypnea of
  the newborn)
TTP (thrombotic
  thrombocytopenic purpura)
T-tube
  T.-t. cholangiogram
  T.-t. cholangiography

tubal
 t. canal
 t. obstruction
 t. patency
tube
 auditory t.
 Bilbao-Dotter t.
 camera t.
 Cantor's t.
 cathode ray t. (CRT)
 Chaoul's t.
 Coolidge's t.
 Crookes' t.
 crystal photomultiplier t.
 discharge t.
 Dobbhoff's t.
 Dotter's t.
 double-focus t.
 electron beam t.
 electron multiplier t.
 electron t.
 endotracheal (ET) t.
 eustachian t.
 fallopian t.
 feeding t.
 gas t.
 Geiger-Müller t.
 glow modular t.
 Hittorf's t.
 hot cathode x-ray t.
 indwelling T-t.
 Kenotron t.
 Leonard ray t.
 Levine t.
 Lilienfeld's t.
 metalix t.
 Miller-Abbott t.
 nasogastric (NG) t.
 oil-cooled t.
 Orthicon t.
 overcouch t.
 photomultiplier t.
 pick-up t.
 Pleur-evac t.
 pleural drainage t.

plumbicon t.
radiopaque intestinal t.
rectifying t.
Rotalix t.
rotating anode t.
self-quenched counter t.
Sengstaken-Blakemore t.
Shiner's t.
stationary anode t.
stomach t.
T-t.
t. angle
t. cooling chart
t. current
t. output
t. rating chart
t. saturation
t. shift
t. travel
t. voltage waveform
thermionic vacuum t.
tracheal t.
tracheostomy t.
triode t.
uterine t.
vacuum t.
valve t.
Vidicon t.
x-ray t.
tube-detector system
tube-object distance
tuber
 t. cinereum
 t. ischii
 t. vermis
tuber, s.
 tubers or tubera, pl.
tubercle
 articular t.
 conoid t.
 Gerdy's t.
 mental t.
 spinous t.
 t. of Chaput
 t. of Lower

tubercle—*Continued*
    tibial t.
    transverse t.
tubercular
tuberculoid lymphadenitis
tuberculoma en plaque
tuberculoma, s.
    tuberculomata, pl.
tuberculomata, pl.
    tuberculoma, s.
tuberculo-occipital
  protruberance line
tuberculosis
    diaphyseal t.
    fibrocavitary t.
    miliary t.
    multinodular t.
    pulmonary t.
    t. sicca
tuberculous
    t. abscess
    t. adenitis
    t. arthritis
    t. colitis
    t. dactylitis
    t. gumma
    t. lymphadenopathy
    t. meningitis
    t. myocarditis
    t. osteomyelitis
    t. pericarditis
    t. spondylitis
    t. synovitis
tuberculum sellae
tuberosity
    deltoid t.
    greater t.
    ischial t.
    lesser t.
    radial t.
    tibial t.
tuberous sclerosis
tubers or tubera, pl.
    tuber, s.

tubo-ovarian
    t. abscess (TOA)
    t. obstruction
    t. opacification
tubular
    t. aneurysm
    t. stenosis
tubulation
tubule
    collecting t.
    distal convoluted t.
    lactiferous t.
    proximal convoluted t.
    seminiferous t.
    uriniferous t.
tuft
    phalangeal t.
    sclerotic t.
    t. fracture
tulip probe
Tulpius, valve of
"tumbling bullet" sign
tumefaction
tumor
    adenomatous t.
    adrenal t.
    benign t.
    biliary t.
    "brown" t.
    carcinoid t.
    carcinomatous t.
    cystic t.
    desmoid t.
    "dumbbell" t.
    epithelial t.
    Ewing's t.
    fibro-osseous t.
    giant cell t.
    glial t.
    glomus jugulare t.
    glomus tympanicum t.
    granular cell t.
    Grawitz's t.
    hourglass t.

"iceberg" t.
islet cell t.
Klatzkin's t.
Krukenberg's t.
malignant mixed t.
mesodermal t.
metastatic t.
mucinous t.
mullerian t.
neurogenic t.
nonseminomatous t.
Pancoast's t.
Perlmann's t.
pharyngeal t.
polycystic t.
postirradiation t.
primary t.
Rathke's pouch t.
serous t.
t. cloud
t. dose
t. dose fractionation (TDF)
t. embolus
t. lethal dose (TLD)
t. necrosis factor (TNF)
t. stain
t. tracer
t. volume
third ventricle t.
ulcerogenic t.
Vanek's t.
"vanishing" t.
Warthin's t.
Wilms' t.
tumor-skin distance
tumoral
t. calcinosis
t. circumscripta
tungsten
tunnel
aorticoventricular t.
carpal t.
cassette t.
cervical t.

cubital t.
flexor t.
inner t.
outer t.
t. projection
t. view
tarsal t.
Tuohy
T. catheter
T. needle
Tuohy-Bost
T.-B. introducer
T.-B. occluder
turbinate (concha, s.; conchae, pl.)
Turcot's syndrome
turf toe injury
turgescence
Turkel needle
turmschadel anomaly
Turner
T. biopsy needle
T. needle
T. pin
Turner's
T.'s phenomenon
T.'s phenotype
T.'s sign
T.'s syndrome
Turner-Fong syndrome
Turner-Kieser syndrome
Turner-like syndrome
Turner-McElvenny pin
turning fracture frame
Turpin's syndrome
turret exostosis
turricephaly
TV fracture
TVC (triple-voiding cystogram)
TVC (true vocal cord)
TVL (tenth value layer)
tween-brain
twelve-pulse three-phase generator

twinge
Twining's
    T.'s line
    T.'s method
    T.'s position
twist
    t. drill
    t. drill catheter
two-compartment system
two-dimensional
    t.-d. echocardiography
      ("two-D echo")
    t.-d. Fourier imaging
    t.-d. Fourier transform
      (2DFT)
    t.-d. Fourier
      transformation imaging
    t.-d. KWE direct Fourier
      imaging
    t.-d. line integral projection
      projection
      reconstruction
    t.-d. modified KWE direct
      ultrasound image
    t.-d. projection
two-emulsion autoradiography
two-point gait
two-stage procedure

two-to-five-second scanner
two-vessel disease
two-way catheter
tylectomy
tylosis palmaris et plantaris
tympanic
    t. antrum
    t. cancaliculus
    t. cavity
    t. membrane (TM)
    t. resonance
    t. ring
    t. sinus
tympanitic
    t. abscess
    t. resonance
tympanocervical abscess
tympanoeustachian
tympanography
tympanohyal
tympanomastoid abscess
tympanosclerosis
tympanostapedial
TyRIA (thyroid radioisotope
    assay)
tyropanoate
tyropanoic acid
Tyson, gland of

Uu

U (uranium)
UAC (umbilical artery
   catheter)
UBI (ultraviolet blood
   irradiation)
UBO (unidentified bright
   object)
UCG (ultrasonic cardiogram)
UGI (upper gastrointestinal)
UGIS (upper gastrointestinal
   series)
UHF (ultrahigh frequency)
UIBC (unsaturated iron-
   binding capacity)
UIP (usual interstitial
   pneumonitis)
UIQ (upper inner quadrant)
ulcer
     anastomotic u.
     aphthous u.
     atheromatous u.
     Barrett's u.
     Curling's u.
     Cushing's u.
     decubitus u.
     diabetic u.
     duodenal u.
     elusive u.
     esophageal u.
     fistulous u.
     follicular u.
     gastric u.
     gastroduodenal u.
     gouty u.
     Hunner's u.
     jejunal u.
     "kissing" u.
     Kocher's dilatation u.

     marginal u.
     Marjolin's u.
     penetrating u.
     peptic u. disease (PUD)
     perforating u.
     prepyloric u.
     pudendal u.
     pyloric u.
     rodent u.
     round u.
     stasis u.
     stomal u.
     stress u.
     sump u.
     u. collar
     u. crater
     u. mound
     u. niche
     varicose u.
ulceration
     "collar button" u.
ulcerative
     u. colitis
     u. multilating acropathy
ulcerogangrenous
ulcerogenic tumor of the
   pancreas syndrome
ulcerogranuloma, s.
     ulcerogranulomata, pl.
ulcerogranulomata, pl.
     ulcerogranuloma, s.
ulceromembranous
ulceromultilating acropathy
Ullrich and Fremerey-Dohna
   syndrome
Ullrich-Turner syndrome
ulna, s.
     ulnae or ulnas, pl.

ulnae or ulnas, pl.
  ulna, s.
ulnar
  u. deviation projection
  u. drift deformity
  u. flexion position
  u. fossa
  u. groove
  u. hemimelia
  u. hypoplasia
  u. ligament
  u. malleolus
  u. nerve
  u. ossicle
  u. styloid fracture
ulnas or ulnae, pl.
  ulna, s.
ulnocarpal ligament
ulnoradial
Ultra-Technekow FM
  generator
Ultracranio T
ultrafast computed
  tomographic scanner
ultrahigh frequency (UHF)
Ultrapaque B
Ultrapaque C
ultraprotraction
ultrasonic
  u. cardiogram (UCG)
  u. cephalometry
  u. echogram
  u. study
  u. tomography
  u. wave
ultrasonogram (USG)
ultrasonography
  A-mode u.
  B-mode u.
  cardiovascular u.
  Doppler u.
  endoscopic u.
  gray-scale u.
  real-time u.

ultrasound (US or U/S)
  ATL (Advanced
    Technology Laboratory)
    real-time u.
  ATL-MK500 u.
  Doppler u.
  NeuroSector real-time u.
  NeuroSector u.
  real-time u.
  u. color flow mapping
  u. imaging
  u. phantoms
  u. propagation parameters
  u. resolution
  u. scanning (USS)
  u. scattering
  waterbath u.
ultraviolet (UV)
  far u.
  near u.
  u. blood irradiation (UBI)
  u. fluorescent dose
  u. fluorescent dosimeter
  u. radiation (UVR)
umbau zones
umbilical
  u. artery catheter (UAC)
  u. canal
  u. catheter
  u. cord
  u. hernia
  u. ligament
  u. thrombosis
  u. vein catheter
  u. venous catheter (UVC)
  u. zone
umbilication
umbilicus
umbo
umbonate
umbra
Umbradil
umbrascopy
Umbrathor

umbrella filter
uncertainty principle
unciform
uncinate
    u. process
    u. process fracture
unco-ossified
uncovertebral joints
uncus of hamate bone
underexposed
underexposure
underhorn
underrange
underreading
underscan artifact
undertoe
undifferentiated
    u. lymphoma
    u. round cell sarcoma
undulating
    u. theory
unerupted teeth
Ungerleider and Gubner
  nomogram
Ungerleider's method
ungual
    u. process
    u. tufts
uniaxial joint
Unibaryt
    U. C
    U. rectal
unicameral cyst
unicornate
unidentified bright object
  (UBO)
unidirectional current
unifocal cyst
unilateral
    u. hyperlucency of the
      lung
    u. mandibulofacial
      dysostosis
    u. nonfunctioning lung
    u. weakness

unilobar
unilocular
    u. cyst
    u. joint
unit
    absolute u.
    Amplatz u.
    Angström u.
    atomic mass unit (amu)
    atomic weight u.
    Bart's abdominoperipheral
      angiography u.
    Behnken's u.
    British Thermal U. (BTU)
    C-arm fluoroscopy u.
    cine CT u.
    decibel (dB) u.
    electromagnetic u.
    electrostatic u. (esu)
    EMI u.
    fundamental u.
    heat unit (HU)
    Holzknecht's u.
    Hounsfield u. (Hu)
    Kienböck's u.
    King-Armstrong u.
    Mache u.
    Magnetrode cervical u.
    Maxwell u.
    monitor u.
    Odelca camera u.
    Optiplanimat automated u.
    Orbix x-ray u.
    Phillips' contact therapy u.
    photodisplay u.
    Polaroid u.
    quantum u.
    roentgen u. (RU)
    uranium u.
    video display u.
    x-ray diffraction u.
    Xu (X-unit)
United States Catheter
  Instrument (USCI)
univentricle

unlabeled ligand
unmodified scatter
Unna-Thost syndrome
unopacified
unsaturated
    u. compounds
    u. iron-binding capacity
    (UIBC)
unsharpness
  subject u.
unstable
unsterile
unsymmetrical
ununited fracture
UOQ (upper outer quadrant)
UPJ (ureteropelvic junction)
upper
    u. gastrointestinal (UGI)
    u. gastrointestinal series
    (UGIS)
    u. inner quadrant (UIQ)
    u. limb cardiovascular
    syndrome
    u. lobe bronchus
    u. respiratory infection
    (URI)
    u. triangle sign
upright
    u. position
    u. view
upside-down
    u.-d. position
    u.-d. stomach
uptake
urachal cyst
uranium (U)
    u. unit
Urbach-Wiethe
  lipoproteinosis
uremic pericarditis
uremic pulmonary edema
ureter
    circumcaval u.
    ectopic u.
    postcaval u.

    retrocaval u.
    retroiliac u.
ureteral
    u. calculus
    u. catheter
    u. jet phenomenon
    u. obstruction
    u. orifice
    u. stent
    u. valve
ureterectasis
ureteric
    u. compression
    u. reflux
ureteritis
    u. cystica
    u. glandularis
ureterocele
ureterocystography
ureteroduodenal
ureterogram
ureterographic catheter
ureterography
ureteropelvic
    u. junction (UPJ)
    u. junction (UPJ)
    obstruction
ureteropyelocaliectasis
ureteropyelography
ureteropyelonephritis
ureterostenosis
ureterovaginal
ureterovesical
    u. angle
    u. junction (UVJ)
    u. junction (UVJ)
    obstruction
    u. reflux
urethan (ethyl carbonate)
urethra
    "spinning top" u.
urethral
    u. abscess
    u. arthritis
    u. catheter

urethral—*Continued*
    u. rheumatism
urethrobulbar
urethrocystogram
urethrocystography
urethrogram
    excretory u.
urethrography
    excretory u.
    injection u.
    retrograde u. (RUG)
urethrovesical differential
  reflux
urge incontinence
uric acid stone
urinary
    u. abscess
    u. catheter
    u. extravasation
    u. tract
    u. tract obstruction
uriniferous tubule
urinoma
Uriodone
uroarthritis
urocyst
uroflowmeter
urogenital
    u. canals
Urografin
    U. 45
    U. 60
    U. 76
urogram
    drip-infusion u.
urography
    ascending u.
    descending u.
    drip-infusion u.
    excretory u. (XU)
    hypertensive u.
    intravenous u.
    oral u.
    percutaneous antegrade u.

    retrograde u.
urokinase protocol
Urokon
urokymography
urologic catheter
Urombrine
Uromiro
Uropac
uropoietic
uroradiology
urorhythmography
Uroselectan B
Urotex
Urotrast
Urov's disease
Urovision
Urovist (diatrizoate
  meglumine, edetate calcium
  disodium)
urticaria
    u. pigmentosa
USCI (United States Catheter
  Instrument) catheter
useful
    u. beam
    u. voltage
user friendly
US or U/S (ultrasound)
USG (ultrasonogram)
USS (ultrasound scanning)
usual interstitial pneumonitis
  (UIP)
uteri or uteruses, pl.
    uterus, s.
uterine
    u. artery
    u. atrophy
    u. canal
    u. carcinoma
    u. cavity
    u. enlargement
    u. fundus
    u. leiomyoma
    u. myoma

u. tilt
u. tube
u. ultrasound
uterocervical canal
uterorectosacral ligament
uterosacral block
uterosalpingogram
uterosalpingography
uterotubal
uterotubography
uteroventral
uterovesical
   u. fistula
uterus, s.
   uteri or uteruses, pl.
uteruses or uteri, pl.
   uterus, s.

UTI-tect bacteriuria diagnostic
   test
utricle
utriculitis
UV (ultraviolet)
UVC (umbilical venous
   catheter)
uveal tract
uveomeningitis
UVJ (ureterovesical junction)
UVR (ultraviolet radiation)
uvula, s.
   uvulae, pl.
uvulae, pl.
   uvula, s.
uvulitis

Vu

V-360-3 CT scanner
V (volt)
"V" sign
V type of ureter
vabra catheter
Vacurette catheter
vacuum
  high v.
  torricellian v.
  v. arthrogram
  v. cassette system
  "v." phenomenon
  v. tube
vagal
vagi, pl.
  vagus, s.
vagina, s.
  vaginae, pl.
vaginae, pl.
  vagina, s.
vaginal
  v. candle
  v. carcinoma
  v. cuff
  v. introitus
  v. prolapse
  v. reflux
  v. vault
vaginogram
vaginography
vagolytic
vagus nerve
vagus, s.
  vagi, pl.
Valdini's
  V.'s method
  V.'s position
  V.'s view

valecula, s.
  valleculae, pl.
valence
  ionic polar v.
  v. bond
  v. electron
  v. shell
Valentine's position
valgus
  cubitus v.
  forefoot v.
  hallux v.
  hindfoot v.
  pes v. (flatfoot)
  talipes v.
  v. deformity
  v. stress film
valleculae, pl.
  vallecula, s.
vallecular sign
valley fever
Valsalva's maneuver
Valvassori's method
valve
  aortic v.
  atrial v.
  attenuation v.
  ball-type v.
  bicuspid v.
  Bochdalek's v.
  colic v.
  dome-shaped v.
  flail v.
  flair v.
  Gibson's v.
  Gott-Daggett v.
  Heister's v.
  Hoboken's v.
  Houston's v.

valve—*Continued*
    ileocecal v.
    Kerckring's v.
    Kohlrausch's v.
    Krause's v.
    Magovern's v.
    Mercier's v.
    mitral v. (MV)
    Nulsen-Spitz v.
    parachute mitral v.
    prosthetic v.
    pulmonary mitral v.
    pulmonary semilunar v.
    pulmonary v.
    pyloric v.
    semilunar v.
    spiral v.
    Spitz-Holter v.
    thebesian v.
    tricuspid v.
    ureteral v.
    v. of Barolius
    v. of Bauhin
    v. of Bidirus
    v. of Hasner
    v. of Krause
    v. of Sylvius
    v. of Taillefer
    v. of Tulpius
    v. of veins
    v. of vermiform appendix
    v. tube rectifier
    Willis' v.
valvula
    v. conniventes
valvula, s.
    valvulae, pl.
valvulae conniventes
valvulae, pl.
    valvula, s.
valvular
    v. calcification
    v. conniventes
    v. regurgitation
    v. sclerosis

    v. vegetation
van Andel
    v. A. catheter
    v. A. dilatation catheter
van Bogaert-Hozay syndrome
van Bogaert-Nyssen-Pfeiffer
    syndrome
van Buchem's
    v. B.'s endosteal
        hyperostosis
    v. B.'s syndrome
van Buren's disease
Van de Graaff generator
van der Hoeve's triad
van der Swan's sign
van Hoorne's canal
van Neck-Odelberg syndrome
van Neck's disease
van Tessel catheter
vanadium
Vance dilator
Vanek's tumor
vanishing tumor
vanSonnenberg
    v. biopsy needle set
    v. catheter
    v. needle
Vaquez-Osler disease
variable
    v. device
    v. dwarfism
    v. resistor
Varian
    V. CT scanner
    V. phased-array
        ultrasonograph V-3000
variation
Varicam nuclear medicine
variceal
    v. hemorrhage
    v. sclerosing procedure
varices
    esophageal v.
varices, pl.
    varix, s.

varicocele
varicography
varicose
    v. aneurysm
    v. ulcer
varicosity
varioliform
varix, s.
    varices, pl.
varus (bent inward)
    cubitus v.
    hallux v.
    humerus v.
    pes v.
    v. deformity
    v. stress film
vas
    v. aberrans
    v. deferens
    v. nervorum
    v. vasorum
vas, s.
    vasa, pl.
vasa, pl.
    vas, s.
VasCath catheter
Vascoray
vascular
    v. anomaly
    v. calcification
    v. collapse
    v. compartment
    v. compression
    v. ectasia
    v. foramen
    v. funnel
    v. groove
    v. murmur
    v. occlusion
    v. ring
    v. sclerosis
    v. sling
vascularity
vasculature
Vasiodone

vasoactive
Vasobrix
vasoconstrictive
vasodilator
vasoepididymography
vasography
vasomotor
vaso-occlusive
vasoparesis
vasopressin
Vasoselectan
vasospasm
vasovagal
    v. attack
Vastine-Kinney
    V.-K. chart
    V.-K. method
vastus
    v. intermedius muscle
    v. lateralis muscle
    v. medialis muscle
Vater's
    V.'s ampulla
    V.'s papilla
V-blade plate
VCG (vectorcardiogram)
VCR (video cassette recorder)
VCU (videocystourethrogram)
VCUG (vesicoureterogram)
VCUG (voiding
    cystourethrogram)
VDA (venous digital
    angiogram)
VDU (video display unit)
vector
vectorcardiogram (VCG)
vectorcardiography
    spatial v.
vectorscope
Veenema needle
vegetations
    bacterial v.
    verrucous v.
vein
    antecubital v.

vein—*Continued*
    aqueductus vestibuli v.
    azygos v.
    basal v. of Rosenthal
    basilar v.
    basilic v.
    Breschet's v.
    Browning's v.
    cephalic v.
    Dandy's v.
    emissary v.
    great anastomotic v.
    great v. of Galen
    inferior mesenteric v.
      (IMV)
    innominate v.
    Johanson's v.
    jugular v. (JV)
    left renal v. (LRV)
    left subclavian v. (LSV)
    levoatriocardinal v.
    medial (basilic) v.
    mesenteric v.
    portal v. (PV)
    Radner's v.
    right renal v. (RRV)
    right subclavian v. (RSCV)
    scalp v.
    superior anastomotic v.
    thebesian v.
    v. of Labbé
    v. of Santorini
    v. of Trolard
    vertical v.
velocity
    closing v.
    v. distribution function
Velpeau's
    V.'s axillary view
    V.'s deformity
vena
    inferior v. cava
    superior v. cava
    v. occipitalis interna

Venable
    V. plate
    V. screw
Venable-Stuck nail
venacavogram
venae magnae cerebri
venereal
    v. arthritis
Venocath catheter
venogram
    intraosseous v.
    splenic v.
venography
    epidural v.
    limb v.
    magnified carotid v.
    mediastinal v.
    peripheral v.
    portal v.
    radionuclide v.
    renal v.
    selective v.
    splenoportal v.
    subtraction v.
venolobar syndrome
venostasis
venous
    clival v. plexus
    v. anastomosis
    v. aneurysm
    v. angiocardiography
      (ACG)
    v. angioma
    v. angle of the brain
    v. aortography
    v. catheter
    v. digital angiogram (VDA)
    v. epidural syncytium
    v. foramen
    v. lake
    v. malformation
    v. murmur
    v. phase
    v. plexus

v. scan
v. sclerosis
v. sinus
v. thrombosis (VT)
ventilation
    alveolar v.
    mechanical v.
    minute v.
    pulmonary v. study
    v. collateralization
    v. scan
    v. study
ventilation-perfusion (VQ or
  V/Q)
    v. imaging study
    v. lung scan
    v. nuclear medicine study
    v. ratio
    v. scan
ventilator-induced
    v. gas
    v. pneumopericardium
    v. pneumoperitoneum
    v. pneumothorax
ventilatory
ventouse
ventrad
ventral
    v. cavity
    v. hernia
    v. pancreas
    v. plate
    v. position
ventricle
    auxiliary v.
    cardiac v.
    cerebral v.
    double-outlet right v.
    fifth v.
    fourth v.
    Galen's v.
    laryngeal v.
    lateral v.
    left v. (LV)

right v.
terminal v.
Verga's v.
ventricular
    v. aneurysm
    v. arrhythmia
    v. canal
    v. chamber
    v. dilatation
    v. ejection fraction (MUGA
      scan)
    v. fibrillation
    v. flutter
    v. hypertrophy
    v. outflow tract
    v. performance studies
    v. prominence
    v. pseudoaneurysm
    v. segment
    v. span
    v. tachycardia
ventriculogram
ventriculography
    cardiac v.
    cerebral v.
    contrast v.
ventriculoperitoneal
    v. shunt
ventriculoradial dysplasia
ventriculoseptal defect (VSD)
ventriculosubarachnoid
ventricumbent
ventrolateral sclerosis
venules
Vepesid (etoposide)
Verbrycke's syndrome
Veress needle
Verga's ventricle
verge
    anal v.
Veri-O-Pake
Veripaque
vermiform
    v. appendix

vermiform—*Continued*
   v. process
verminous
   v. abscess
   v. aneurysm
vermis
   cerebellar v.
vermography
Verner-Morrison syndrome
Vernet's syndrome
verrucous
   v. carcinoma
   v. vegetations
Versatrax pacemaker
vertebra
   abdominal v.
   basilar v.
   biconcave v.
   block v.
   "butterfly" v.
   Calvé's v. plana
   cervical v.
   cleft v.
   coccygeal v.
   "codfish" v.
   cranial v.
   dorsal v.
   "fish" v.
   "H" v.
   herniated v.
   "ivory" v.
   lumbar v.
   occipital v.
   odontoid v.
   sacral v.
   "sandwich" v.
   thoracic v.
   tricuspid v.
   v. plana
   v. plana osteonecrotica
   v. prominens
   wedge-shaped v.
vertebra, s.
   vertebrae or vertebras, pl.

vertebrae or vertebras, pl.
   vertebra, s.
vertebral
   v. "rugger jersey"
   v. angiography
   v. angle
   v. aponeurosis
   v. arch
   v. arch projection
   v. arteriography
   v. arthritis
   v. bodies
   v. collapse
   v. column
   v. dislocation
   v. epiphysitis
   v. foramen
   v. fusion
   v. hemangioma
   v. joint
   v. notch
   v. ossification
   v. osteochondritis
   v. syndrome
   v. vein
vertebras or vertebrae, pl.
   vertebra, s.
vertebrated catheter
vertebrobasilar
   v. angiography
   v. arteriography
   v. magnification
   v. system
vertebrochondral
vertebrocostal
vertebrofemoral
vertebrosacral
vertebrosternal
vertex
   v. projection
   v. view
vertical
   v. axis
   v. heart

v. line of Ombredanne
v. ray
v. vein
verticomental projection
verticosubmental
    v. position
    v. projection
vertigraphy
verumontanum
Vesalius
    bone of V.
    foramen of V.
Vesell's syndrome
vesica
    v. prostatica
    v. urinaria
vesica, s.
    vesicae, pl.
vesica-fellea
vesicae, pl.
    vesica, s.
vesical
vesicle
    auditory v.
    cervical v.
    graafian v.
    multilocular v.
    prostatic v.
    seminal v.
vesicoureteral
    v. junction
    v. obstruction
    v. reflux
    v. regurgitation
vesicoureteric reflux
vesicoureterogram (VCUG)
vesicovaginal (V-V)
vesicular resonance
vesiculogram
    seminal v.
vesiculography
vesiculotympanic resonance
vestibula, pl.
    vestibulum, s.

vestibular
    v. fold
    v. window
vestibule
    Gibson's v.
    Lerche's v.
vestibulocerebellar tract
vestibulocochlear
vestibulo-ocular
vestibulospinal tract
vestibulourethral
vestibulum, s.
    vestibula, pl.
viable
Viamonte's classification
vibrating-reed electrometer
vibration
Vibrio
    V. fetus
vibrocardiography
vibrophonocardiography
Victoreen
    V. dose
    V. dosimeter
    V. R-meter
video
    v. cassette recorder (VCR)
    v. character generator
        model 660
    v. disk recorder
    v. display camera
    v. display unit
    v. tape recorder (VTR)
    v. tape study
videocystourethrogram
    (VCU)
videodensitometric
videodisk
videognosis
videotape study
vidian
    v. artery
    v. canal
    v. nerve

Vidicon
    V. camera
    V. tube
Vierordt's sphygmograph
view-aliasing artifact
view-sampling artifact
view-streak artifact
viewbox
viewing monitor
viewpoint
views
    Albers-Schönberg v.
    Andrus v.
    anteroposterior (AP) v.
    anterosuperior (AS) v.
    AP (anteroposterior) v.
    apical v.
    Arcelin's v.
    Arcelin-Stenver v.
    AS (anterosuperior) v.
    "ball catcher" v.
    basilar v.
    Bertel's v.
    biplane v.
    blow-out v.
    Bossing occipital v.
    Breuerton's v.
    Bucky v.
    Cahoon's v.
    Caldwell's v.
    Chamberlain's v.
    Chaussé's v.
    Clayton-Johnson v.
    Cleopatra v.
    "coalition v."
    comparison v.
    coned-down v.
    craniocaudal v.
    cross-sectional v.
    cross-table lateral v.
    cross-table v.
    decubitus v.
    dens v.
    dorsal v.

    Dutt's v.
    expiration v.
    first-pass v.
    frog-leg v.
    frontal v.
    Haas' v.
    Hampton's v.
    Henschen's v.
    Hickey's v.
    Hirtz' v.
    Hughston's v.
    jackknife v.
    Johnson and Dutt v.
    Judet's v.
    Kasabach's v.
    lateral (L) v.
        l. left v.
        l. oblique
        l. recumbent
    Law's v.
    lordotic v.
    May's v.
    Mayer's v.
    mediolateral v.
    notch v.
    oblique v.
    open-mouth odontoid v.
    open-mouth v.
    overcouch v.
    Owen's v.
    panoramic v.
    Panorex v.
    pantomographic v.
    parallax v.
    pillar v.
    Pirie's v.
    pivot v.
    plantar v.
    plantodorsal v.
    posterioanterior v.
    posterior sagittal v.
    posterior v.
    posterolateral v.
    profile ray v.

radiographic v.
recumbent v.
Rhese's v.
right lateral (RL) v.
Runström's v. (mastoid)
Schüller's v.
"scottie dog" v.
scout v.
Settegast v. of the knee
sitting v.
skyline v.
soft-tissue v. (STV)
squat v.
Stenver's v.
stereoscopic v.
stress v. (ankle joint)
submentovertex v.
submentovertical v.
sundown v.
sunrise v.
superoinferior v.
swimmer's v.
tainted v.
tangential v.
targeted field of v.
Titterington's v.
Towne's v.
true lateral v.
tunnel v.
upright v.
Valdini's v.
Velpeau's axillary v.
vertex v.
von Rosen's v.
Waters' v.
"weight-bearing" v.
vignetting
villard
villi, pl.
    villus, s. (noun)
villonodular
    v. adenoma
    v. synovitis
    v. tenosynovitis

villous adenoma
villous (adj.)
villus, s. (noun)
    villi, pl.
Vim-Silverman needle
Vineberg's procedure
vinyl catheter
viral
    v. hepatitis
    v. infection
    v. particle
    v. pneumonia
Virchow's
    V.'s angle
    V.'s gland
    V.'s node
    V.'s plane
Virchow-Seckel syndrome
Virden catheter
Virgin hip screw
viris, pl.
    vis, s.
virus
    respiratory syncytial v.
      (RSV)
vis, s.
    viris, pl.
viscera
    abdominal v.
    thoracic v.
viscera, pl.
    viscus, s.
visceral
    selective v. aortography
    v. angiography
    v. aortography
    v. arteriography
    v. muscle
    v. peritoneum
    v. pleura
viscerocranium
viscerocystic
    retinoangiomatosis
viscerography

visceromegaly
visceroptosis
viscid
Visciodol
Visco Rayopake
viscosity
viscus, s.
    viscera, pl.
visibility of detail
visible radiation
Vistec x-ray detectable sponge
visual
    v. acuity
    v. evoked potential
    v. pathway
visualization
    contrast-enhanced v.
    double-contrast v.
    gas-obstructed v.
visualize
vital node
Vitallium
    V. plate
Vitamin B_{12} (Co 57) radioassay
  kit
vitelline
    v. cyst
    v. duct
    v. sac
vitreous
    detached v.
    v. abscess
    v. body
    v. hemorrhage
vocal
    v. cord
    v. resonance
Vogt's bone-free projection
Voice RAD
voiding
    v. cystogram
    v. cystourethrogram
      (VCUG)
    v. sequence

volar
    v. angulation
    v. aspect
    v. ligament
    v. plate
    v. plate fracture
    v. projection
Volkmann's
    V.'s canal
    V.'s contracture
    V.'s deformity
    V.'s disease
    V.'s paralysis
Vollmer's patch test
volt (V)
Volta effect
voltage
    forward-biased v.
    full-wave rectified v.
    half-wave rectified v.
    inverse v.
    root-mean-square (RMS)
      v.
    v. amplifier
    v. compensator
    v. drop
    v. regulator
    v. waveform
volume
    atomic v.
    molar v.
    tumor v.
    "v. averaging" artifact
    v. imaging
volumetric
voluntary
    v. effort
    v. muscle
Voluter test (V-test)
volvulus
    midgut v.
    sigmoid v.
vomer
    v. bone

v. ridge
vomerobasilar canal
vomeronasal cartilage
vomerovaginal canal
von Bezold's abscess
von Gierke's
    v. G.'s disease
    v. G.'s syndrome
von Gies' joint
von Hippel-Lindau disease
von Pirquet's
    v. P.'s cutireaction
    v. P.'s test
von Recklinghausen's
    v. R.'s disease
    v. R.'s osteitis
von Rosen's view
von Saal pin
Voorhoeve's dyschondroplasia
vortex
    v. of heart

voxel
voxel-volume
    v.-v. element
VQ or V/Q (ventilation-perfusion) (Q = quotient)
VQR (ventilation-perfusion ratio) (Q = quotient)
Vrolick's type of osteogenesis imperfecta
VSD (ventricular septal defect)
VT (venous thrombosis)
V-test (Voluter test)
VTR (video tape recorder)
vulvar
    v. canal
vulvouterine canal
vulvovaginal anus
V-V (vesicovaginal)
VWD (pulsed-wave Doppler)
V-Y procedure

Ww

W (wehnelt)
  W. rays
Waardenburg's
  acrocephalosyndactyly
  syndrome
Waelsch's syndrome
wagonwheel
  w. fracture
  w. separation
Wagstaffe's fracture
Wainwright plate
Walcher's position
Waldenström's
  W.'s disease
  W.'s macroglobulinemia
  W.'s overlap
Waldeyer's sheath
Walker's
  W.'s magnet
  W.'s sarcoma
wall sign
Wallenberg's syndrome
Wallgren's disease
Walther catheter
Walther's
  W.'s fracture
  W.'s oblique ligament
wandering
  w. abscess
  w. gallbladder
  w. kidney
  w. spleen
Warburg effect
wart
  plantar w.
Warthin's tumor
wash-in (WI)
  w.-i. phase

wash-out (WO)
  w.-o. phase
  w.-o. pyelogram
  w.-o. pyelography
  w.-o. study
  w.-o. test
Wassermann-positive
  pulmonary infiltration
water
  activated w.
  body w.
  regional extravascular lung
  w.
  w. path scanning
  (ultrasound)
  w. proton
  w. range
  w. siphonage test
  w. soluble
waterbath ultrasound
"waterfall" stomach
"water-lily" sign
Waterhouse, technique of
Waters'
  W.' method
  W.' position
  W.' projection
  W.' view
Waters-Waldron position
watershed infarctions
Waterston shunt
Waterston's operation
Watson-Jones cannulated nail
watt-hour
watt-second
wattmeter
wave
  alpha w.

wave—*Continued*
    beta w.
    dicrotic w.
    diffraction w.
    electromagnetic w.
    light w.
    positive rolandic sharp w.
    sine w.
    "standing" w.
    theta w.
    tricrotic w.
    ultrashort w.
    ultrasonic w.
    w. amplitude
    w. motion
    w. theory
    w. velocity
wave-particle duality
waveform
wavelength
    Compton's w.
    de Broglie's w.
waxy
    w. degeneration
    w. liver
    w. spleen
WBR (whole body radiation)
WBS (whole body scan)
web
    esophageal w.
    laryngeal w.
    tracheal w.
Web tibial bolt
webbed
    w. fingers
    w. neck
    w. toes
    w. trigger finger
Weber
    W. catheter
Weber's
    W.'s classification
    W.'s syndrome
Weber-Dimitri syndrome

wedge
    w. arteriogram
    w. arteriography
    w. sign
    w. vertebra
Wedge's filter
wedge-and-groove joint
wedge-shaped
    w.-s. defect
    w.-s. field
    w.-s. lesion
    w.-s. phalanx
    w.-s. vertebra
wedged
    w. lateral portals
    w. pair
wedging
Wegelius-Lind sign
Wegener's
    W.'s granuloma
    W.'s granulomatosis
    W.'s osteochondritis
Wehlin's method
wehnelt (W)
weight
    atomic w. unit
weight-bearing
    w. position
    w. view
weight-holding
weight-sharing
weighted
    T1 w.
    T1-w. coronal image
    T1-w. sagittal image
    T2 w.
Weill-Marchesani syndrome
Weinberg-Himelfarb syndrome
Weingarten's syndrome
Weismann-Netter syndrome
Weitbrecht's ligament
Welch's abscess
Welin's technique
well counter

well-defined
    w. density
    w. fracture
Wenger slotted plate with nut
Wermer's syndrome
Werner's syndrome
Wernicke's area (brain)
West's
    W.'s lacunae
    W.'s lacunar skull
West-Engstler skull
Westberg's space
Westcott needle
Westermark's sign
Westmark's sigmoid
Westphal-Strümpell syndrome
wet
    w. film
    w. lung disease
    w. reading
wetting agent
Weyers'
    W.' dysostosis acrofacilis
    W.' polyatresia
Weyers-Thier syndrome
whalebone filiform catheter
Wharton's
    W.'s duct
Wheatstone stereoscope
wheeze and crackle
whiplash
Whipple's procedure
whipworm colitis
whispering resonance
whistle-tip catheter
whistling face syndrome
white
    w. hot
    w. kidney
    w. line of Fraenkel
    w. line of Toldt
    w. radiation
White catheter
Whitman fracture frame

Whitnall's ligament
whole-body
    w.-b. counter
    w.-b. irradiation
    w.-b. proton magnetic
      resonance imaging
      system
    w.-b. radiation (WBR)
    w.-b. scan (WBS)
    w.-b. scanner
Wholey catheter
whorled pattern
WI (wash-in)
Wiberg's angle
wide-angle tomography
widened Lippe's loop sign
Wiedemann's syndrome
Wiedemann-Beckwith
  syndrome
Wigby-Taylor
    W.-T. method
    W.-T. position
Wiljasalo's index
Wilkie's syndrome
Williams'
    W.' elfin facies syndrome
    W.' method
    W.' position
    W.' syndrome
Williams-Campbell syndrome
Willis'
    W.' antrum
    W.' valve
Willis, circle of
willow fracture
Willson torque wire guide
Wilms'
    W.' nephroblastoma
    W.' tumor
Wilson
    W. chamber
    W. cloud chamber
    W. plate
    W. spinal fusion plate

Wilson—*Continued*
    W. spinal plate
Wilson's
    W.'s fracture
    W.'s syndrome
Wilson-Mikity syndrome
Wimberger's
    W.'s line
    W.'s sign
Winchester's disk or disc
Winchester-Grossman
    syndrome
winding
window
    aortic w.
    aorticopulmonary w.
    bone w. technique
    cochlear w.
    oval w.
    radiation w.
    round w.
    vestibular w.
    w. level
    w. width
Winer catheter
winged
    w. catheter
    w. scapula
Winslow, foramen of
wire
    address w.
    Copan's w.
    ground w.
    guide w.
    hot w.
    Kirschner's w. (K-wire)
    tantalum w.
    w. suture
wire guide
    Amplatz w. g.
    Coons interventional w. g.
    Cope Mandril w. g.
    Lunderquist exchange w.
        g.

Lunderquist-Ring torque
    w. g.
Moses curved safe-T-J w.
    g.
Ring intravascular torque
    w. g.
Rosen curved safe-T-J w.
    g.
Willson torque w. g.
wire-loop lesion
Wirsung, duct of
Wisconsin
    W. kVp test cassette
    W. timing and mA.s test
        tool
Wise's time density factor
Wishard catheter
within normal limits (WNL)
Witzel
    W. catheter
    W. enterostomy catheter
WL symphalangism-
    brachydactyly syndrome
WNL (within normal limits)
WO (wash-out)
Wolf
    W. catheter
Wolf's method
Wolf-Marshak maneuver
Wolfenden's position
Wolff's law
Wolff-Parkinson-White
    syndrome
wolffian duct
wolfram
Wolfring's glands
Wolman's familial lipoidosis
wooden resonance
wooden-shoe
    w.-s. configuration
    w.-s. heart
Woodruff catheter
worm
    w. abscess

w. aneurysm
WORM (write once, read
  many)
wormian bone
"wormy" appearance
Worth's generalized cortical
  hyperostosis
woven-silk catheter
Wratten 6B filter
Wright knee plate

Wrisberg's ligament
wrist
  tennis w.
  w. joint
write once, read many
  (WORM)
wryneck
WT syndrome
Wurd catheter
Wyburn-Mason syndrome

Xx

X (Kienböck's unit)
X (transverse)
X axis
X-Baryt
X-iodol
X-Prep
X-omat
X-radiation
x-ray (roentgen rays)
    discrete x.
    grid controlled x.
    hard x.
    monoenergetic x.
    polyenergetic x.
    soft x.
    x. beam
    x. bremsstrahlung
    x. characteristic
    x. circuit
    x. detector
    x. diffraction unit
    x. emission spectrum
    x. energy
    x. exposure fog
    x. film latitude
    x. generator
    x. image
    x. in plaster (XIP)
    x. jacket
    x. K-characteristic
    x. magnification
    x. orthovoltage
    x. out of plaster (XOP)
    x. photon
    x. pinhole camera
    x. remnant
    x. spectra
    x. spectrometer

    x. spectrum
    x. synchronization
    x. table
    x. therapy (XRT)
    x. tube
    x. tube housing
    x. tube rating chart
X-Y plotter
xanthochromic
xanthofibroma
xanthogranuloma
xanthogranulomatous
    pyelonephritis (XGP)
xanthoma
xanthomatoses, pl.
    xanthomatosis, s.
xanthomatosis, s.
    xanthomatoses, pl.
xanthomatous biliary cirrhosis
xanthosarcoma
XC (excretory cystogram)
XC (excretory cystography)
Xe (xenon)
Xeneisol
xenon (Xe)
    x. 127
    x. 133
    x. gas
    x. scan
xenophor femoral prosthesis
xerogram
xerography
xeromammography
xeroradiogram
xeroradiography
xerosialography
xerosis
xerostomia

xerotomography
XGP (xanthogranulomatous
    pyelonephritis)
XIP (x-ray in plaster)
xiphisternal joint
xiphisternum
xiphocostal
xiphoid
    x. cartilage
    x. process
XL (inductive reactance)
XO syndrome
XOP (x-ray out of plaster)

XRT (radiotherapy)
XU (excretory urogram)
XU (excretory urography)
Xu (X-unit)
Xumbradil
XX and XY Turner phenotype
    syndrome
XXXXY syndrome
XXY syndrome
xylene
Xylocaine (lidocaine)
xylose
XYY syndrome

Yy

Y (yttrium)
Yankauer catheter
yaws
    y. dactylitis
Y-axis
Yb (ytterbium)
Yb-169-DTPA
Y-bone plate
Y-cartilage
yellow ligament
Yersinia
yersiniosis
Y-ligament
yoke
    alveolar y.

    sphenoidal y.
young female arteritis
    syndrome
Youssef's syndrome
Y-shaped gallbladder
ytterbium (Yb)
    y. chloride (Yb-169)
    y. pentetate sodium
    y. (Yb-69) DTPA
yttrium (Y)
    y. oxysulfide
    y.-90
Yune-Klatte catheter
Y-ureter
Y-Y line

Zz

Z line of the esophagus
Z lines
Z rib
Zahn
    line of Z.
    rib of Z.
Zancolli's procedure
Zanelli's
    Z.'s method
    Z.'s position
Zang's space
Zanosar (streptozocin) (SZ)
Zavala lung biopsy needle
Zavod catheter
Zeeman's hamiltonian function
Zeis, gland of
Zellweger-Bowan syndrome
Zellweger's syndrome
Zenker's
    Z.'s pouch
    Z.'s diverticulum
zero potential
zero-field splitting
zeugmatography
    Fourier transformation z.
Zickel
    Z. device
    Z. nail
Zigmor modification
Zimm's artery
Zimmer pin
Zimmer's
    Z.'s method
Z-impedance
zinc (Zn)
    z. cadmium sulfide
    z. chloride (Zn-65)

z. peroxide
z. sulfide
Zinn
    anulus of Z.
    tendon of Z.
zinostatin (neocarzinostatin)
zipper (on bone scan)
zirconium (Zr) (with niobium-95)
Zizmor's method
Zn (zinc)
Zollinger-Ellison syndrome
zonal gastritis
zone
    epigastric z.
    focal z. (FZ)
    hemorrhoidal z.
    hypogastric z.
    Looser's tranformation z.
    subcostal z.
    Trümmerfeld's z.
    umbau z.
    umbilical z.
    z. plate
zonogram
zonography
    stereoscopic z.
zonular space
zoom
    z. factor
    z. lens
    z. reconstruction
zoomed image
Zr (zirconium)
Zuckerkandl's
    Z.'s body
    Z.'s fascia

Z.'s organ
Zuelzer
    Z. hooked plate
    Z. plate
Zwahlen's syndrome
zwitterion
zygapophyseal joint
zygapophyses, pl.
    zygapophysis, s.
zygapophysis, s.
    zygapophyses, pl.
zygia, pl.
    zygion, s.
zygion, s.
    zygia, pl.
zygodactyly
zygoma (jugal, malar, or cheek)
zygoma, s.
    zygomata, pl.
zygomata, pl.
    zygoma, s.

zygomatic
    z. arch
    z. bone
    z. fossa
    z. process
zygomaticofacial foramen
zygomaticofrontal suture
zygomaticomaxillary suture
zygomatico-orbital
zygomaticosphenoid
zygomaticotemporal
    z. canal
    z. suture
zygomaticus
    z. major
    z. minor
zygomaxillare
zygopophyseal joint
zymogen

APPENDIX 1: SAMPLE REPORTS

VENTILATION-PERFUSION LUNG SCAN

The patient breathed to full inspiration 15 mCi of xenon-133 gas. At this time, static scintiphotos were taken in the posterior projection. Following this, the patient rebreathed the xenon into a closed collection system, during which time serial wash-out photos were made. Then 4 mCi of Tc-MAA was injected intravenously, and the lungs were imaged in multiple projections.

At full inspiration, there is marked irregular underventilation of both lower lung fields. Xenon appears uniformly distributed in the upper lung fields. During wash-out, there is mild diffuse trapping in both lower lung fields. There is very marked, irregular underperfusion of both dependent lung fields, corresponding to regions of marked ventilatory abnormality and, therefore, nonspecific. There is a subsegmental perfusion abnormality in the anterior left upper lobe.

Impression. Abnormal ventilation-perfusion lung scintigram, as described above. The perfusion abnormalities occur in regions of abnormal ventilation. Although these are consistent with pulmonary emboli, the probability is indeterminate.

BONE SCAN

Following the intravenous injection of 20 mCi Tc-MDP, a whole-body bone survey was performed.

There is focal increase in uptake in the body of approximately, the D-2 vertebra (as well as D-11) and in what appears to be the upper aspect of L-1. There is also intense focal increase in uptake in the right posterior eleventh rib and the right anterior fifth rib. There is focal increase at the proximal left clavicle. These findings are nonspecific, but are consistent with myelomatous involvement. With the exception of the upper dorsal vertebral abnormality, they have all appeared since the most recent study performed (date).

There is intense increase in uptake in what appears to be the proximal aspect of the right femoral head. There is much less intense increase in uptake in the left femoral head. These findings are not obviously myelomatous in nature and may simply represent severe degenerative change. They have appeared since the most recent study.

Impression. Abnormal Tc-MDP bone survey, as described above, with interim change.

EXAMINATIONS

1. Fluoroscopically guided biopsy of the left retroperitoneum.
2. Insertion of percutaneous nephrostomy catheter.
3. Dilatation of left ureteral stricture.
4. Insertion of left ureteral stent.

Technique. Following appropriate premedication and with intravenous fluids in progress, the patient was brought to the Radiology Department and placed in the prone position on the examining table. The left lumbar region was prepared and draped in the usual fashion. With 2% Xylocaine for local anesthesia, a Chiba needle was introduced into the collecting system and contrast agent was injected. Utilizing the contrast agent within the ureter as a marker, a TruCut biopsy needle was advanced under fluoroscopic control and directed to the area of stricture involving the ureter. Several biopsy specimens were obtained immediately adjacent to the area of stricture. These were submitted in formalin for histologic evaluation.

Subsequently, a guide wire was introduced via the Chiba needle and directed into the proximal ureter. Over the wire, an angiographic catheter was then advanced, and the combination of catheter and wire was then directed into the ureter. The guide wire was then advanced into the distal ureter and, thereafter, into the bladder. Over the wire, a series of smaller dilators was passed until a balloon dilatation catheter could be positioned at the level of the stricture. This was inflated and deflated several times under fluoroscopic control. Subsequently, a #8 French ureteral stent was advanced over the wire and positioned with the distal portion coiled within the bladder and the proximal portion coiled within the collecting system. Finally, a #12 French nephrostomy catheter was inserted over the wire and coiled within the renal pelvis. This catheter was attached to an external drainage system, and a sterile dressing was applied.

The patient tolerated the procedure well and was returned to his room in an unchanged condition at the conclusion of the examination.

Radiographic Findings

1. Stricture of the left midureter with biopsy obtained.
2. Balloon dilatation of the stricture with insertion of ureteral stent and temporary insertion of nephrostomy catheter.

EXAMINATION

Splenoportogram and therapeutic embolization of splenic artery. **Technique.** Following appropriate premedication and with intravenous fluids in progress, the patient was brought to the Radiology Department and placed in the supine position on the examining table. A preliminary scout film was obtained for correction of technical factors. Thereafter, the left lateral abdominal wall was prepared and draped in the usual fashion.

With 2% Xylocaine for local anesthesia, a Chiba needle was introduced into the substance of the spleen under fluoroscopic control. Manual injection of contrast agent was then performed with serial films obtained in the AP position. The needle was then repositioned and withdrawn until a branch of the splenic artery was entered. A small-caliber guide wire was then advanced through the Chiba needle and directed through the splenic artery to the level of the celiac axis. Over this wire a series of small dilators was passed until an angiographic catheter could be advanced and positioned within the proximal portion of the splenic artery. Injection of contrast agent was performed, and serial films were obtained in the AP position.

With the catheter tip at the level of the proximal splenic artery, a series of Gianturco coils was extruded from the catheter as it was slowly withdrawn to the level of the splenic hilum. The catheter was then withdrawn to the level of the outer margin of the spleen, where the catheter track was then embolized with a single Gianturco coil and with Gelfoam sponge. A sterile dressing was applied upon removal of the catheter.

The patient tolerated the procedure well and was discharged to her room in an unchanged condition.

Angiographic Findings

1. The splenoportogram reveals obliteration of the splenic vein with identification of multiple enlarged varicosities, predominantly in the fundus of the stomach with an enlarged left gastric vein feeding into the portal venous system.
2. Satisfactory cannulation of the splenic artery was achieved with embolization of this vessel from its origin at the celiac axis to the level of the splenic hilum.

EXAMINATION

Needle Biopsy of Right Lung
Technique. Following appropriate premedication, the patient was brought to the Radiology Department and placed in the supine position on the examining table.

An area of increased density associated with the lower lung zone was identified by fluoroscopy and marked on the surface of the patient's skin. This area was then prepared and draped in the usual fashion.

With 2% Xylocaine for local anesthesia, a Chiba needle was introduced and advanced under fluoroscopic control. The needle was directed into the area of density at the lung base. This was seen to deform easily upon approach of the needle, suggesting that it might represent entrapment of fluid. A specimen was obtained from this area and submitted in formalin for histological evaluation. A needle was then reintroduced and directed into the pleural compartment, where fluid was aspirated and submitted for cytological evaluation, as well as evaluation of protein, sugar, cells, etc.

The patient tolerated the procedure well, and a postbiopsy film revealed a small pneumothorax. Follow-up films of the chest will be obtained. The patient was asymptomatic at this time.

EXAMINATION

Abscess Drainage and Fluoroscopy

Technique. After using ultrasound to localize a fluid collection in the right upper quadrant of the abdomen, the patient was prepared and draped in the usual manner.

Under local anesthesia and monitoring with medications by the CRNA, a 23-gauge needle was placed via a right flank approach into a fluid collection in the right upper quadrant. Blood-tinged, straw-colored serous fluid was obtained and sent to the laboratory for aerobic and anaerobic cultures and Gram stain.

A guide wire was placed through the needle; and after successive dilatation catheters had been placed through the track, a #12 French Cope-type drainage tube was placed with its tip coiled in the cavity. After this was secured in place, contrast was injected into the abscess cavity and an overhead film showed delineation of the cavity. The drainage tube was then connected to a collection bag.

Impression. Successful placement of the #12 French Cope drainage tube via a right flank approach in a right upper quadrant fluid collection.

EXAMINATIONS

1. Thoracic aortogram.
2. Selective right bronchial arteriogram.
3. Therapeutic embolization of right bronchial artery.

Technique. Following appropriate premedication and with intravenous fluids in progress, the patient was brought to the Angiography Department and placed in the supine position. The right inguinal region was prepared and draped in the usual fashion and, with 2% Xylocaine for local anesthesia, a radiopaque polyethylene catheter was inserted into the right common femoral artery utilizing the Seldinger technique.

The catheter was advanced centrally under fluoroscopic control and positioned within the distal portion of the aortic arch. A test injection of contrast agent was administered without incident, and then pressure injection of contrast agent was performed with serial digital subtraction images obtained in the AP position. The catheter was then exchanged over a guide wire for a selective end-hole catheter, which was positioned within an identified right bronchial artery that was increased in size. The guide wire was advanced through the catheter and into the bronchial artery. Over this wire, the catheter was then advanced well into the bronchial vessel. Once again, contrast agent was injected and serial digital subtraction images obtained. Subsequently, a combination of Gelfoam and Ivalon pledgets was injected into the right bronchial artery under fluoroscopic control. Follow-up injections were performed with digital subtraction images demonstrating successful occlusion of this vessel and its branches. Thereafter, the catheter was removed and hemostasis achieved by direct compression over the puncture site.

The patient tolerated the procedure well and was discharged to his room in unchanged condition.

Angiographic Findings

1. Enlarged right bronchial artery. The left bronchial system appears small and there is no predominant left bronchial artery identified.
2. Injection of the bronchial vessel on the right demonstrates filling of multiple irregular vessels with a central area that may represent extravasation involving the region of the right upper lobe.
3. Satisfactory occlusion of the bronchial vessel was demonstrated.

DIGITAL VASCULAR IMAGING SCAN OF HEAD, NECK, AND AORTIC ARCH

A central venous catheter was placed from the right antecubital venous approach, and the tip of the catheter was placed into the right atrium. Digital vascular images of the aortic arch, common carotid bifurcations, and skull base circulation were obtained.

Images of the aortic arch demonstrated a prominent, but normal "ductus bump" (remnant of the fetal ductus arteriosus). The aortic arch was otherwise normal in contour and caliber. The proximal brachiocephalic vessels were somewhat tortuous, but no stenotic lesions were identified. The origins of the vertebral arteries were tortuous, but no stenotic lesions were identified.

Images of the common carotid bifurcations demonstrated normal contour and caliber bilaterally. There was no evidence of significant plaque or stenotic disease. The left cervical vertebral artery was somewhat larger than the right. Simultaneous antegrade flow was noted.

Images of the skull base circulation demonstrated a normal appearance to the carotid siphons, supraclinoid segments, and the M1 and A1 segments bilaterally. There was no shift of midline. The basilar artery was tortuous and mildly ectatic. However, no stenosis was identified.

Impression:

1. Mild tortuosity of the proximal brachiocephalic vessels: as well as the basilar artery.
2. Otherwise unremarkable digital vascular imaging of the head, neck, and arch.

EXAMINATIONS

1. Left femoral arteriogram.
2. Therapeutic urokinase infusion.
3. Follow-up angiogram through existing catheter.

Technique. The patient was brought to the Angiography Department on an emergency basis with intravenous fluids in progress. The left inguinal region was prepared and draped in the usual fashion. With 2% Xylocaine for local anesthesia, a small-caliber catheter was introduced into the left common femoral artery. A test injection of contrast agent was administered without incident, following which pressure injection of contrast agent was performed with serial films obtained over the pelvis, left thigh, left knee, and left lower leg.

Thereafter, utilizing a torque control wire, the orifice of the thrombosed left femoropopliteal graft was localized and entered with the wire. The catheter was then directed into the orifice of this graft. The guide wire was passed to the level of the popliteal, and the inner thrombus was partially macerated. Thereafter, the catheter was exchanged over the wire for a #5 French catheter positioned within the proximal portion of the bypass graft. Urokinase infusion was begun at 4000 units/minute. A follow-up angiogram was performed at approximately one hour with overhead films being obtained following the pressure injection of contrast agent. A sterile dressing was then applied with the catheter left in position, and the patient was discharged to the Intensive Care Unit with infusion of urokinase in place.

The patient was returned at approximately four hours following inception of urokinase infusion for follow-up arteriogram. Pressure injection of contrast agent was performed via the indwelling catheter. At the conclusion of this procedure, the patient was returned to the Intensive Care Unit with the catheter in place.

Angiographic Findings

1. The initial arteriogram revealed complete occlusion of the left femoropopliteal graft, which appears to be diffusely thrombosed. There was evidence of proximal occlusion of the native superficial femoral artery, and there was decreased flow to the level of the left calf.
2. At one hour, there was evidence of recanalization of the most proximal portion of the femoropoplital graft. At four hours, there was evidence of almost complete lysis of underlying thrombotic material with good visualization of the graft, the popliteal trifurcation vessels, and the vessels of the foot.

COMPUTERIZED TOMOGRAPHIC SCAN OF BRAIN

Axial images of the brain are obtained after the intravenous administration of contrast. Thin-section, axial-plane images are obtained, traversing the petrous portions of the temporal bones.

The internal auditory canals are within normal limits for size. There is no evidence of focal bone erosion at the petrous apices on either side. The cerebellopontine angle cisterns are symmetric. Small linear densities traverse the right cerebellopontine angle cistern. These are felt to represent computer artifacts secondary to beam hardening.

It is not possible to entirely exclude a minimal intracanalicular or juxtacanalicular neoplasm, and this would be better evaluated on thin-section MRI or possibly on air CT cisternography. There is, however, no definite evidence seen to indicate the presence of an intracranial neoplasm on this examination.

The cerebral ventricles are normal in size, shape, and position. There is no midline shift. There is no extra-axial collection. There are no focal parenchymal abnormalities seen.

The mastoid air cells are normally aerated bilaterally, as are the middle ear cavities. The ossicles are in normal position. The sphenoid, ethmoid, and frontal sinuses are normally aerated.

Conclusion

1. Small linear artifacts traversing the cerebellopontine angles preclude the detection of very small juxtacanalicular neoplasms.
2. Otherwise negative CT scan, as described.

COMPUTERIZED TOMOGRAPHIC SCAN OF LUMBAR SPINE

CT scan of the lumbar spine from the upper sacrum to L-2 is performed with serial axial slices.

The preliminary scout views reveal evidence of moderate rotoscoliosis and extensive spondylosis in the lumbar spine.

On the axial slices, there is a vacuum effect of the L5-S1 disk space. There is considerable lateral bulging of the disk. This appears to extend into the left foramen and could compress the ganglion of the fifth lumbar root on the left. There is very mild indentation upon the dural sac. There are osteophytes projecting from the adjacent vertebral bodies and apophyseal joints, but there is no definite compression of the neural structures by the osteophytes.

There is moderate, diffuse bulging of the L4-5 disk space with indentation upon the dural sac. The lateral bulges do not appear to significantly extend into the left foramen. There may be slight extension into the inferior aspect of the right foramen. The osteophytes at this level appear to be anterior and lateral to the neural structures. A small vacuum phenomenon is seen within the disk space and minor degenerative apophyseal joint disease is noted.

At L3-4 there is diffuse bulging of the disk space in all directions, though it does maintain some concavity against the dural sac. No significant involvement of the foramina is seen. The large osteophytes appear to be anterior and lateral to the neural structures. Minor degenerative apophyseal joint disease is seen.

At L2-3 there is vacuum effect within the disk space and there is diffuse bulging of the anulus in all directions, though it does maintain a concavity against the dural sac. The foramina do not appear to be significantly involved. The osteophytes, by and large, are anterior and lateral to the neural structures. Minor degenerative joint disease is seen.

Conclusion

1. Extensive lumbar spondylosis, degenerative disease, and scoliosis.
2. Bulging of all the lumbar disk spaces. There is a possibility of compression of the nerve root ganglion of the fifth root on the left from a far lateral bulge of the L5-S1 disk space.

COMPUTERIZED TOMOGRAPHIC SCAN OF SINUSES

The head is examined in the axial and coronal planes, and axial images were obtained from the hard palate through to the frontal sinuses. Coronal images covered the paranasal air sinuses. Comparison is made to a previous examination done on (date).

There is evidence of a surgical defect involving the medial walls of the maxillary sinuses. There is fluid or mucosal thickening in the left maxillary sinus; this was present on the previous examination and has not changed significantly. The right maxillary sinus appears clear. There is normal aeration of the right ethmoid air cells and the right frontal sinus on this examination.

The inferolateral wall of the right frontal sinus is better corticated on this study. There is no definite evidence of bone destruction on the right side. The right ethmoid air cells are normally pneumatized. The sphenoid sinus outlines normally.

There is fluid or mucosal thickening and opacification of the anterior ethmoid cells on the left side with opacification of the cells of the frontoethmoid junction and the left frontal sinus. These changes have progressed since the previous examination.

There is no evidence of soft tissue density within the orbits. The muscle tone appears normal, and the extraocular muscles have a normal appearance. The optic nerves outline normally.

Impression

1. Compared to the previous examination done (date), there has been clearing of the right frontal sinus and the right ethmoid air cells.
2. There is opacification of the anterior ethmoid air cells on the left side, as well as the left frontal sinus. These changes have progressed since the previous examination on (date).

MAGNETIC RESONANCE SCAN OF ABDOMEN

Clinical Information: Abnormal liver function tests; abnormal CT scan.

A CT scan of the abdomen was performed here on (date), and an unusual area of high attenuation was seen near the dome of the liver along its posterior surface. The gallbladder was also noted to be in an unusual position along the posterolateral aspect of the liver and extending lateral to the right kidney.

No previous MRI scans have been performed. For today's examination, scans were made first in the axial projection from the diaphragm and continuing down through the liver using 10-mm thick slices. The scans were performed with T1-weighted proton, and T2-weighted spin-echo sequences. Additional scans were then made through the right abdomen in the sagittal plane, again with T1-proton, and T2-weighted spin-echo sequences.

The overall size of the liver was normal, and the margins were slightly lobulated. The signal intensity of the liver was quite remarkably low on all the scan sequences. The signal intensity of the liver was much lower than that of the spleen or kidneys, and this would suggest the possibility of iron deposition within the liver. Hemochromatosis must be ruled out.

I cannot see a definitive abnormality on the MRI scan that corresponds to the area of increased attenuation seen on the CT study. I do not see a focal mass within the liver. The gallbladder was again seen to be in an unusual posterior position and it has a normal signal intensity, which was midlevel on the T1 scans and very high on the T2 scans. The spleen, kidneys, and the pancreas have a normal appearance, and I do not see evidence of adenopathy or ascites.

Impression. The liver has a very low signal intensity; rule out hemochromatosis.

MAGNETIC RESONANCE SCAN OF CHEST

Clinical Information: Heart murmur. Cardiac ultrasound showed a right atrial mass measuring 2×3 cm. Patient underwent repair of coarctation of the aorta prior to age two years.

The examination is tailored to evaluate for a possible right atrial mass and a series of sequences performed. T1-triggered impulses are obtained, as well as nontriggered and triggered FLASH. Triggered T2 images are also made. All of these images are made in the axial plane, and a series of coronal slices also made.

I believe the area of sonographic abnormality is demonstrated on axial images (stores 8, 15, and 22). On coronal images, the area of suspected abnormality is noted on stores 56 and 49. The area of abnormality is adjacent to the tricuspid valve in the right atrium along its anterior wall. It has a high signal similar to fat and may be prominent fat in the aortoventricular groove.

The ascending aorta is prominent when compared with the descending aorta. A specific study for coarctation is not obtained with the patient in the LAO position. I would like to do another magnetic resonance examination to evaluate for possible recurrent or residual coarctation.

The left ventricular wall appears prominent, but this may not be a significant finding in view of the fact that I cannot tell if the gated images are obtained during systole or diastole.

I have reviewed this case with Dr. Blank at The University of Health Science Center and with Dr. Jones. Both are familiar with the patient's echocardiograms. We feel that the area in the right atrium could be a myxoma, but it is atypical for a myxoma and could be an unusual anatomic anomaly. It is difficult to be definitive about further evaluation on this patient. Perhaps repeat ultrasound studies looking for interval growth might be performed.

MAGNETIC RESONANCE SCAN OF BRAIN

Axial images of the brain have been obtained using proton density and T2-weighted image parameters. T1-weighted axial images were also obtained, traversing the cerebellopontine angles.

There is artifact related to patient motion on the T1-weighted axial images through the cerebellopontine angles. As a result, a very small intracanalicular or juxtacanalicular neoplasm cannot be excluded. There is, however, no evidence seen to indicate a cerebellopontine angle neoplasm on either side. The cerebellopontine angle cisterns are symmetric. The brain stem is normal in size and configuration.

There is a moderate degree of diffuse brain atrophy, manifested by enlargement of the cerebral and cerebellar sulci, associated with a mild degree of diffuse ventriculomegaly. There are multiple small focal areas of abnormal signal intensity imaged within the periventricular white matter of both cerebral hemispheres. These are more conspicuous in the right parietal lobe, in the left subinsular region, and along the roofs of the lateral ventricles. These are compatible with multiple small foci of lacunar-type infarction of indeterminate age.

There is no evidence for mass effect or focal edema. There is no evidence of an intracranial neoplasm.

Incidentally noted is a small focus of mucosal thickening in the inferior margin of the left maxillary sinus, most likely a result of sinusitis.

A small, somewhat linear focus of increased signal in the inferomedial aspect of the petrous portion of the left temporal bone is felt to represent paradoxical, flow-related enhancement within a portion of the internal jugular vein at this site.

Conclusion

1. There is a mild degree of diffuse brain atrophy.
2. Multiple foci of lacunar-type infarction are imaged, as described.
3. A small amount of mucosal thickening is imaged at the inferior margin of the left maxillary sinus.

MAGNETIC RESONANCE SCAN OF LEFT KNEE

Serial images of the left knee are obtained in the sagittal and coronal planes, utilizing T1-weighted and three-dimensional gradient imaging techniques.

There is no evidence of joint space effusion, and there is no evidence of fracture or destructive lesion involving the distal femur, the proximal tibia, or the patella. The menisci appear intact. The articular cartilage appears uniform with no focal areas of disruption, and there are no erosive changes of underlying bone identified. The posterior cruciate ligament appears intact and unremarkable.

The anterior cruciate ligament occupies a normal position and appears grossly intact. However, there is a small, rounded structure adjacent to the base of the distal attachment of the anterior cruciate. This structure is located posterior to the transverse ligament and has an intermediate intensity. The differential considerations include a pedunculated, partially detached fragment of the anterior cruciate ligament or a small cyst or cartilaginous loose body within the joint space.

The examination is otherwise unremarkable.

MAGNETIC RESONANCE SCAN OF LUMBAR SPINE

Clinical History: Left leg pain; low back pain.

Technique

1. Sagittal 5 mm interleaved slices, slightly overlapped, TR 0.5, TE 16, as well as TR 2.3, TE 35, and 90, covering segment from S1 to the lower margin of T11.
2. Axial 5 mm orthogonal slices, TR 1.5, TE 30, and 80. These are also interleaved.

Findings. There is very mild bulging of the L5-S1 disk space without evidence of deformity of the dural sac or the foraminal structures.

There is focal protrusion or herniation of the L4-5 disk space deforming the dural sac in the midline and to the left of midline. No definite involvement of the foramina is seen.

There is slight to moderate diffuse bulge of the L3-4 disk space, slightly indenting the dural sac. The foraminal structures are normal. The L2-3 disk and foramina are also normal.

There is loss of signal intensity in the L3-4 and L4-5 disk spaces on the T2-weighted images. There is no evidence to suggest bony canal stenosis. There is a suggestion of degenerative apophyseal joint disease at L5-S1 on the right with some posterolateral indentation upon the dural sac.

Conclusion

1. Posterolateral protrusion or herniation of the L4-5 disk on the left.
2. Moderate diffuse bulge of the L3-4 disk space.
3. Mild bulge of the L5-S1 disk space.
4. Suggest degenerative apophyseal joint disease at L5-S1 on the right with slight compression of the dural sac from the posterolateral aspect.

APPENDIX 2: PHYSICAL CONSTANTS OF THE ELEMENTS

Element	Symbol	Atomic number	Atomic weight
Actinium	Ac	89	227.0278*
Aluminum	Al	13	26.98154
Americium	Am	95	(243)
Antimony	Sb	51	121.75
Argon	Ar	18	39.948
Arsenic	As	33	74.9216
Astatine	At	85	(210)
Barium	Ba	56	137.373
Berkelium	Bk	97	(247)
Beryllium	Be	4	9.01218
Bismuth	Bi	83	208.9804
Boron	B	5	10.81
Bromine	Br	35	79.904
Cadmium	Cd	48	112.41
Calcium	Ca	20	40.08
Californium	Cf	98	(251)
Carbon	C	6	12.011
Cerium	Ce	58	140.12
Cesium	Cs	55	132.9054
Chlorine	Cl	17	35.453
Chromium	Cr	24	51.996
Cobalt	Co	27	58.9332
Copper	Cu	29	63.546
Curium	Cm	96	(247)
Dysprosium	Dy	66	162.50
Einsteinium	Es	99	(252)
Erbium	Er	68	167.26
Europium	Eu	63	151.96
Fermium	Fm	100	(257)
Fluorine	F	9	18.998403
Francium	Fr	87	(223)
Gadolinium	Gd	64	157.25
Gallium	Ga	31	69.72
Germanium	Ge	32	72.59
Gold	Au	79	196.9665
Hafnium	Hf	72	178.49
Helium	He	2	4.00260
Holmium	Ho	67	164.9304
Hydrogen	H	1	1.0079
Indium	In	49	114.82
Iodine	I	53	126.9045
Iridium	Ir	77	192.22
Iron	Fe	26	55.847
Krypton	Kr	36	83.80
Lanthanum	La	57	138.9055
Lawrencium	Lr	103	(260)
Lead	Pb	82	207.2
Lithium	Li	3	6.941
Lutetium	Lu	71	174.967
Magnesium	Mg	12	24.305
Manganese	Mn	25	54.9380
Mendelevium	Md	101	(258)
Mercury	Hg	80	200.59

Element	Symbol	Atomic number	Atomic weight
Molybdenum	Mo	42	95.94
Neodymium	Nd	60	144.24
Neon	Ne	10	20.179
Neptunium	Np	93	237.0482*
Nickel	Ni	28	58.70
Niobium	Nb	41	92.9064
Nitrogen	N	7	14.0067
Nobelium	No	102	(259)
Osmium	Os	76	130.2
Oxygen	O	8	15.9994
Palladium	Pd	46	106.4
Phosphorus	P	15	30.97376
Platinum	Pt	78	195.09
Plutonium	Pu	94	(244)
Polonium	Po	84	(209)
Potassium	K	19	39.0983
Praseodymium	Pr	59	140.9077
Promethium	Pm	61	(145)
Protactinium	Pa	91	231.0359*
Radium	Ra	88	226.0254*
Radon	Rn	86	(222)
Rhenium	Re	75	186.207
Rhodium	Rh	45	102.9055
Rubidium	Rb	37	85.4678
Ruthenium	Ru	44	101.07
Samarium	Sm	62	150.4
Scandium	Sc	21	44.9559
Selenium	Se	34	78.96
Silicon	Si	14	28.0855
Silver	Ag	47	107.868
Sodium	Na	11	22.98977
Strontium	Sr	38	87.62
Sulfur	S	16	32.06
Tantalum	Ta	73	180.9479
Technetium	Tc	43	(98.9062)
Tellurium	Te	52	127.60
Terbium	Tb	65	158.9254
Thallium	Tl	81	204.37
Thorium	Th	90	232.0381*
Thulium	Tm	69	168.9342
Tin	Sn	50	118.69
Titanium	Ti	22	47.90
Tungsten	W	74	183.85
Unnilhexium**	Uah	106	(263)
Unnilpentium**	Unp	105	(262)
Unnilquadium**	Unq	104	(264)
Uranium	U	92	238.0289
Vanadium	V	23	50.9415
Xenon	Xe	54	131.30
Ytterbium	Yb	70	173.04
Yttrium	Y	39	88.9059
Zinc	Zn	30	65.38
Zirconium	Zr	40	91.22

Based on 1979 IUPAC Atomic Weights of the Elements.
A value given in parentheses denotes the mass number of the longest-lived isotope.
*Atomic weight of most commonly available long-lived isotope.
**The elements, as well as their symbols, are not yet internationally recognized.

APPENDIX 3: COMPUTER GLOSSARY

abort. To stop or discontinue the operation of a program before completion.

adapter. A printed circuit board, q.v., that allows an external option to be plugged into the system board.

alphanumeric. A system of characters or programming language that includes only roman numbers, letters, and punctuation marks.

ALT. A key that, when depressed in conjunction with the regular alphanumeric keys, changes the signals normally sent to the CPU, q.v.

analog. A continuous scale subject to visual judgment and interpretation. The typical clock, with hour and minute hands, is an analog device. SEE: *digital.*

ASCII. *American Standard Code for Information Interchange.* An agreed-upon system that assigns specific code numbers to all numerals, letters, and punctuation marks and permits communication between all machines, regardless of make or model.

AT. *advanced technology.* A computer model that uses a chip developed for processing data at high speeds. SEE: *chip; clock.*

backup disk. SEE: *disk, backup.*

BASIC. *Beginner's All-purpose Symbolic Instruction Code.* A widely used programming language that uses English words to enter commands, q.v., via the keyboard into the CPU, q.v. These commands are interpreted internally by the machine itself into numeric codes necessary for execution of a program.

baud rate. A unit of telegraphic signaling speed used to indicate the rate of transmission of data from a computer to a distant site by use of a special device, usually attached to a telephone, called a modem. A baud is one pulse per second.

binary system. A numbering system particularly well suited to use by computers. All of the information placed into a computer is in binary form; i.e., numbers made up of zeros and ones (0's and 1's). In this system each "place" in a binary number represents a power of 2; i.e., the number of times 2 is to be multiplied by itself. Ex.: the binary number 1000 indicates that the first zero to the right is 1×2^0 which is zero; the next zero to the left indicates 0×2^1 and, again, that is zero; the next zero represents 0×2^2 (i.e., 2×2) but, again the value is zero; the one in the next, and last, place to the left represents 1×2^3 or $1 \times 2 \times 2 \times 2$, or 8. The numerical value is the sum of each of these calculations; in this case, this is 8. Next, calculate the value of 101010. The first zero to the right from the initial example will be equivalent to zero;

the next digit to the left, a one, indicates 1×2^1 which is 2; the next digit, a zero, represents 0×2^2 (i.e., $0 \times 2 \times 2$) or zero; the next digit, a one, represents 1×2^3 (i.e., $1 \times 2 \times 2 \times 2$) which is 8; the next digit, a zero, indicates 0×2^4 and, again, zero times something is zero; the next and last digit is a one and stands for 1×2^5 (i.e., $1 \times 2 \times 2 \times 2 \times 2 \times 2$) which is 32. Again, we add all of these values and find that the number 101010 in binary notation is equal to 42 (i.e., $32 + 8 + 2$).

BIOS. *basic input/output system.* System that oversees how data is channeled into and out of the CPU.

bit. Abbreviation for *binary digit.* Computers work with binary numbers made up of zeros and ones (0's and 1's). A bit is a single number in a binary digit. SEE: *binary system; byte.*

board. SEE: *circuit board.*

boilerplate. To read into a file text that has been prepared and stored in another. Boilerplating is convenient for forms, headings, addresses, and text that is repeated often.

boot. To turn on a computer.

    b., cold. Starting a computer by throwing its main switch.

    b., hot or b., warm. Reinitiation of a program or machine system without turning off the main power switch.

break. A program interrupt; a temporary halt. A program can usually be continued from its interrupt point. SEE: *abort.*

buffer. A temporary storage area for data. It is inserted between a sending and receiving device and can typically be used between a CPU and printer. All data can be fed into a buffer that will continue to feed those data into the printer, thus freeing the computer for other tasks.

bug. A faulty datum or program instruction that causes malfunction of the computer.

bulletin board. A message system usually accessible by modem, q.v. It allows users, q.v., a wide range of informational services. Users may advertise, receive, and store electronic mail, or contact other users interested in various subjects.

bus. The main data transmission line of the CPU which sends all data and instructions from one section of memory or operating system to another.

byte. A bit, q.v., is a single number in a binary digit. Bits used by a computer are grouped into larger units. A group of eight bits is called a byte. SEE: *binary system; bit.*

cable. A collection of conductors used to connect the CPU to its peripherals, q.v. Wires can be bundled, twisted, or arranged as flat cable with all wires in line next to each other.

call up. To bring stored data onto the screen.

card. SEE: *circuit board.*

carriage return. ABBR: <CR>. The key that indicates the decision to accept and perform a command or recently typed information. Until <CR> is used, alterations to entered data can be made or the entire command canceled. Also called <ENTER>, q.v.

cartridge. An insertable device containing data or program information; often used with CPUs to extend their memory capacity, provide automatic startup of specific programs, or provide other functions not part of the initial machine.

cathode ray tube. ABBR: CRT. Euphemism for the monitor or screen. A special vacuum tube that transforms electronic signals into visible images (letters, numbers, pictures) on a phosphorescent screen.

character set. Binary numbers transmitted from or to the CPU and interpreted as alphanumeric characters, graphics characters, q.v., or control codes, q.v. SEE: *alphanumeric.*

chip. An integrated circuit measuring no more than 1/10 in. square. Complete electronic subsystems or operating systems can be included in a single chip.

circuit board. A hard, plastic, sometimes glass-reinforced board on which all circuit components are mounted and electrically "wired" to each other by printed copper paths. Numerous types of boards allow graphics representation, color capability, boost of storage capacity, and other features to a computer. SYN: *card.*

clock. An electronic timing device that sets the pace at which data manipulation takes place. Typical clock speeds are 4, 8, and 10.5 megahertz. SEE: *hertz.*

clone. A less-expensive, off-brand duplicate of a widely used computer system, usually capable of reading most application software.

codes. SEE: *control codes.*

cold boot. SEE: *boot.*

color graphics adapter. ABBR: CGA. A plug-in circuit board that permits images to be presented in monochrome or color on a color monitor or screen. A CGA can display characters in 16 choices of background color and eight choices of foreground color.

color monitor. SEE: *monitor.*

command. Instruction issued to the computer asking for execution of a specific task.

command driven. A type of program that allows a user to pick commands which will perform a desired action.

communications. The sending and receiving of signals between two computers usually connected to each other via a telephone line.

communications adapter. A board placed in a computer which allows communications with other devices.

compatibility. The ability of one computer to run a program generated on or written for another.

computer. An electronic device for storing and retrieving numerical or textual information; and, in the case of numerical or mathematical data, for processing and analyzing it. In medicine and in biological sciences in general, the use of computers has made it possible to store on and retrieve from small disks quantities of data that would require an inordinate amount of space if stored in conventional files.

c., digital. Computer that processes information in the form of discrete digits or units.

c., laptop. A very small, portable computer containing its own power supply and (usually) disk drive. SYN: *portable computer.*

c., mainframe. Major computer installation requiring one or more very large cabinets. Mainframe computers are fixed in place.

c., micro-. Computer in which all equipment fits on a desk and is readily transportable to another location. Internal memory capacity for most microcomputers is often 640K and is connected to floppy disk drives or hard disk drives, q.v., of 10 megabytes or more. SYN: *PC (personal computer).*

c., mini-. Computer whose physical and computing size is between that of a mainframe computer, q.v., and a microcomputer, q.v. The CPU is usually a floor model cabinet with disk drives of several hundred megabyte capacity. Minicomputers may be moved if necessary.

computer-assisted design. ABBR: CAD. The use of computer systems to assist in designing two-dimensional objects. This may occur in plastic surgery to reshape body parts, such as the face; or in orthopedics to design replacement parts, such as an artificial hip.

configuration. The manner in which hardware and software is programmed and arranged in order to operate a system or network.

connector. A polarized termination at the end of a cable permitting insertion into a peripheral. SEE: *cable.*

console. The monitor, q.v., or screen, q.v.

constant. A single letter or letter combination that can represent many different numerical values as a program is executed. Each constant will hold the last value assigned to it until that value is deliberately changed.

continuous forms. Perforated, connected, paper forms that continuously feed through a printer.

control codes. Codes used to send instructions to the printer or other peripherals; a system of symbols that represents information contained in a computer data bank.

cps. *cycles per second.* SEE: *hertz.*

CPU. *central processing unit.* The basic box or cabinet containing all a computer's circuit boards. The CPU handles I/O, q.v., manipulation and calculations, and temporary data storage (RAM, q.v.). When turned off, the CPU by itself does not store data created by the user.

crash. Sudden and unexpected program termination that may cause a computer to hang up and require a cold reboot. SEE: *hangup.*

CTRL. The major code command key that generates a different set of keyboard signals when used in conjunction with regular (white) keys. SEE: *ALT.*

cursor. A flashing line or small square on the monitor that moves each time a key is struck and indicates where the next keystroke will appear. The cursor can also be used to indicate onscreen position in a document.

daisy wheel. A central hub that has several dozen spokes radiating from it and is inserted into the printer. At the end of each spoke is a complete letter and, when struck by the printer's hammer, one complete gapless letter is formed on the paper. SEE: *dot matrix.*

data. Plural of datum: one piece of information. In order of increasing size: bit, byte, word, line, paragraph, page. Data may be alphabetical, numerical, or graphics instruction, operated on with all conventional mathematical functions. Data can also be words and phrases, in which case it is called word processing.

database. A collection of data, either numerical or textual, that has been keyed in and stored on disk or other storage medium. A database is usually created in a specific format, allowing easy insertion of future additions.

data processing. Manipulation of pieces of information to achieve a desired result.

debug. The review of a program or procedure to discover and correct a malfunction or flaw.

decimal. Arithmetic to the base 10 in which numbers have locational value; each one-

column move to the left being equivalent to multiplication by 10. Other systems used in computer work are base 2 (binary), base 8 (octal), and base 16 (hexadecimal, q.v.). SEE: *binary system.*

default. A set of assumed values that will be used in calculations and operations, unless changed by the operator. Rebooting always restores the default values.

default disk drive. Unless otherwise reprogrammed by a user, the disk drive deferred to by a computer for file search.

destination drive. The drive on which incoming data is received. When copying with two drives, the destination drive is usually, but not always, the B: drive.

device name. Names and conventional abbreviations assigned to all computer system components. Major components are central processing unit (CPU), keyboard (KBD), monitor/console (CON), printer (PRN) or line printer (LPT), and communications port (COM).

digital. Method of counting in discrete, full-number steps, i.e. 1, 2, 3, 4, without fractions or segments less than unity. Ex.: digital watch. SEE: *analog.*

digital radiography. Radiography using computerized imaging instead of the conventional film or screen imaging.

directory. ABBR: DIR. A listing of all the filenames presently in working order on a disk. Also called "CATALOG" in some computers.

   d., root. The main segment of a directory.

   d., sub-. Directory which branches off from the root directory.

disk, diskette. A round, plastic or metal platter coated with a magnetic medium and used for storage of data. A disk's particles are reoriented only when information is written to them. Disks are inserted into a disk drive, q.v., and interchanged as needed. SEE: *format.*

   d., backup. A precautionary or safety disk used to duplicate information from a master disk. Backup disks are usually used for archiving or storage purposes and to insure against damage to or loss of the master disk.

   d., destination. Disk that receives information from another source or disk. SYN: *source disk.* SEE: *destination drive.*

   d., double-density or d., double-sided. A magnetically treated disk that enables storage of data on both sides.

   d., floppy. A thin, very flexible, plastic platter inside a stiff, cardboard, protective jacket which spins at 300 rpm. SEE: *disk;*

high density.

d., hard. A nonremovable disk sealed in an airtight metal case within the CPU. A hard disk spins at 3600 rpm for faster data transfer.

d., protected. A floppy disk whose square notch is taped over, making writing to the disk impossible. Data on a protected disk can be read and used but not altered.

d., single-density or d., single-sided. A magnetically treated disk enabling storage of data on one side only.

d., source. Destination disk, q.v.

disk capacity. The informational storage capacity of a disk, measured in sectors, tracks, and recorded bytes per sector. Sectors × tracks × bytes per track = disk capacity. A floppy disk's, q.v., normal data storage capacity is approximately 360,000 bytes. A hard disk, q.v., can typically hold 10 to 40 megabytes of data. SEE: *high density.*

disk controller. Electronic circuitry enabling a disk drive to perform the four vital functions listed. SEE: *disk drive.*

disk drive. A mechanical device within the CPU that spins the disk; provides timing and lateral head movement to locate proper disk sector; lowers/raises the read/write head; and transfers data to or copies data from a disk. In most machines, drives are designed as A:, B:, C:, and D:, but may also be called 0, 1, 2, and 3.

display. Visual imaging of numbers, letters, and graphic characters on the monitor screen.

document. Any body of text that is typed and stored in a file.

documentation. Manuals, instruction books, literature, and how-to-do-it information in the form of a program or help menus that provide guidance and know-how to a user.

DOS. *disk operating system.* A type of software that provides the basic set of instructions to a computer on the method for executing programs. A computer's built-in "startup" program has only enough instruction to allow its managing the DOS that has to be installed separately from a special floppy disk.

dot matrix. An arrangement of "pins" punched by a printer's print head which form letter patterns. SEE: *draft mode; printer, NLQ.*

double-sided. SEE: *disk, double density.*

download. To transfer and save a program or data *from* a computer at a remote location. SEE: *upload.*

draft mode. One row of pins (out of the three in a 24-pin printer) used to form printed let-

ters which increases production speed considerably but leads to a reduction in letter quality. SEE: *dot matrix; printer, NLQ.*

drive. SEE: *disk drive.*

drive, logged. The currently active disk drive, indicated to the user by a prompt, q.v.

EBCDIC. *extended binary coded decimal interchange code.* An eight-bit character code.

edit. To change the text of a program, instruction set, or contents of a file.

EGA. *enhanced graphics adapter.* A plug-in circuit board offering a much wider range of color choices than the color graphics adapter, q.v. when used with a suitable color monitor. On-screen definition is considerably sharper because the pixels, q.v., are smaller and more numerous.

electronic mail. Information sent from one computer to another via telephone. Data being sent will be visible on both computer screens at the same instant and can be filed away on disk for future use by the remote machine. SEE: *bulletin board; modem.*

enter. Written: <ENTER>. A key which is the official "do it" command. Prior to pressing this key, issued instructions can usually be changed or canceled. Also called carriage return (<CR>), q.v.

EOF. *end of file.* 1. A control character that designates the end of a file. 2. Condition occurring when the computer has read the last record of a data file.

error message. A message from the CPU indicating faulty instructions have been entered. This message will often enumerate the types of mistakes made and query the user for new and better instructions complying with the CPU's rigid set of input techniques.

escape. ABBR: ESC. A key that permits the user to abandon a particular routine in progress, erase an entered message, return to an earlier menu, or "escape" from a troublesome situation. Activating this key does not always allow one to escape from the situation.

EXE. An extension, q.v., (.EXE) used to indicate an EXEcutable file. This type of file can be run from the prompt, q.v., without typing in the extension.

exit. To discontinue a program and stop the operation in progress.

extension. Three letters following the period at the end of a filename. Extensions may indicate that the file is run from DOS (ready); others may indicate that BASIC must be loaded prior to running a file. Extensions can also indicate that the file is part of a commercial word processing or database management program. Some extensions serve a specific function (e.g., .COM); others are descriptive (e.g., .BAS) or totally optional (e.g., .TXT). SEE: *filename.*

external. SEE: *internal/external.*

eye-gaze communicator. An electronic device that allows a person to control a computer by looking at words or commands on a video screen. A very low intensity light shines into one of the user's eyes. Reflections from the cornea and retina are picked up by a TV camera. As the direction of gaze moves, the relative position of the two reflections changes, and this information is used by the computer to determine the area at which the user is looking. The computer then executes the command.

file. 1. Data stored as a single unit. 2. To enter and store data as a file for retrieval.

filename. An assigned name given to a collection of data enabling the user to retrieve a file by name. Filenames may have a main segment of up to eight characters followed by a period (.) and up to three more characters called the extension, q.v. SYN: *filespec.*

fixed drive. SEE: *disk, hard.*

flip-flop. A circuit that yields as an output one of two possible conditions: either high (1) or low (0). Used in memory circuits and counters.

floppy disk. SEE: *disk, floppy.*

format. 1. To install the primary divisions and structure required for storage and retrieval on a new disk. 2. The structural arrangement (sectors and tracks) of a disk. A new disk is a total blank. Formatting divides it into sectors (like pie slices) and tracks (annular rings) so that files can be started at known intersections and their locations labeled for future retrieval. SEE: *disk capacity.*

form feed. Motion of the printer platen, q.v., which brings the paper to the end of the page. Generally used with continuous paper forms that cause each new page to start at exactly the same location.

freeze. SEE: *hangup.*

function keys. Programmable keys that cause specific instructions or routines to be executed. The keys are usually gray rather than white and are labeled F1 to F12. Various software programs may assign differing functions to these keys, and striking nonnumbered gray keys in conjunction with a numbered function key may alter their function. Ex.: When struck directly, a key may be programmed to turn on boldfacing; yet the same key, when struck together with the shift key, may open a window into another file.

game port. An outlet on the CPU that is both

electronic and physical and permits the attachment and use of a joystick, q.v.

garbage. The appearance of useless screen presentation in the form of random letters, numbers, and graphical symbols in total disarray.

garbage in, garbage out. ABBR: GIGO. An expression indicating that what is entered into the computer by a user is ultimately what will be produced regardless of computer capability or processing sophistication. If information, coding, or programming is invalid or incorrect, what emits from the system will be invalid or incorrect.

GIGO. *garbage in, garbage out,* q.v.

glitch. SEE: *bug.*

graphics card. A board enabling display of graphic images.

graphics characters. Visual symbols and patterns sent to the screen which form a picture.

graphics mode. Mode of computer representation that may include lines and boxes, circles, diamonds, miniature drawings, symbols, and special shapes, as well as tints and shadings.

hangup. Situation in which the computer becomes totally inoperative. The screen is frozen, and there may be no response to a keystroke or other user input. Any working data not previously saved to a peripheral, q.v., is lost. To rectify hangup, the computer may need to be completely turned off and then cold booted, q.v.

hard copy. Physically printed material produced by the lineprinter. SEE: *printout.*

hard disk drive. An airtight metal case within the CPU which contains the hard disk. SEE: *disk, hard.*

hardware. Term usually referring to the CPU, monitor, keyboard, and printer, as well as any add-on circuit boards or other devices installed in or connected to the computer. SEE: *software.*

height. The size of the rectangular opening on the front of the CPU.

  h., full. The complete extent of the rectangular opening on the front of the CPU. Originally, only one disk drive would fit into the slot, but presently two half-height drives may be located in the same space.

  h., half. Disk drive that is one-half the height of the rectangular opening on the front of the CPU.

Hercules® card. A special plug-in circuit board, q.v., (card) that permits the production of elaborate graphics pictures onscreen.

hertz. ABBR: Hz. A unit of frequency equal to one cycle/second.

hexadecimal. In computers, a number system using the base sixteen rather than base two (binary) or ten (decimal).

high density. Disk density in which the magnetic medium is packed more tightly and with more magnetic particles than a single density disk; thus, additional data can be stored in the same physical space on a disk. SEE: *disk capacity.*

hot boot. SEE: *boot.*

hub ring. Reinforcement of the inner annulus of a floppy disk to safeguard against wear from the disk drive mechanism that grasps the disk at the inner annulus in order to spin it.

IC. *integrated circuit.* A tiny, specially treated silicon chip, q.v., on which complicated electronic circuits have been produced. Chips are often less than ⅛ in. square.

initialize. To return equipment or program back to its original state. SEE: *default.*

inkjet. SEE: *printer, inkjet.*

input. Data that flows into the equipment, usually the CPU.

install program. A program that prepares applications software for use.

interface. 1. Device that enables two normally noncompatible circuits or parts to function together. 2. A physical connection between two pieces of equipment. 3. A program step or steps permitting data flow from one point to another.

internal/external. Hardware, such as a modem, that may be available as a stand-apart unit (external) or a plug-in module (internal) and whose installation requires opening the CPU case.

I/O. *input/output.* Transfer of data between the CPU and its peripherals.

jack. Plug, q.v.

jacket. Stiff cardboard envelope lined with a dust-catching material to protect and support the enclosed thin plastic disk.

joystick. A device with a control handle. When manipulated by hand, the joystick causes direct responsive lateral or vertical motion of the cursor. SYN: *paddle.*

justification. Text alignment at the right margin, usually achieved by the addition of small spaces between words. Many computers have automatic justification capability that may be turned on or off by a user.

K, KB. *kilobyte.* 1024 bytes (2 raised to the power of 16). A 64K CPU has a total memory of 65,536 bytes.

key. A button on the keyboard, q.v., that controls input to a computer.

keyboard. ABBR: KBD. The typewriterlike arrangement of letters and numbers on which input information or control codes are typed.

keypad. A secondary grouping of keys to the right of the typewriter keyboard similar to that of an adding machine and containing numbers and several special keys, such as directional arrows. SYN: *numberpad.*

laptop. SEE: *computer, laptop.*

laser. Acronym for *light amplification by stimulated emission of radiation.* A device that emits intense heat and power at close range. The instrument converts various frequencies of light into one small and extremely intense unified beam of one wavelength radiation.

LCD. *liquid crystal display.* 1. A light-sensitive display showing alphanumeric characters. 2. A computer screen readout system.

LED. *light-emitting diode.* A semiconductor device requiring very little current to generate a visible light output and used to emit the glowing figures or symbols on a computer screen. The LED is most often red but can also be amber or green.

letter quality. SEE: *printer, letter quality.*

line feed. 1. A function that rotates the printer platen and places the next line on the paper underneath the preceding one. 2. Movement of the cursor on the monitor, which causes it to drop down one line.

lineprinter. SEE: *printer.*

list. A programming command that causes the computer to project on the monitor all instructions, usually numbered lines, contained within a program.

load. To insert data into the memory section of the CPU; transfer program information or instructions from disk or tape into the console memory. SEE: *download; RAM; upload.*

lockup. SEE: *hangup.*

loop. One or several instructions that are repeated a specified number of times before proceeding to the follow-on step.

   l., infinite. A set of instructions that double back on themselves without an exit instruction and cause computer hangup, q.v.

LPT 1, 2. *lineprinter 1, lineprinter 2.* Designations telling the CPU where to route information for hard copy output.

M, MB. *megabyte.* 1,048,576 bytes.

mainframe computer. SEE: *computer, mainframe.*

manual. Printed instructions that provide procedural and operational information and guidance. SEE: *documentation.*

matrix. The arrangement of pixels, q.v., or picture elements that make up the computerized image.

MEDLARS. *Medical Literature Analysis and Retrieval System.* A modem-accessible, 24-hour retrieval system of the National Library of Medicine. MEDLARS offers multiple databases, some of which include information on the history of medicine and related sciences, registry of toxic effects of chemical substances, and cancer research projects.

MEDLINE. *MEDLARS on-line.* The bibliographic database of MEDLARS, q.v.

mega-. 1. Combining form that means great or large. 2. Indicates one million (10^6) when used in combination with terms indicating units of measures; thus, megaton is one million tons.

memory. The area in a computer where processing information is stored. SEE: *storage.*

memory map. Listing of the location of various types of information in the computer.

menu. A list of options and commands shown onscreen that permit the user to pick a particular program operation.

menu-driven. Programming technique that permits the user to make all required choices from the menu, q.v., shown on the monitor. Selecting appropriate numbers or letters from the menu will help lead the user through the necessary commands. SEE: *user friendly.*

MeSH. *medical subject headings.* The National Library of Medicine's medical language thesaurus offered through MEDLINE, q.v.

message. A statement from the program appearing onscreen to inform the user of a mistake or to ask for additional information.

microcomputer. SEE: *computer, micro-.*

microprocessor. Silicon chip, q.v., of major proportions containing enough circuitry and power to perform the bulk of a computer's vital functions.

minicomputer. SEE: *computer, laptop; computer, mainframe; computer micro-.*

modem. *modulator-demodulator.* Device that allows data to be transmitted in serial form over conventional phone lines.

monitor. A cathode ray tube, q.v., similar to a TV screen on which all input received from peripherals (keyboard, modem, disk, cassette) is visually recorded.

mono, monochrome. Display of only a single color, equivalent to a black-and-white TV set. Mono computer screens are generally smoke gray, green, or amber.

motherboard. The main circuit board, q.v., in the CPU which contains the microprocessor and other primary circuits. It also has expansion slots into which add-on circuit boards are easily inserted.

mouse. A hand-manipulated device that generates electrical signals relative to its mo-

tion. Signals are interpreted by the CPU to reflect corresponding motion of a cursor, arrow, or other indicator on the monitor screen.

multiplexor. In computers and instrumentation, a circuit that allows a single processor to sample multiple input channels by sequencing them.

MUMPS. *Massachusetts General Hospital Utility Multi-Programming System.* A programming language designed to handle complex data, such as patient records.

nano-. Prefix indicating one-billionth (10^{-9}) of the unit following. Thus a nanogram is one-billionth (10^{-9}) of a gram.

NLQ. *near letter quality.* SEE: *printer, NLQ.*

number pad. Keypad, q.v.

OCR. *optical character reader,* q.v.

operating system. SEE: *DOS.*

optical character reader. ABBR: OCR. Device that automatically reads printed or handwritten characters and transfers the information into data adaptable to computer processing.

output. Any data that flows from the computer to a peripheral device.

paddle. SEE: *joystick.*

parallel, parallel interface. The most common interface between computers and printers in which several (usually eight or more) signals are transmitted over an equal number of wires simultaneously.

password. An identification code or name that allows a user access to a computer program or computer-related service such as a bulletin board, q.v.

PC. *personal computer.*

peripheral. Any piece of equipment added on to the basic computer set (CPU, monitor, keyboard). Major peripherals include printer, spooler, modem, joystick, mouse.

pitch. The number of characters per inch.

pixel. *picture element.* The smallest area on the screen that can be illuminated or darkened, i.e., turned on or off. The higher the number of pixels, the sharper the definition of alphanumeric characters or graphic presentations.

platen. The roller of a typewriter or printer that rotates to move paper through the machine.

plotter. Equipment that utilizes one or more drawing pens and generates a graphic or pictorial image on paper.

plug. Device which permits two or more signal or power lines to be connected.

port. An input/output connection through which data flow can be directed.

portable. SEE: *computer, laptop.*

power supply. The means by which adequate

current is supplied to drive all connected circuits and disk drives.

print enhancement. A special print feature in word processing programs, such as boldface or underline.

printer. A keyless device, similar to a typewriter, that prints the output of data from a computer. Also called lineprinters, printers are available in four styles: dot matrix, near letter quality (NLQ) dot matrix, daisy wheel, and laser. SEE: *daisy wheel; dot matrix; laser.*

    p., dot matrix. Printer using an arrangement of "pins" punched by a printer's print head. Dot matrix printers have nine, 18, or 24 pins that generate the characters. Many dot matrix printers now use a three-row staggered arrangement of 24 pins to eliminate the obvious dot pattern of each letter. High-quality printers permit two modes of operation: draft mode and near letter quality (NLQ).

    p., inkjet. Printer generating characters by squirting tightly spaced dots of ink.

    p., letter quality. Printer utilizing character formation from a dot matrix printer but very closely approaching the quality of letters produced by a typewriter or a daisy wheel printer.

    p., NLQ. near letter quality. Printer producing characters by a dot matrix printer which approaches the quality of a typewriter or daisy wheel printer, though some of the dot formation is still discernible.

    p., 9-pin/18-pin/24-pin. Dot matrix printer, q.v.

print modes. The style and appearance of the printed character.

printout. A printed copy of computer data, programs, or screen images. SYN: *hard copy.*

print screen. A command that transfers all text and graphic symbols presently visible on the monitor screen to the lineprinter for hard-copy, q.v., output.

program. A set of step-by-step instructions telling the computer which actions to take in a predetermined sequence.

PROM. *programmable read-only memory.* Manufacturer or user-specified stored data that cannot be erased, reprogrammed, or lost.

prompt. A standard symbol that appears on-screen, indicating the computer is ready to receive commands. In an IBM® personal computer and its clones, q.v., the prompt is a greater than symbol (>) which can often be changed to any other character desired by the user.

QWERTY keyboard. Standard typewriter key arrangement in which the letters QWERTY appear in the second row of the upper left side.

ragged right. Text appearing without right justification, q.v.

RAM. *random access memory.* Segment of the CPU's internal memory that is available to the user for programs, data manipulation, and storage. RAM can be changed at will as often as desired. All changes made to RAM are lost when the machine is turned off.

read. To call up, q.v., copy, or move information from a disk or other source into a computer's memory.

read-only memory. ABBR: ROM. The portion of a computer's memory that contains permanent instructions as opposed to random access memory (RAM), which holds the temporary instructions (a program).

REMark. Information added to program lines that serves as a reminder or help but is not used by the program when it runs.

remote access. A mode in which a user can control unattended terminals in another location.

resolution, low, medium, high. The size of dots used in generating the image on the screen or by the printer. The more dots in a given area, the higher the resolution and the clearer and sharper the image.

retrieve. 1. To gather data from storage, i.e., a disk or tape, and insert it into the CPU's own memory core. 2. To restore a program or command either deliberately or inadvertently deleted.

return. Carriage return, q.v.

ROM. *read-only memory,* q.v.

run. 1. To operate a program or computer routine. 2. A command to indicate the beginning of program operation in which each step is executed in the order listed in the program.

save. To send and store information from memory to a disk.

screen. The image-generating segment of the monitor.

screen-print. SEE: *print screen.*

scroll. Moving on-screen text in any direction, usually up or down.

sector. The smallest division of a diskette track. SEE: *disk capacity.*

serial. The sequential performance of two or more actions in one device.

setup. Preparation of the computer system for operation.

slot. The multiconductor socket into which circuit boards, q.v., can be plugged.

software. Programs, q.v., written for computer use. Ex.: games, word processing, data processing, graphics, flight simulators, etc.

source disk. SEE: *disk, destination.*
special (gray) keys. Function keys, q.v.
spreadsheet. A program designed as an electronic worksheet. Numbers and formulae appear in columns and rows in a mathematical relationship; and, when one number is changed, the spreadsheet will recalculate the figures.
storage. 1. Device that can store data. 2. A floppy or hard disk.

    s., primary. Location of data and program storage used during processing.

    s., secondary. Location of data and program storage not being used during processing.

store. 1. To place data in a device for storing purposes. 2. To keep data in a device for storing purposes.
subdirectory. SEE: *directory, sub-.*
syntax. Precise rules for the formation of "grammatical" commands as dictated by the "language" in use by the computer.
system. The basic computing equipment: a CPU, keyboard, and monitor.
system variables. Variables provided by an operation system.
telecommunications. The transmission of data over telephone lines. SEE: *modem.*
terminal. Computer device capable of receiving and displaying data.
track. Annular ring on a disk divided into sectors on which program information or data or both can be stored. A double-density disk, q.v., has 40 such parallel tracks. SEE: *disk capacity; sector.*
tree. A DOS function used to denote the structure of a directory of files. SEE: *directory.*
upload. To transfer and save a program or data *to* a computer at a remote location. SEE: *download.*

user. Anyone who operates a computer.
user friendly. A program or computer that offers guides and menus to aid the user in operation.
utility program. A program that makes operation of a computer easier, faster, and less bothersome.
V. *volts.*
value. A character, word, or number.
video cards. Plug-in boards that determine proper operation of the corresponding monitors.
voice recognition. Capability of utilizing audio input to translate sounds into computer-recognizable electronic signals for data and word processing purposes.
warm boot. SEE: *boot.*
word processing. The use of software to manipulate, edit, write, and print text.
word wrap. Automatic movement of lines of text to a consecutive line without the necessity of striking a return key. Words appear to "wrap" around the screen while being typed.
worksheet. A spreadsheet file.
wrapping (line). SEE: *word wrap.*
write. To copy data from the memory onto a disk or other storage device.
write protect. To prevent the storage of information on a diskette. SEE: *disk, protected.*
WYSIWYG. *what you see is what you get.* Hard copy printout that is an exact duplication of what appears onscreen. The term applies particularly to graphics characters which sometimes do not print out the same as those that appear on the monitor.
XT. An expanded version of the original IBM® personal computer model with greater internal memory and generally improved performance.

APPENDIX 4: FRACTURES

Fractures

Type	History	Pathology	Complications	Hemorrhage	Color of Area	Treatment	Transportation
Com-minuted	Injury due to crushing blow.	Bone is broken into two or more fragments.	Malunion; unstableness; infection.	Occurs in area of injury.	Discoloration is delayed. Appears in area of deeper bones.	Splint before transportation. Replacement of fracture. Occasionally requires open reduction.	Splint and traction.
Compound	Fall or accident.	Injury where either one or both fragments are through the skin.	Infection; hemorrhage; shock.	May or may not hemorrhage.	Slight to marked increase in ecchymosis.	Immediate debridement in hospital. Antitetanus therapy.	Cover with sterile dressing. Maintain traction. For leg fracture use Thomas splint.
Greenstick	Fall or accident. (In children)	Fracture is incomplete but there is bowing of the bone.	Complete fracture; deformity.	Probably no hemorrhage will occur.	Discoloration may be slight or it may be marked.	Splint for preparation for transportation. Reduction of the curvature and place in cast.	Splint.
Impacted	Crushing force causing fracture. Fragments telescoped.	One fragment is jammed into another.	Deformity; loss of function; pain; osteomyelitis.	Occurs in area of injury.	Discoloration according to extent of bone injury. It may be delayed.	Traction must be made while reduction and proper cast is fitted to hold extremity in place.	Splint and traction.
Simple	Fall or accident.	A complete fracture with no fragments.	Pressure on the blood supply; malunion; osteomyelitis.	Subcutaneous or capillary.	Slight to marked increase in ecchymosis.	Splint before preparation for transportation. Reduction (depending	In splint.

Fractures (Continued)

Type	History	Pathology	Complications	Hemorrhage	Color of Area	Treatment	Transportation
						upon skill of operator).	
Transverse and Spiral	Sudden twisting violence exerted upon extremity.	Fracture line across the bone. Fracture through the bone or around it.	Malfunction; loss of function; cutting of blood supply; infection of bone.	Frequently occurs around area of fracture.	Same as compound fracture.	Depending on site. Splint and traction.	Traction and immobilization.
Ankle (Potts Fracture)	A sudden or forceful wrenching of the lower end of tibia and fibula.	Fracture of the lower ends of the fibula and tibia. Foot is displaced outward. Impairment of tissues, vessels, etc., from trauma.	Dislocation and sprains may occur simultaneously.	May or may not hemorrhage. Discoloration.	Slight or marked areas of ecchymosis.	Immobilize immediately by pillow splint or rigid splint.	Keep limb well supported with slight elevation.
Back	Occurs after jackknife fall and other accidents.	Usually crushing body of vertebrae.	Paralysis and shock (depending upon location of the fracture).	None in surrounding tissues.	Usually no change in color of the skin.	Extreme care in preparation and transportation. Rigid support. Place in hyperextension for 8 weeks. Body cast.	Place and secure in prone position. Keep patient in hyperextension. Restrain if necessary. Rigid stretcher or improvision.
Coccyx	Falling into sitting position.	Fracture may be from sacral region or from tip of coccyx.	Constant pain; abscesses; osteomyelitis.	None in surrounding tissues.	No change in color of the skin.	Hot sitz bath after 24-48 hours of cold applications to area. Rest in bed. Perform coccygectomy if not cured.	Carry patient on rigid stretcher. Keep in dorsal recumbent position.
Femur or Thigh	Usually sudden and severe trauma to thigh.	Bone and nerve injury; paralysis and permanent disability.	Deformity and shortening of the limb where an endocrine disturbance is present; severance of nerves and blood vessels; paralysis and gangrene.	May or may not hemorrhage. Discoloration may be delayed.	Slight to marked increase in ecchymosis.	Splint to leg and body. Keep patient flat. Provide and retain traction. Watch for shock.	Use rigid stretcher. Keep leg in traction until ready for reduction.

Fractures (Continued)

Type	History	Pathology	Complications	Hemorrhage	Color of Area	Treatment	Transportation
Forearm and Colles' Fracture	Result of a twisting force upon the lower arm or wrist, or from violence exerted upon the arm in preventing the body from falling.	Fracture and displacement of the radius. Tip of styloid process of ulna broken off. Backward displacement of radius.	Trauma and swelling of tissues. Dislocations and sprains.	Slight. Increased if fracture is not immediately immobilized.	Slight to marked.	Rigid splint, arm support with a sling.	Place in a sling after splinting.
Hip	Usually found in elderly people.	Fracture through neck or through trochanter or both.	Loss of function; deformity and shortening.	Hemorrhage but not in large amounts.	Ecchymosis but it may be delayed.	Traction; Smith-Peterson Nail.	Place in Thomas Splint as improvised.
Humerus	Result of a twisting force or blow upon upper arm.	Injury to the osseous structures. Trauma and lacerations of tissues, muscles, etc., if compound fracture.	Severance of nerves and blood vessels; temporary deformity.	Slight. Increased if compound fracture.	Slight or marked areas of discoloration.	Immobilize immediately by splint or sling (weight of forearm usually provides the necessary traction).	Keep arm in sling or splint.
Neck	Diving into pools; auto wrecks; accidents.	Break extends through body of vertebrae or the laminae.	Paralysis (total or partial). Death.	None noted in the tissues.	No change in color of the skin.	Keep neck in hyperextension. Place rolled blanket under shoulders. Minor fracture needs traction for 5-6 weeks. Major (with cord injury) cast or collar for 10-12 months.	Patient must not move the neck under any circumstances. Keep neck and head hyperextended. Restrain if necessary. Rigid stretcher or improvision for rigidity.
Pelvis	A blow or crushing force.	Bone impairment; involvement of sacral nerves. Paralysis, torn ligaments, and lacerated muscles.	Rupture of bladder and rectum; deformity and shortening of limb; sprain of pelvic joints.	Same as in compound fracture. Discoloration may be delayed.	Same as in compound fracture if compound. Otherwise delayed.	Keep in dorsal recumbent position; after reduction keep prone. Reduction of fragments; symptomatic treatment.	On rigid stretcher in dorsal recumbent position. Keep body extended

Skull	Fall or blow upon the skull.	In VAULT. Little or no intracranial trauma. Linear fracture may be overlooked. In BASE. Serious compression in brain. Concussion injury to vital cranial nerves.	Concussion; paralysis of limbs of the body; infection of brain; compression of brain. Extent and nature determined by location of injury. Dangers of pressure upon the brain.	Bleeding (bright) from mouth and ears. Clots on the brain.	Ecchymosis over the mastoid process	Place in dorsal recumbent position. Watch for infection. Allow skull base fractures to bleed. Limit fluids.	Place on rigid stretcher. Keep flat. Keep patient quiet.

493

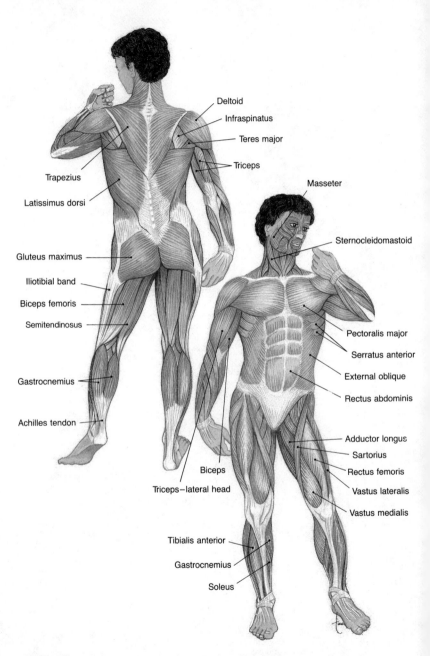

FIGURE I–1. Anterior and posterior views of the major muscles.

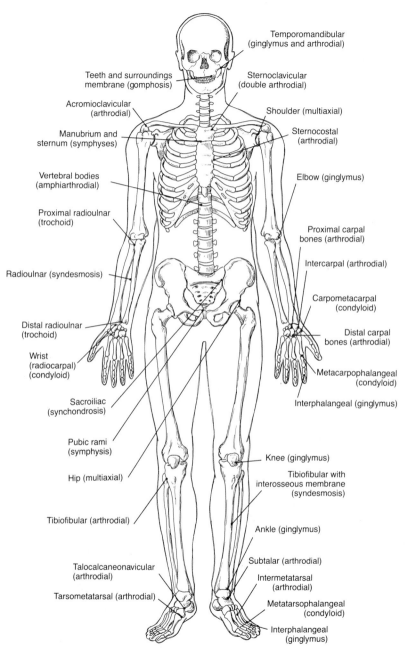

FIGURE I–2. Anterior view of the skeleton.

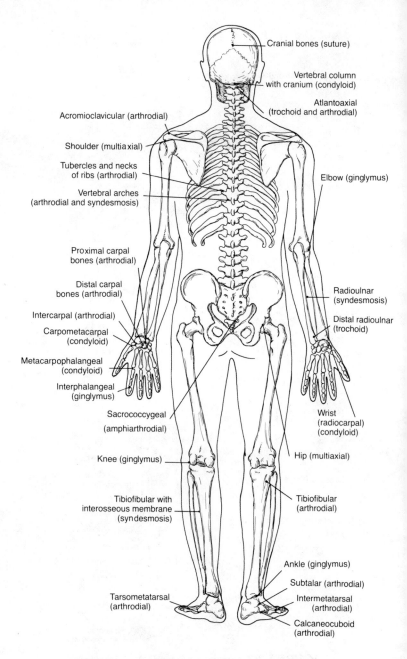

Cranial bones (suture)

Vertebral column with cranium (condyloid)

Atlantoaxial (trochoid and arthrodial)

Acromioclavicular (arthrodial)

Shoulder (multiaxial)

Tubercles and necks of ribs (arthrodial)

Vertebral arches (arthrodial and syndesmosis)

Elbow (ginglymus)

Proximal carpal bones (arthrodial)

Distal carpal bones (arthrodial)

Intercarpal (arthrodial)

Carpometacarpal (condyloid)

Metacarpophalangeal (condyloid)

Interphalangeal (ginglymus)

Sacrococcygeal (amphiarthrodial)

Knee (ginglymus)

Tibiofibular with interosseous membrane (syndesmosis)

Radioulnar (syndesmosis)

Distal radioulnar (trochoid)

Wrist (radiocarpal) (condyloid)

Hip (multiaxial)

Tibiofibular (arthrodial)

Ankle (ginglymus)

Subtalar (arthrodial)

Intermetatarsal (arthrodial)

Calcaneocuboid (arthrodial)

Tarsometatarsal (arthrodial)

FIGURE I–3. Posterior view of the skeleton.

VERTEBRAL COLUMN

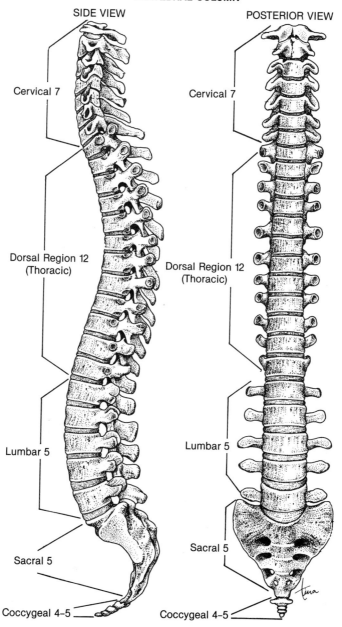

SIDE VIEW

POSTERIOR VIEW

Cervical 7

Cervical 7

Dorsal Region 12
(Thoracic)

Dorsal Region 12
(Thoracic)

Lumbar 5

Lumbar 5

Sacral 5

Sacral 5

Coccygeal 4–5

Coccygeal 4–5

FIGURE I–4. Lateral and posterior views of the vertebral column.

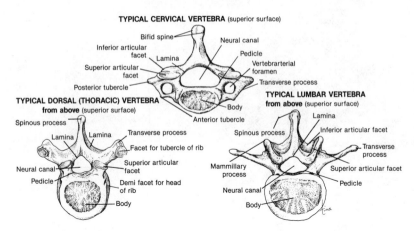

FIGURE I–5. Views of dorsal, cervical, and lumbar vertebrae.

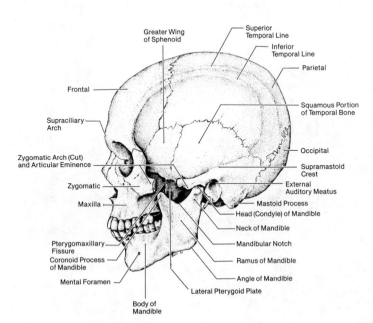

FIGURE I–6. Lateral view of the skull.

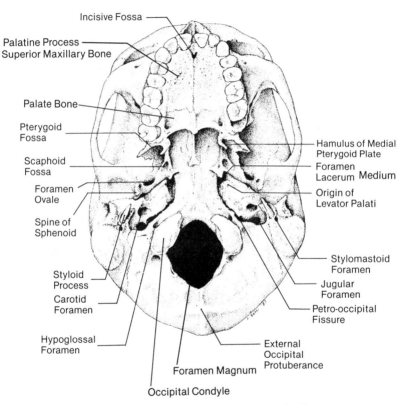

FIGURE I–7. Inferior view of the skull.

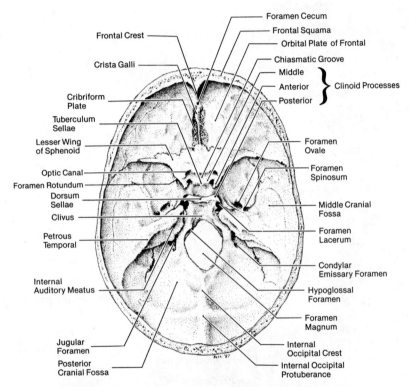

FIGURE I-8. Superior view of the internal skull floor.

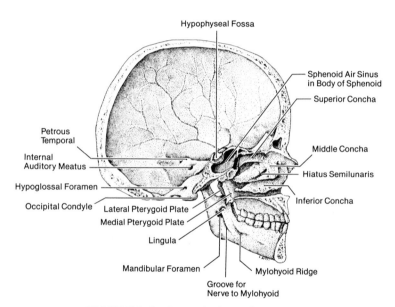

Hypophyseal Fossa

Sphenoid Air Sinus
in Body of Sphenoid

Superior Concha

Petrous
Temporal

Middle Concha

Internal
Auditory Meatus

Hiatus Semilunaris

Hypoglossal Foramen

Inferior Concha

Occipital Condyle

Lateral Pterygoid Plate

Medial Pterygoid Plate

Lingula

Mandibular Foramen

Mylohyoid Ridge

Groove for
Nerve to Mylohyoid

FIGURE I–9. Lateral view of the skull.

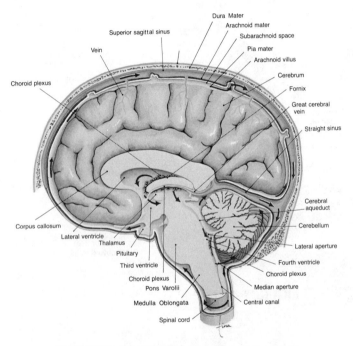

FIGURE I–10. Medical aspect of the brain.

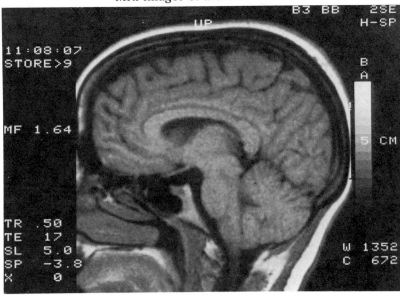

FIGURE I–11. Sagittal plane image with short TR of 0.5 sec. and a single spin echo of 17 msec.

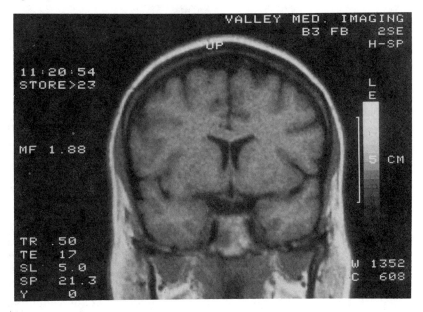

FIGURE I–12. Coronal plane with short TR of 0.5 sec. and a single spin echo of 17 msec.

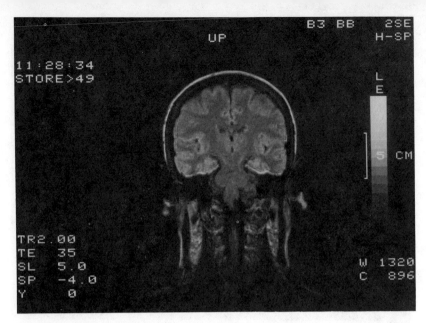

FIGURE I-13. Coronal plane using long TR of 2.0 sec. and multiple spin echos of 35-90 msec.

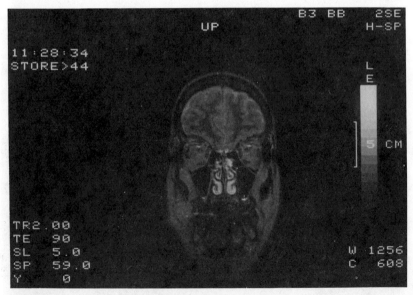

FIGURE I-14. Coronal plane using long TR of 2.0 sec. and multiple spin echos of 35-90 msec.